INTERPRETING RESEARCH IN
SPORT AND EXERCISE SCIENCE

INTERPRETING RESEARCH IN
SPORT AND EXERCISE SCIENCE

Randy Hyllegard
Kansas State University

Dale P. Mood
University of Colorado

James R. Morrow, Jr.
University of North Texas

First Edition
with 50 illustrations

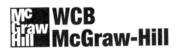
WCB McGraw-Hill

Boston   Burr Ridge, IL   Dubuque, IA   Madison, WI   New York   San Francisco   St. Louis
Bangkok   Bogotá   Caracas   Lisbon   London   Madrid
Mexico City   Milan   New Delhi   Seoul   Singapore   Sydney   Taipei   Toronto

WCB/McGraw-Hill

A Division of The **McGraw·Hill** *Companies*

Vice President and Publisher: James M. Smith
Senior Acquisitions Editor: Vicki Malinee
Developmental Editor: Brian Morovitz
Project Manager: Deborah L. Vogel
Production Editor: Karen L. Allman
Manufacturing Supervisor: Theresa Fuchs
Designer: Pati Pye

Printed in the United States of America
Composition by Shepherd, Inc.
Printing/binding by The Maple-Vail Book Manufacturing Group

Library of Congress Cataloging in Publication Data

Hyllegard, Randy.
    Interpreting research in sport and exercise science/Randy
Hyllegard, Dale P. Mood, James R. Morrow, Jr.—1st ed.
        p.   cm.
    Includes bibliographical references and index.
    ISBN 0-8016-7932-X
    1. Sports medicine—Research. 2. Exercise—Research. I. Mood,
Dale. II. Morrow, James R., 1947- . III. Title.
RC1210.H9   195
617.1'027'072—dc20   95-39006
                                                      CIP

98 99 00 / 9 8 7 6 5 4 3 2

Preface

This textbook is designed to prepare students in the field of sport and exercise sciences to read and interpret research reports effectively. Our goal is to present the information in an interesting and relevant fashion. Our assumption is that students should first develop a knowledge of how research is conducted and reported. Students armed with this knowledge and interest in developing further skills in this area can then focus on learning to execute specific experimental designs and conduct data analysis.

ORGANIZATION

The organization of this textbook mirrors the organization of a research report and is divided into four main sections: *The Introduction and Literature Review, Methods, Results,* and *Discussion.* The Introduction and Literature Review section includes Chapters 1 through 4. Chapter 1 provides an introduction to the development of knowledge through research and emphasizes the role of theories in the research process. Chapter 2 presents sources for research questions and describes different types of research conducted in sport and exercise sciences. Chapter 3 discusses the most common methods for disseminating research findings and provides information on how a research manuscript is prepared for publication. Chapter 4 contains both a discussion of the traditional information resources housed in a university library as well as a discussion on emerging information resources such as the Internet and the World Wide Web. The Methods section begins with Chapter 5 and ends with Chapter 9. The goal of this section is to present information about common research methods and procedures used in sport and exercise sciences. In Chapter 5 information on sampling procedures, variables, variance, and research validity is presented. Chapter 6 introduces the process of simple experimental design. Chapter 7 continues the discussion on experimental design by describing complex experiments. Chapter 8 reviews qualitative research methods. This section concludes with Chapter 9, which provides information and examples of a wide range of research methods including surveys, epidemiological methods, meta-analysis, and others. The Results section includes chapters 10 and 11. Chapter 10 contains discussions on measurement issues and descriptive data analysis methods. Chapter 11 focuses on statistical methods used to support research findings. The Discussion section consists of Chapter 12 and contains information on research proposals, ethical issues, and conducting research. Appendices include a sample survey analysis of variance source tables, and the Library of Congress classification system.

PEDAGOGICAL FEATURES

Each chapter includes several features intended to aid student learning.

Key Terms—Each chapter begins with a list of terms that are the key concepts that students should understand.

Learning Goals—A list of learning goals also appears at the beginning of each chapter; these are connected to the key terms. Each of these goals represents an important concept in the chapter.

Examples from the Literature—We have included many abstracts, tables, figures, and sections of text from a variety of journals publishing sport and exercise science research reports. These examples serve two purposes: first, to illustrate a concept with an example from the literature and second, to provide the student with a sense of the breadth of sports and exercise science research.

Chapter Summary—The chapter summary reviews the main concepts and topics presented in the chapter.

Exercises—Each chapter offers exercises and learning activities designed to reinforce the concepts presented in the chapter.

INSTRUCTOR'S MANUAL

An Instructor's Manual is available to qualified adopters of this book. Supplemental materials presented in the Instructor's Manual include:

- Exercises and assignments
- Transparency masters
- Testbank of potential questions

ACKNOWLEDGMENTS

The assistance and support of the many individuals who contributed to the writing and production of this text are gratefully acknowledged. Specifically, we would like to thank Mary McElroy for contributing Chapter 8: Qualitative Research. We would also like to thank the many journal publishers and authors who granted permission to reproduce Abstracts, Tables, Figures, and sections of text in this book. In particular, Maureen Weiss from the *Research Quarterly for Exercise and Sport* for her 3 Editor's Viewpoint articles.

Special recognition goes to our reviewers: Karen DePauw, Washington State University; Gerald Hyner, Purdue University; Ron McBride, Texas A&M University; and Laurette Taylor, University of Oklahoma. Their comments and suggestions were very helpful.

Several other people also contributed to the writing of this textbook. We would like to thank Mitsi Hulsing, Kathy Walden, Katherine Moore, Karen Hennessy, and Phyllis Bailey who made many helpful additions, suggestions, and who also helped produce some of the illustrations. We also thank Luke Patrick and David Dzewaltowski for the section on multi-dimensional scaling. We also acknowledge the contributions of the many students who are too numerous to mention individually for helping over the years in formulating ideas and for making suggestions. We would like to thank everyone at Mosby-Year Book who encouraged us and assisted in the production of the text including Vicki Malinee, Brian Morovitz, Michelle Turenne, and Christy Wells.

Finally, the authors would like to thank their wives and families for their patience and sacrifice during the time this book was being written. A task such as this becomes far more time consuming than one might originally imagine.

Randy Hyllegard
Dale P. Mood
James R. Morrow, Jr.

Contents in Brief

Detailed Contents

INTERPRETING RESEARCH IN
SPORT AND EXERCISE SCIENCE

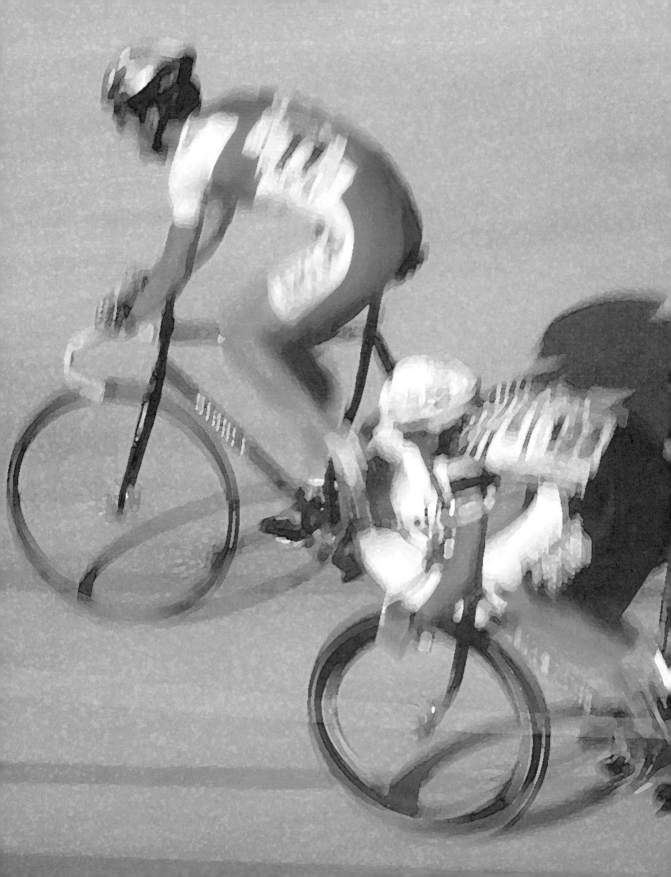

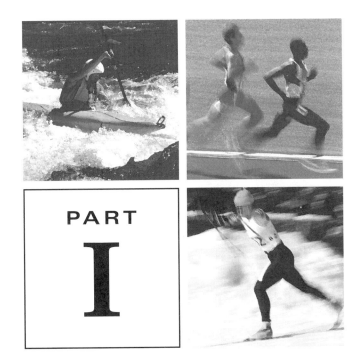

Introduction and Literature Review

PART I

The Scientific Process

CHAPTER 1

LEARNING GOALS

After reading this chapter you will be able to:

1 Describe why studying research methods is valuable; both academically and in daily life.

2 Identify the subdisciplines that form sport exercise sciences.

3 State the six steps in research.

4 Define and explain the term *theory*.

5 Differentiate between a theory and a hypothesis.

6 Describe the different levels of knowledge.

7 Explain the difference between inductive reasoning and deductive reasoning.

TERMS

Research
Theory
Empiricism
Hypothesis
Deduction
Induction

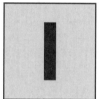

n 1903, the scientist and engineer Simon New-comb wrote an article entitled *The Outlook for the Flying Machine* in which he argued that mankind would never build a useful airplane (Newcomb, 1903). Based on the fact that birds have brains and nervous systems, which enable them to flap their wings and thus fly, Newcomb concluded that a machine could not be built with the physical and cognitive abilities needed to fly. Newcomb further argued that a machine could not be built that could support the weight of passengers and still fly, and that even if such a machine could fly, it could not land safely (Figure 1.1).

Newcomb's beliefs were disproven within the year when on December 17, 1903, Orville and Wilbur Wright successfully flew the first engine-powered airplane at Kitty Hawk, North Carolina. This landmark event not only dispelled previously held notions but also initiated the science of aeronautics,

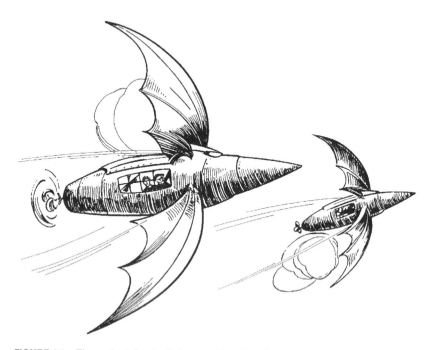

FIGURE 1.1 The outlook for the flying machine. Two fanciful flying machines, one has twice the lineal dimensions of the other. It has eight times the weight, but only four times the carrying capacity, its own weight included. (Professor Simon Newcomb, LL. D.)

which eventually led to the development of passenger and military aircraft such as the Concorde and the F-117A stealth fighter that we are familiar with today. Only 66 years after the Wright brothers flew less than 100 yards, Apollo 11 landed on the moon. Today, space shuttle flights are almost routine. It is remarkable to think that the developments in aeronautics that led to these events occurred in less than 100 years.

The Wright brothers' success is one example of how human knowledge and understanding of the world is continually challenged by new discoveries, findings, insights, and inventions. Such advancements are generally not accidental but the result of directed research, hard work, and a quest for new knowledge. It is through such endeavors that we further our understanding of the world we live in and change the manner in which we live.

Research plays an important role in expanding our knowledge and understanding of human movement. As a student, your understanding of the principles of research will provide you with a strong foundation for classroom learning and individual research projects.

ORGANIZATION OF THE TEXTBOOK

Research reports are normally organized to follow a standard format. The organization of this textbook mirrors that of a typical research report and is divided into four main sections: *Introduction and Literature Review, Methods, Results,* and *Discussion* with each section divided into chapters. The introduction section presents information on the philosophy of research, research reports, and information resources. The methods section focuses on experimental design. The results section discusses how to interpret the statistics found in research reports. The discussion section presents topics and concepts that the researcher must consider when conducting research.

RESEARCH IN SPORT AND EXERCISE SCIENCES

Sport and exercise science is a relatively young academic discipline with roots in both the social and natural sciences. In a series of articles Newell (1990a; 1990b) and Slowikowski and Newell (1990) discuss the state of sport and exercise science at institutions of higher education. One issue they discuss is the lack of a common name among departments in the field. Examples include The Department of Exercise and Movement Sciences (University of Oregon), The Department of Kinesiology (Kansas State University, University of Colorado, University of Maryland, and others), The Department of Sport and Exercise Science (Oregon State University), and The Department of Health and Human Performance (Iowa State University).

This lack of a common name illustrates the evolving nature of the discipline. Historically, sport and exercise research took place in the physical education department at most universities or colleges. These departments also normally trained educators in physical education and conducted a wide variety of activity and fitness classes. Many traditional physical education departments have redefined their mission and increased the emphasis on research while decreasing the emphasis on training educators. Name changes are intended to reflect the new emphasis on academics and research.

Sport and exercise sciences are divided into several overlapping subdisciplines including: *adapted physical education,* where physical activities and sports are modified to meet the needs of the disabled; *biomechanics,* where the principles of mechanics are applied to sports and movement; *exercise physiology and biochemistry,* which emphasize the analysis of chronic and acute physiological adaptations to exercise; *growth and development,* where physical and psychological maturation and aging are related to movement; *sport history,* which traces important developments in sports and athletics; *sport nutrition,* where the impact of nutrition on athletic performance is studied; *sport sociology,* which examines the impact of sports and athletics on society; *measurement and evaluation,* in which the statistical techniques and procedures for evaluating movement are developed and assessed; *motor behavior,* which is further divided among *motor learning, motor control,* and *sport psychology,* where the conditions that affect the acquisition and production of skilled motor behaviors are studied.

WHY STUDY RESEARCH METHODS?

Several factors probably contributed to your reasons for enrolling in a research methods course. Students usually give the pragmatic reasons such as completing a required course, earning credit hours toward graduation, or satisfying admission requirements for graduate or professional schools. Departments offer a research methods course for several reasons (see the box below). A research methods course can enhance your understanding of other courses such as exercise physiology, biomechanics, or motor behavior. Sport and exercise sciences is a research-based discipline, and the chances are high that your professors will present information from a research perspective. In addition, a research methods course will help you read and interpret scientific journal articles. When researchers write journal articles, they assume that the reader has a certain level of familiarity with research fundamentals. A research methods course will not necessarily help you understand the contents of an article—that depends on your knowledge of a given subject. However, a research methods course will help you appreciate and understand the research process in a general sense, and that knowledge can be applied to a wide range of subjects.

Top 10 Reasons for Studying Research Methods

10 To gain credit hours toward graduation.

 9 To meet entrance requirements for graduate or professional school.

 8 To help you complete assignments for your classes.

 7 To help you understand information presented in classes.

 6 To help you understand your textbooks.

 5 To help you understand the research process.

 4 To help you understand research reports.

 3 To distinguish factual information from quasi-factual information and opinion not based in fact.

 2 To develop your own research skills.

 1 To develop a more critical thought process.

A research methods course will also help you distinguish factual information from quasi-factual information and opinions not necessarily grounded in facts. Each day we are exposed to large amounts of information from a wide range of sources. The researcher tends to view this information with a critical eye and asks questions about the information before accepting it as fact.

One way to fine tune your ability to distinguish between different types of information is to carefully examine product advertisements. Companies, often advised by their advertising agencies, invest considerable amounts of time and money trying to convince us to choose one product over another. As a careful consumer, we need to be able to separate advertising claims from facts (Table 1.1). Three strategies are commonly used in many advertisements that are intended to convince us that one product is superior to another or that a product is effective. These strategies include using parity claims, statistical information, and testimonials. Let's look at some examples of each.

Parity claims

A parity claim is the careful wording of an advertisement that gives the reader the impression that one product is superior to another, when actually the wording means that two products are essentially equal. An advertisement for the pain medication Advil is worded, "Nothing is proven more effective or longer lasting than Advil." The phrase, "Nothing is proven more effective or longer lasting . . ." is easily interpreted by the consumer as stating that Advil is the *most* effective and the *longest* lasting pain reliever. However, examine the wording carefully: The key words in the ad are *more* and *longer*. The wording actually means that other pain medications are as *equally as effective* and last *equally as long* as Advil. Advil is not more effective or longer lasting than other comparable pain medications. The subtle wording of the advertisement makes it appear that the product is better than competing products, when actually it is only just as good as other products.

The Oral-B toothbrush is advertised with the slogan, "You can buy a fancier toothbrush. But you can't buy a more effective one." Do you see the parity claim? Similar to the Advil ad, the claim, "But you can't buy a more effective one"

TABLE 1.1 Techniques Used in Advertising

Technique	Questions to raise
Power words to gain attention	
"Strengthens immune system"	Is this possible? Will it help treat AIDS?
"Helps . . ."	Does it? What way? How much?
"Fights . . ."	How? Is it effective?
"Provides relief three times longer"	Longer than what? Why not four times?
"Free . . . money back"	What is free? Is this a come-on? What do you pay for?
"It's natural"	Is anything natural? Meaning? Is it better? More expensive?
"Amazing breakthrough"	Who says? What evidence? How effective?
"Less salt, fat, calories"	Than what? Than previous product? Is it still high?
"Cholesterol-free"	Is it undesirably high in fat?
Misleading comparisions to encourage consumers to jump to conclusions	
"Contains twice as much . . ."	As what? Is it better? More economical?
"Wrinkle eraser"	Does it really erase? Or cover temporarily?
"Isn't it time you tried . . ."	Why? Because everybody does?
"Contains X"	What is X? What does it do? Is it better than the ingredient(s) of competing products?
"Up to 8-hour relief"	What is "up to"?
"Fast-acting" "Inexpensive"	How does it compare to other products?
"Guaranteed purity, potency, and quality"	Does the product work?
"Clinically proven safe and effective"	What's the evidence?
Imagery to appeal to emotion	
"Quiet world is like taking a vacation from tension"	Will it help you escape from problems? The real world?
"Beautiful people, places, things"	Will the product help you achieve this?
"The Marlboro man"	Is smoking macho or stupid?
"Look younger instantly"	How quickly? Possible? Temporary? Aren't most products? Qualifications?
"Created by research scientist (or specialist)"	What is? Why secret? Does it work?
"Miracle beauty secret, no surgery" "Used extensively in Europe?"	Why not in United States? Not FDA approved?

From Cornacchia HJ and Barrett S: Consumer health: A guide to intelligent decisions, St Louis, 1993, Mosby.

implies that the Oral-B is the most effective toothbrush available. It actually says that the Oral-B is equally as effective as other toothbrushes. Battery manufacturers have long used the same strategy: Duracell advertisements say, "No other battery lasts longer." This means that Duracell batteries last just as long as the competition, but not necessarily any longer.

Table 1.1 lists a number of common techniques used in advertising.

Testimonials

A testimonial is defined as a statement providing evidence in support of a claim. An old joke among statisticians and researchers is the saying that 10 testimonials and 50 cents will get you a cup of coffee. The point is, we should regard testimonial evidence cautiously. Strength and fitness magazines offer prime examples of testimonial-based advertisements. Chief among these are products promoted to accelerate strength gains. Various protein supplements and other products claim they will help build muscle fast and the advertisements use before-and-after photographs of individuals who show considerable muscular development. Even though those people shown in the photographs may have actually gained muscle mass, they do not necessarily represent what will happen to the average individual under similar conditions. For example, some people have a genetic predisposition for muscular hypertrophy caused by weight training, but most do not. The claim that these products are equally effective for all people is not necessarily valid.

Statistical information

A third way advertisements try to appear objective or scientific is to give statistical information. Whenever reading advertisements that contain a lot of statistical information, keep in mind Mark Twain's famous axiom, "There are lies, damn lies, and statistics"—the point being that statistics can be made to say just about anything. Advertisements for skin care products are notorious for using statistics to support their claims. The problem is that the statistics given are usually difficult to evaluate and interpret and therefore largely meaningless. The advertisement for Revlon Results night cream is a prime example. The advertisement claims,

"Instantly skin's moisture is boosted by over 600%!" Or, "In just one week, fine dry lines and wrinkles are reduced by over 38%!" The questions we have to ask ourselves are where do these numbers come from and exactly what comparisons are being made? Unfortunately, these advertisements do not provide enough information for the reader to clearly evaluate the statistics. Because only incomplete information is provided, the statistics lose impact for the aware reader. Our purpose is not to criticize these products. Our intention is show that we should use our critical thinking skills when evaluating information, commercial advertisements included.

Perhaps the best reason for taking a research methods course is to develop your own research and critical reading skills. Many students continue their education in graduate and professional programs and often find themselves either assisting in research projects or conducting their own projects. There are also a number of undergraduate opportunities to participate in research projects. These can range from laboratory assignments, independent studies, practicums, and/or research assistantships. The more you know about research methods, the better off you will be as you begin your research. Research can be described as an attitude and a process that results in progressive learning and knowledge building.

GAINING KNOWLEDGE

The main goal of research is the gathering and interpreting of information to answer questions. This basic principle is true in all academic areas, and sport and exercise sciences is no exception. Below are a few sample questions under investigation by researchers in sport and exercise sciences:

- Does aerobic exercise inhibit the natural aging process?
- How knowledgeable are children today in the areas of physical fitness, diet, and exercise?
- Under what practice conditions are motor skills most effectively acquired and retained?
- What type of diet is best for athletic performance?
- Why does strength training actually increase muscular strength?

- What is the relationship between physical activity and health?
- What factors affect peoples' choices of recreational activities?

Questions like these and many others provide researchers in sport and exercise sciences with the problems and ideas they work with to advance the body of knowledge in this discipline.

Researchers may not be any more curious than anyone else, but they are willing to work hard to answer questions. In the early 1500s, Nicolaus Copernicus spent countless nights carefully observing and recording objects in the heavens to develop his controversial (at the time) explanation of planetary motion. Galileo, in the late 1500s, painstakingly timed balls rolling down inclined planes to study gravity. During the 1950s, Franklin Henry, in his laboratory at the University of California, initiated a considerable amount of research on skilled motor behaviors. Copernicus, Galileo, and Henry each used a similar process to gain knowledge: (1) ask a new question; (2) make initial observations; (3) conduct a systematic investigation; (4) analyze the new information; (5) interpret the findings; and (6) integrate the findings with previous knowledge. This basic research cycle has been followed by generations of researchers either intuitively or through formal training. In the story of Adam and Eve, Mark Twain (1938, 73) shows how Eve uses the six-step process to investigate the world:

> I scored the next great triumph for science myself: [1]*to wit, how the milk gets into the cow.* Both of us had marveled over that mystery a long time. [2]*We had followed the cows around for years—that is, in the daytime—but never caught them drinking a fluid of that color.* And so, at last we said they undoubtedly procured it at night. Then we took turns and watched them by night. The result was the same—the puzzle remained unsolved. . . . One night as I lay musing, and looking at the stars, a grand idea flashed through my head, and I saw my way! . . . [3]*deep in the woods I chose a small grassy spot . . . making a secure pen; then I enclosed a cow in it. I milked her dry, then left her there, a prisoner.* There was nothing there to drink— she must get milk by her secret alchemy, or stay dry.
>
> All day I was a fidget, and could not talk connectedly I was so preoccupied; but Adam was busy trying to invent the multiplication table, and did not notice. Toward

sunset he had gotten as far as 6 times 9 are 27, and while he was drunk with the joy of his achievement and dead to my presence and all things else, I stole away to my cow. My hands shook so with excitement and with dread failure that for some moments I could not get a grip on a teat; then I succeeded, and the milk came! [4]*Two gallons. Two gallons, and nothing to make it out of.* I knew at once the explanation: [5]*The milk was not taken in by the mouth, it was condensed from the atmosphere through the cow's hair.* I ran and told Adam, and his happiness was as great as mine, and his pride in me inexpressible.

Presently he said, `Do you know, you have not made merely one weighty and far-reaching contribution to science, but two.'

And that was true. By a series of experiments we had long ago arrived at the conclusion that atmospheric air consisted of water in invisible suspension; also, that the components of water were hydrogen and oxygen, in the proportion of two parts of the former to one of the latter, and expressed by the symbol H_2O. My discovery revealed the fact that was still another ingredient—milk. [6]*We enlarged the symbol to $H_2O, M.$*

THEORIES

The basic goal of science is to develop a body of knowledge based on facts. However, the road leading to facts can be a bumpy one with occasional wrong turns, conflicting and confusing signs, and unpredictable stops and starts. To help guide the journey to facts, researchers often rely on theories. The term **theory** is defined as a set of related statements that explain a set of facts. Researchers in all disciplines use theories to help them describe, predict, and explain events or behaviors. For example, between A.D. 130 and 200, the Greek physician Galen theorized that the nervous system operated on the same basic principles as the circulatory system. Galen suggested that axons and nerve bodies were hollow, and a clear fluid termed *animal spirits* flowed throughout the nervous system. Muscle contractions occurred when these animal spirits flowed through the nervous system to muscles producing the particular movement. Galen's theory was largely accepted until the early 1700s when the Dutch anatomist Van Leeuwenhoek examined tissue cross sections with the newly invented microscope. He found evidence that nerve fibers were not hollow as Galen had suggested, thus bringing Galen's theories into doubt. In the late 1700s, the Italian inventor Galvani conducted experiments with static electricity on frog legs. Galvani showed that muscles would twitch when the nerve axon was stimulated with an electrical charge. Galvani recognized the importance of the relationship between electricity and muscle contractions and theorized that electricity played an important role in the function of the nervous system. This discovery initiated an entirely new way of investigating and understanding the nervous system.

You might think that Galen's animal spirits theory was a poor theory. This is not necessarily the case. Researchers argue that the only bad theories are those theories that cannot be shown to be incorrect. When the results of empirical tests support a theory, it is strengthened. A theory is weakened when tests fail to find results predicted by the theory. It is commonly believed that researchers *prove* theories. Most researchers believe that theories are never proven. There are only competing theories of differing levels of acceptance. One reason absolute proof is difficult to achieve is because we can never know what knowledge the future may hold. Theories are accepted originally for a variety of reasons, the most important of which is the theory's ability to explain behavior. Many of today's theories will eventually be replaced or modified by better theories sometime in the future. Galen's animal spirits theory of the nervous system endured for hundreds of years because there was little evidence demonstrating it false. With the development of the microscope and the harnessing of electricity, the technological innovations needed to bring Galen's theory into doubt became available.

The Functions of Theories

Theories serve two general roles in the development of knowledge: (1) they help *organize* information and facts about events or behaviors, and (2) they are used to *make predictions* that provide the basis for new research. Theoretical research is commonly regarded as one of the most valuable forms of research because it is based on specific predictions.

The ability to unify information and predict future knowledge is a particularly powerful attribute.

Evaluating Theories

Three factors help researchers judge the merits of competing theories: precision, simplicity, and testability. *Precision* is how accurately a theory describes behavior or makes predictions. Precise theories are favored over imprecise theories. *Simplicity* of a theory refers to the number of qualifiers or special conditions that must be met before a theory can be used to make accurate predictions. For example, a theory that needs three qualifiers to explain behavior is less desirable than a theory that explains the same behavior with no qualifier. Occam's razor is the name given to a principle that implies explanations should be kept as simple as possible with the fewest number of assumptions. *Testability* refers to the extent to which **empirical** methods may be used to gather evidence about a theory. Without the benefits of astronomical instruments, the Big Bang Theory could not be tested and therefore would be of little theoretical value. A theory that holds no promise of being empirically tested serves little useful purpose. This is not to say that futuristic theories are of no value. Some of Einstein's ideas concerning space and time, for example, were expressed prior to the development of the technology needed to test them. Many forward-looking individuals develop ideas and theories beyond the capabilities of the current technology to adequately assess them. Galen's view of the central nervous system went unchallenged for several centuries because of technological limitations. The key element is the promise for future knowledge or technology that will help test new theories.

Theories in the News

The discussion of theories is not limited to the classroom or to research reports. It is quite common to hear someone mention a theory on television, or to read about a theory in a newspaper or magazine. The next time you hear an explanation based on a theory, pay close attention and try to decide if the term is being used correctly. The theories presented in the following sections were found in popular magazines.

The ultra-violet light theory for the mysterious disappearance of frogs

Biologists have noticed an alarming reduction in the number of frogs and related amphibians in many environments. One theory explaining this phenomenon is a thinning of the ozone layer in the upper atmosphere. A consequence of a thinner layer of ozone is an increase in the amount of ultraviolet light passing through the upper atmosphere and reaching the surface of the earth. This increase in ultraviolet light is thought to be harmful to amphibians. To test this theory, a researcher at Oregon State University designed an experiment in which frog eggs were exposed to different amounts of ultraviolet light. Some eggs were exposed to natural sunlight; other eggs were partially shielded from natural sunlight and thus exposed to lower levels of ultraviolet light. Following an exposure interval, the researchers counted the number of eggs produced in each of the ultraviolet conditions and found that the eggs exposed to natural sunlight produced fewer tadpoles than the eggs shielded from sunlight. The biologist suspected that because the eggs float in ponds near the surface as they gestate, they are exposed to direct sunlight and that the high levels of ultraviolet light damage the eggs, causing fewer eggs to fully develop thus reducing the number of tadpoles. This evidence supports the theory that as the ozone layer thins, increasing exposure to ultra-violet light may be harmful to amphibians and possibly other species.

Two social theories for inappropriate rising intonation

Some have noticed an increasing amount of so-called inappropriate rising intonation at the end of declarative sentences. Correctly used, rising intonation indicates that the speaker is asking a question. For example, when asking the question, "Does class meet in Carlson Gym?" the voice rises on the word *Gym* to help the listener identify the remark as a question. A declarative statement with inappropriate rising intonation might be, "It looks like the basketball team will have a good record *this year.*" In this example, the rising intonation on the words *this year* is not appropriate. Inappropriate rising intonation is particularly common among adolescent females and is sometimes referred to as "val speak."

Let's suggest a couple theories that might help us explain this behavior. Our first theory proposes that individuals use rising intonation when speaking to authority figures as an approval-gaining device. The theory is based on the assumption that adolescents are sometimes unsure of themselves and express their need for approval by completing most sentences as if they were a question. Psychological or emotional factors are said to be the basis for this speech pattern. Our second, and competing, theory argues that rising intonation is little more than a trendy speech pattern currently in vogue among adolescents (similar to popular slang expressions). Adolescent behaviors are strongly influenced by peers in areas such as dress, music, and hair styles. In addition, adolescents like to probe the limits of their parents' tolerance. This theory therefore suggests that adolescents, being adolescents, speak this way mainly because their friends do the same and also because parents and teachers disapprove.

As researchers, we could develop a series of studies investigating this speech pattern. Eventually, the weight of the evidence would support one theory over the other and that theory would gain acceptance.

Three theories for the origin of HIV

Research on viruses, including Human Immunodeficiency Virus (HIV), the virus associated with Aquired Immunodeficiency Syndrome (AIDS) is an important issue. One question under investigation is determining the origin of viruses. Researchers have theorized three possibilities. One theory suggests that new viruses develop through a gradual evolutionary change in an older virus. Thus the current HIV may be a more potent form of an older HIV. A second theory suggests a virus that affected only one species might begin to affect another species. Consequently, the immunodeficiency virus originally infecting monkeys could be the origin for HIV. A third theory argues that a very rare virus might seem new when it suddenly emerges in larger numbers of victims. Some have argued that HIV is actually ancient but was extremely rare until the late 1960s or early 1970s when behavioral changes began to expose more people to the virus.

Each of these theories provides a basis for research into the origin of viruses. The advantage of theoretical research is that predictions can be tested empirically and the theory most strongly supported by evidence is favored over competing theories.

THEORIES IN SPORT AND EXERCISE SCIENCES

There are many, many theories in sport and exercise sciences. You will no doubt learn several theories in your classes. A few examples follow.

Delayed-Onset Muscle Soreness

Delayed-onset muscle soreness (DOMS) is muscle soreness that occurs about 24 to 48 hours after strenuous eccentric exercise. Symptoms are stiffness and pain in the muscles lasting for 2 or 3 days following exercise. Several theories have been suggested to explain the cause of DOMS. These include the *connective tissue damage theory* (Komi and Buskirk, 1972), the *muscle tear theory* (Frieden, Kjorell, and Thornell, 1984), and the *muscle spasm theory* (de Vries, 1966) (see the box on p. 19). The connective tissue damage theory suggests that strenuous exercise places stress on the connective tissue surrounding muscles that results in small tears. These tears result in inflammation in the connective tissue and thus the soreness. The muscle tear theory proposes basically the same idea, the difference being that the tissue damage occurs in the muscle fibers rather than in the connective tissue. The muscle spasm theory, as you might suspect, attributes DOMS to localized spasms. The spasms increase muscle tension, and reduce the range of motion, thus leading to the stiffness and soreness.

The Benefits of Random Practice

Random and blocked practice schedules have been studied extensively by motor learning researchers. When using a blocked practice schedule, the learner practices one skill over many identical practice trials. For example, you might hit a 7-iron 15 or 20 times before switching to a different club. With a random practice schedule, you would hit one 7-iron shot,

The Effects of Static Stretching and Warm-Up on Prevention of Delayed-Onset Muscle Soreness

David M. High, Edward T. Howley, and B. Don Franks

It has been suggested in the lay literature that static stretching and/or warm-up will prevent the occurrence of Delayed-Onset Muscle Soreness (DOMS). The primary purpose of this study was to determine the effects of static stretching and/or warm-up on the level of pain associated with DOMS. Sixty-two healthy male and female volunteers were randomly assigned to four groups: (a) subjects who statically stretched the quadriceps muscle group before a step, (b) subjects who only performed a stepping warm-up, (c) subjects who both stretched and performed a stepping warm-up prior to a step test, and (d) subjects who only performed a step test. The step test (Asmussen, 1956) required subjects to do concentric work with their right leg and eccentric work with their left leg to voluntary exhaustion. Subjects rated their muscle soreness on a ratio scale from zero to six at 24-hour intervals for 5 days following the step test. A $4 \times 2 \times 2$ ANOVA with repeated measures on legs and Duncan's New Multiple Range post-hoc test found no difference in peak muscle soreness among the groups doing the step test or for gender ($p > .05$). There was the expected significant difference in peak muscle soreness between eccentrically and concentrically worked legs, with the eccentrically worked leg experiencing greater muscle soreness. We concluded that static stretching and/or warm-up does not prevent DOMS resulting from exhaustive exercise.

From High DM, Howley ET, and Franks BD: Research Quarterly for Exercise and Sport 60(4):357-361, 1989.

then maybe one 3-wood shot, followed by one 5-iron, and so on. This type of practice is termed random because the practice order is continually varied. Research has shown that when practicing several related skills such as different golf club hits or badminton serves for example, skills are most effectively learned following a random practice schedule (Goode and Magill, 1986). Two similar theories provide an explanation for the benefits of random practice: the elaboration theory and the memory reconstruction theory. The elaboration theory argues that random practice helps the learner better discriminate the subtle differences between similar skills (Shea and Morgan, 1979). These differences are *elaborated* in memory, or made more distinct. Because each skill is

The Contextual Interference Effect for Skill Variations from the Same and Different Generalized Motor Programs

Hiroshi Sekiya, Richard A. Magill, Ben Sidaway, and David I. Anderson

Magill and Hall (1990) hypothesized that the contextual interference (CI) effect is found only when task variations to be learned are governed by different generalized motor programs (GMPs). The present experiments examined their hypothesis by requiring subjects to learn variations of a tapping task that had either different (Experiment 1) or the same (Experiment 2) relative timing structure. In each experiment, subjects (N = 36) performed 270 acquisition trails with knowledge of results (KR) in either a blocked or a serial order. One day later, subjects performed 30 retention trials without KR. In data analyses, errors due to parameter modifications were dissociated from errors due to GMP construction to examine which process was responsible for the CI effect. In both experiments, parameter learning created a CI effect while GMP learning failed to produce a CI effect. In the light of these findings, a modification is proposed to the Magill and Hall (1990) hypothesis that takes into account these distinct processes in motor learning.

From Sekiya H, et al.: Research Quarterly for Exercise and Sport 65(4):330-338, 1994.

more distinct, the learner is better able to produce them (see the box above).

The memory reconstruction theory, on the other hand, suggests that when practicing skills, action plans are constructed in memory. When practicing randomly, the learner constructs an action plan, is forced to forget it, and develops a new action plan for the next skill. This process of action plan construction, forgetting, and action plan construction results in effective learning (Lee and Magill, 1985).

MENTAL PRACTICE

The term *mental practice* refers to the cognitive rehearsal of physical skills. Novices learning a skill and experts preparing for competition both have experimented with various mental practice techniques (see the box on p. 21). Research has shown that mental practice, especially when combined with physical practice, is an effective learning tool (Hird, Landers, Thomas, and Horan, 1991).

A Comparison of Mental Practice Techniques as Applied to the Developing Competitive Figure Skater

Shawna L. Palmer

This study investigated the influence of two distinct mental practice techniques on figure skating performance. Twelve prenovice and novice level competitive figure skaters each performed two figures which were assessed as a pretreatment measure. In Phase I the subjects were assigned to one of three groups: Martin self-talk technique, paper patch technique, or a no-treatment control group. Following a 4-week period of using the assigned technique, a second performance assessment revealed no significant differences between the Martin group and the control group, while the paper patch group showed significant improvements over both. In Phase 2 a multiple-comparison-across-subjects design was used. A third assessment was completed after an additional 4-week period which demonstrated that a significantly greater number of skaters using the paper patch technique improved in performance. This study reveals the importance of investigating the efficacies of different types of mental practice when applied to specific sporting or performance activities.

From Palmer SL: The Sport Psychologist 6(2):148, 1992.

The benefits of mental practice have been explained by two theories: the neuromuscular theory and the cognitive theory. The *neuromuscular theory* asserts that when mentally practicing a motor skill, the motor system is responding, but at levels too low to generate overt movements. In other words, the motor system is sending the same instructions to the musculature that it would during normal movements, but below the threshold necessary for physical movement (Hale, 1982). In effect, mental practice activates the motor system as it would during actual movements and thus benefits performance.

The *cognitive theory* suggests that mental practice helps the learner better understand the goals of the movement and thus makes practice more effective. With mental practice, the learner develops a clearer understanding of the movements. Evidence for this theory comes from studies where subjects practice tasks that have a low mental demand or a high mental demand. If the cognitive explanation is true, the subjects in the high mental demand condition should benefit the most from mental practice, which was found by Ryan and Simons (1983).

As you can see in the previous examples, a theory serves as a tentative explanation for a particular behavior or event. Theories are valued because they allow researchers to ask questions and classify findings or knowledge within a specific framework.

HYPOTHESES

If a theory is a statement that organizes a set of related facts, a research **hypothesis** is a prediction stemming from a theory. For example, the Big Bang theory of the birth of the universe suggests that the universe originated with a vast explosion of matter. One research hypothesis based on this theory predicts that if the universe did indeed begin with an explosion, then the universe should be expanding. If astronomical observations find evidence of an expanding universe, the theory would be strengthened. A hypothesis from the muscle tear theory of DOMS might predict an increase in metabolic by-products found in the blood associated with muscle tissue repair processes.

LEVELS OF KNOWLEDGE

The term *science* is derived from the Latin word *scientia* meaning having knowledge. The development of scientific knowledge has several levels beginning with the description of behavior, then building toward the prediction of behavior, the control of behavior, and the explanation of behavior. For example, since heart disease is a serious problem today, let's look at how cardiovascular disease research progresses from the simplest level of description to the more difficult level of explaining.

Research to Describe

Cardiovascular disease accounts for over 50% of the total deaths in the United States. We know this because various agencies gather information on mortality rates and causes of death. This information makes no attempt to predict who is most susceptible to cardiovascular disease or to explain the causes of cardiovascular disease. Nevertheless, this research is important because comparisons can be made with past measurements so that trends or unusual occurrences can be identified.

Research to Predict

An important step forward in the advancement of knowledge is demonstrating the relationships among variables. If behaviors or events are found to be systematically related to one another, then prediction becomes possible. For example, research has shown that we are more susceptible to cardiovascular disease if certain risk factors are present. These risk factors include elevated blood lipids, hypertension, cigarette smoking, physical inactivity, obesity, diet, personality type, and stress levels among others. We can predict the likelihood that someone may be vulnerable to cardiovascular disease depending on the level of each of these factors. As you can see, prediction is more powerful than description. Description only tells us how things are, prediction can tell us what is likely to happen. In research, as in life, predictions are not always accurate. One of the goals of research is to make increasingly accurate predictions by better defining the relationships among variables.

Research to Control

If we understand how events are related to each other, we can begin to control events. By changing our behavior, for example, we can affect cardiovascular disease risk factors (decrease dietary fats, stop smoking cigarettes, increase the amount of exercise activity, reduce stress levels, and so forth). In order to control, we must understand relationships so we can affect variables to produce the intended results. We can change our diet and exercise patterns to control blood lipids and weight.

Research to Explain

Although behaviors may be predicted and controlled, we still may not understand why events occur. The issue here is *why* do these risk factors increase the likelihood of cardiovascular

Diet and Coronary Heart Disease: Beyond Dietary Fats and Low-Density-Lipoprotein Cholesterol

Gary E. Fraser

Traditonally, the effects of diet on coronary heart disease have been attributed to the effects of medium-chain fatty acids, soluble fiber, and dietary cholesterol on serum low-density-lipoprotein (LDL) cholesterol concentrations. We review evidence here that many other dietary substances may affect risk, often via mechanisms not involving LDL-cholesterol concentrations directly. Such substances include phytosterols, tocotrienols, arginine, and antioxidant vitamins. The effects of diet on high-density-lipoprotein-cholesterol concentrations, triglycerides (fasting and postprandial), oxidized LDL particles, prostaglandins, and endothelium-derived relaxing factor are described. Finally, an illustration of some epidemiologic associations between diet and coronary disease events is made from the Adventist Health Study data.

From Fraser GE: American Journal of Clinical Nutrition 59(suppl):1117S-23S, 1994.

disease? It is known, for example, that diets high in cholesterol and saturated fats are associated with atherosclerosis, the buildup of fatty deposits or plaques in the coronary arteries, and this is linked to cardiovascular disease (see the box above).

The American Heart Association estimates that a person with a blood cholesterol level above 250 milligrams per 100 milliliters of blood has about three times the risk of cardiovascular disease as a person with cholesterol below 200 milligrams. An understanding of the mechanism by which fatty deposits and plaques develop would help explain why high fat diets lead to atherosclerosis. Explanatory knowledge is more difficult to develop than predictive, control, or descriptive knowledge because it requires an understanding of cause and effect relationships.

DEDUCTIVE AND INDUCTIVE REASONING

Deductive reasoning is commonly defined as the method of logically drawing conclusions. Observations of general facts are shaped to explain specific occurrences. For example, one could deduce:

Reasonable men adapt to the world.
Unreasonable men expect the world to adapt to them.
Therefore, all progress is made by unreasonable men.

In a sense, this statement functions as a theory; it identifies certain behaviors and then makes a prediction. One problem with the deductive method is many of the assumptions made about behavior may be difficult to test and may, in fact, be wrong. What evidence is there to support the claim that reasonable men adapt to the world? It is difficult to positively support a claim such as this.

Inductive reasoning is generally just the opposite of deductive reasoning. Many researchers emphasize empirical observations (data) and view science as working from data to theory. Put another way, observations progress from specific to general. One limitation of the inductive method is that empirical observations are tied to the conditions under which they are made. In other words, facts or theories are limited to circumstances under which they are drawn.

Historically both inductive and deductive methods have contributed to the development of knowledge. Each method also has advantages and disadvantages. Generally, however, inductive methods are preferred because of a reliance on empirical observations.

SCIENTIFIC AXIOMS

The scientific acquisition of knowledge is based on a series of philosophical axioms, principles or assumptions that govern the foundations of knowledge. The axioms are general in nature but provide a basis from which knowledge is developed.

Amorality

The scientific development of knowledge is neither moral nor amoral; it simply contributes to the knowledge base. The issue of amorality can be controversial because some research methods are considered morally wrong by certain groups. Animal rights groups, for example, have raised strong objections to the use of animals in research. Another example is the knowledge gained in weapons research. There are strong objections to the application of science to develop effective methods of conducting war. The morality of the methods or the application of knowledge may be debated, but knowledge itself is morally neutral.

Caution—maintains that scientists be careful when gathering data and drawing conclusions. A single finding usually does not satisfy the cautious researcher; findings gain weight when they are replicated or are found to apply well in other situations.

Consistency—argues that the universe is orderly and remains constant for long periods of time. If the universe frequently underwent fundamental changes, then knowledge accumulated over time would not be worthwhile.

Determinism—the cause for all events can be determined and takes place for certain reasons.

Empiricism—knowledge should be based on observations in the real world and should not be based on logical arguments, opinion, or intuition.

Intelligibility—when systematically studied, the physical world can be understood by humankind.

Objectivity—scientists must remain impartial when making observations and giving interpretations. It is also acknowledged that all scientists are subject to human emotions and failings and so should actively strive to maintain objectivity.

Parsimony—all things being equal, the simplest and most concise of two competing explanations is preferred.

Physical reality—space, time, and matter are real and not imaginary. Since they are real, they are subject to study and understanding.

Quantifiability—what exists, exists to the extent that it can be observed and measured. Some phenomena such as x-rays or chemical components may require special equipment to make observations or measurements.

Skepticism—knowledge, no matter how carefully developed, remains open to criticism or challenge. Knowledge is not absolute and is always in a state of flux.

SUMMARY

Research is an important procedure for the development of new knowledge. However, in a sense, the research process is a philosophy as well as a method. Our experiences with research teach us to examine the world with an inquiring eye. An understanding of the research process is essential in scientific disciplines such as sport and exercise sciences. In addition, as a consumer of general information, research skills help us understand how to separate facts and theories from opinions, unsubstantiated conjecture, and inaccuracies.

Theories are one of the most important tools the researcher has to generate new knowledge. Theories allow us to test our questions by providing a framework for knowledge and a method for making predictions that can be tested with further research. A prediction arising from a theory is termed a hypothesis.

EXERCISES

1 Look through some magazines such as *Time* or *Newsweek* for a recent theory. Give the name of the theory and describe the behaviors or events that it explains.
2 Search through one of your textbooks for any discussions of specific theories. List two predictions that could be made from one of the theories found in your text.
3 Search for a parity claim, a testimonial, and a meaningless statistic in some popular magazines. Which of these three advertising methods did you find most often?

Research: Questions and Types

2

CHAPTER

LEARNING GOALS

After reading this chapter you will be able to:

1 Describe the main function of the Introduction and Literature Review sections of a research report.

2 Explain the purpose of the references presented in the Introduction of a research report.

3 Discuss why new research questions are important for the advancement of knowledge.

4 Explain how theories are used to ask new research questions.

5 Describe how the findings from a single research study can lead to the development of new research questions.

6 Explain the differences between using theories to ask new questions and asking new questions based on practical problems.

7 Explain the differences between basic research and applied research.

8 Differentiate between qualitative research and quantitative research.

9 Identify the characteristics of descriptive research and experimental research.

10 Explain the differences between longitudinal research and cross-sectional research.

TERMS

Basic research
Applied research
Qualitative research
Quantitative research
Descriptive research
Experimental research
Longitudinal research
Cross-sectional research
Human research
Animal research

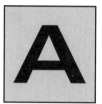s you learned in Chapter 1, research reports are customarily divided into four sections: the Introduction and Literature Review, Methods, Results, and Discussion. In this chapter, we will discuss the Introduction and Literature Review section, common sources for research questions, and several categories of research.

THE INTRODUCTION AND LITERATURE REVIEW SECTION OF A RESEARCH REPORT

The Introduction and Literature Review section of a research report serves two main functions: (1) to present a discussion of the question under investigation, and (2) to present a review of the literature relevant to the question. The first goal of the Introduction and Literature Review section is to describe the question under investigation. Although the actual statement of the question may appear near the end of the section, the purpose of the Introduction is to establish the foundation for the question. In effect, the Introduction sets the stage for the remainder of the report by presenting the question, by discussing the current known facts, and by showing how the investigation will contribute to the body of knowledge.

The second goal, reviewing the literature, is accomplished in part by citing previously published reports and providing references for those reports. In fact, one of the most important features of the Literature Review is the references. Providing references in a research report serves three important functions: (1) they help a reader distinguish between facts, speculation, and questions discussed in the report, (2) they provide a reader with the source for factual information, and (3) they provide the location of a report in a book or journal. With this information, you can locate reports in the library.

The length of the Introduction and Literature Review section can vary widely from just a couple of paragraphs in some reports to a lengthy chapter in other reports such as a dissertation. The Introduction and Literature Review in most journal articles is relatively short—typically from two or three paragraphs to a few pages. Journals commonly allot only a limited number of pages for a given report, so authors are encouraged to be concise. Conversely, when a graduate student writes a thesis or dissertation, the Introduction section is normally relatively lengthy. When writing a thesis or dissertation, there are no page number limitations, so students are encouraged to elaborate.

Notice in the Introduction section of the Hooper (1994) report, how the researchers discuss the issue of overtraining in general terms, provide references for published reports (in this example the numbers indicate a specific reference found at the end of the original report), and then conclude the section by stating the specific research question (see the box below).

Markers for Monitoring Overtraining and Recovery

Sue L. Hooper, Laurel Traeger Mackinnon, Alf Howard, Richard D. Gordon, and Anthony W. Bachmann

Overtraining has been the term to describe both the process of excessive training and the resulting condition of "staleness" or "burnout" (2,4). Overtraining is considered to occur in response to large volumes and/or high intensities of training with inadequate recovery periods between workouts. Although it is generally agreed that staleness is characterized by chronic fatigue and poor performance (8,20,25), few attempts have been made to quantify these factors. In addition, there is no general agreement on the objective markers of overtraining (8,11,25). Parameters that have been studied as possible markers of staleness include resting and/or post-exercise heart rate (HR) and blood pressure (BP) (4,26,29), resting and exercise oxygen consumption (VO_2) (4,10,29), and blood levels of various enzymes (13,28) and hormones (1,10,13). To date, these parameters have either shown inconsistent responses, or where trends have appeared, there are too few studies reported to make definite conclusions. Hence, a diagnosis of staleness has been based largely on subjective assessment. Furthermore, athletes have been classified as either stale or not stale when in fact the condition is on a continuum.

Staleness has been identified in a variety of athletes including basketball players (26), boxers (29), cyclists (3,11), gymnasts (29), rowers (3), swimmers (3,16), track and distance athletes (1,14,13), and wrestlers (16). The identification of easily monitored, reliable indicators of overtraining may aid in the diagnosis and prevention of staleness in a wide variety of athletes.

Continued.

From Hooper SL, et al.: Medicine and Science in Sports and Exercise 27:106-112, 1995.

**Markers for Monitoring Overtraining
and Recovery—cont'd**

The recovery of athletes from the fatigue of intense training has not been studied in detail, although coaches have long used the technique of tapering (a gradual reduction in training load) to allow the athlete to recover from intense training and thus optimize performance during competition. It is currently unknown whether tapering provides sufficient recovery to reverse the effects of overtraining and facilitate achievement of peak performance. Moreover, markers for monitoring the recovery of the athlete during the taper do not appear to have been studied in detail.

The purpose of this study was to measure a wide range of parameters during a 6-month swimming season (during training, tapering, and shortly after competition) in order to determine which parameters could be used to monitor overtraining and recovery.

RESEARCH QUESTIONS

The research process is similar to an engine in a car—both need a constant supply of fuel to keep running. Questions are the fuel that power research. When reading a research report, you may find yourself wondering where new questions come from. Determining the source of a question, however, is not necessarily easy; it's like asking where a writer gets an idea for a novel. If you ask your professors where they get their ideas for new research questions, they will probably tell you they get them from their own research, from presentations given at meetings, and from reading research reports written by colleagues. In general, however, most new research questions originate form three sources: theories, previous research, or practical problems (see the box on pp. 33-34).

Theories

Recall from Chapter 1 that one of the important functions of theories is to help researchers ask new questions. One way researchers ask new questions is by making predictions based on a theory. After making a prediction, the study is conducted and the findings are compared with the prediction. If the

Editor's Viewpoint: Why Ask "Why?"

Maureen R. Weiss

As Editor I repeatedly encounter several universal comments made by reviewers across all disciplinary areas served by *RQES*. These involve questions of "why?"—especially as they relate to content in the Introduction section. *Why* is conceptual or theoretical rationale not provided? *Why* are certain variables included in the study design? *Why* is the research question important; specifically, how does it extend beyond present knowledge? Without exception, reviewers in areas such as motor control/learning, physiology, pedagogy, biomechanics, and psychology are asking these questions. In turn, my question as an editor is "why ask 'why'?"

Each section of an article—Introduction, Method, Results, Discussion—is scrutinized by reviewers for accuracy, clarity, and contribution to the literature. However, there is little doubt in my mind that poor introductions increase the possibility of rejection. *Why?* Without a sound rationale, a systematic presentation of previous research, a logical progression of ideas that culminate in the purpose statement, and hypotheses that emanate directly from theory and research, the author will probably not convince the reviewers that the study is a meritorious one that will extend the boundaries of knowledge. Moreover, the Introduction colors the reviewer's impression of the author's rigor in reviewing the literature, thoughtfully considering theoretical underpinnings, and logically arriving at a research question that elicits and "ah hah! I see!" reaction from reviewers. Even when a study is well designed and data are analyzed appropriately, I have witnessed votes of unacceptability that are primarily based upon comments about a poorly organized and poorly written Introduction.

To illustrate these points, I refer to different categories of examples that cut across several papers. The first category pertains to the conceptual rationale for the study. One type of error is what I call an "overexclusive error." This occurs when the author fails to adequately describe the underlying theoretical principles that are driving the research question. The reader, left to read between the lines, comes away without a clear picture of how the question is derived from the theory. In essence, the author has not described relevant aspects of the conceptual framework in enough detail. A second type of error is an "overinclusive error." In this instance, the author describes so many facets of the theory that the presentation lacks focus. That is, the reader is so overloaded with information that the salient theoretical aspects driving the study are lost. The author spends too much time describing details and not enough time directing attention to the specific parts of the theory to be tested. A third error—typically a fatal one—is lack of a theoretical or conceptual rationale whatsoever. Even if the study is primarily descriptive in nature, such as during the early stages in the development of a particular research area, a sound rationale for conducting the study must be communicated. To increase the probability of favorable reviewer responses, authors should clearly, concisely, and systematically describe their conceptual framework, synthesize research that has tested the theory or model, and propose hypotheses that logically follow from the theory and research just described.

The second category of examples concerns the rationale for why certain variables are included in the design of a study. One frequent problem is introducing an independent variable (for example, gender, age) in the Method or Results sections without previously explaining

Continued.

From Weiss MR: Research Quarterly in Exercise and Sport 65(1):iii-iv, 1994.

Editor's Viewpoint: Why Ask "Why?"—cont'd

why this variable is theoretically relevant. For example, if prior theory and research provide no reason to expect that males and females should differ, then why incorporate gender as an independent variable? On the other hand, if theory and research consistently identify gender as a salient variable, then why is it not being examined or at least included in a preliminary analysis? In sum, key variables implemented to test theoretical predictions should be justified in the Introduction. Variables that are described in the Method or Results sections should not come as a total surprise to the reviewer.

The final category of examples pertains to how the research question contributes to the knowledge base by going beyond previous research. It is not enough to simply describe and explain the theoretical framework and justify the key variables. Authors need to ensure that their expressed purpose, questions, and study design clearly convey how the study will extend beyond the existing knowledge base in the research area. The question to be answered is "What does this study do that is different from previous research?" If the answer to this question is unclear, then the author needs to step back and reevaluate how to make a convincing argument for the merit of the study. In extending previous research, the author should communicate exactly how or which aspect of the study goes beyond previous literature.

In sum, authors can maximize the probability that their manuscripts will receive favorable reviews by writing a coherent Introduction that contains the elements just described. Reviewers should be able to follow the conceptual basis of the study, understand how the study uniquely contributes to the literature. I recommend that authors carefully consider the following questions when writing and editing their papers prior to submission:

- Have I presented a theoretical or conceptual rationale for the study?
- Is the discussion of the conceptual basis focused? That is, did I describe and explain the relevant aspects of the theory in a concise manner?
- Did I review the pertinent empirical literature on the topic?
- Did I omit any key references or recently published studies on the topic?
- Did I justify the inclusion of key variables?
- Did I present a logical progression of ideas that leads to the purpose of the present study?
- Did the hypotheses emanate logically from theory and research?
- Did I specify how the present study extends the knowledge base?

This Viewpoint is the first in a series of installments devoted to issues surrounding the peer review process, including characteristics of good article submissions as well as characteristics of constructive reviews of research articles. The Introduction is the reviewer's first encounter with the manuscript—its readability, theoretical grounding, review of literature, purpose, and hypotheses. To enhance the receptiveness of reviewers to your manuscript, I recommend that you consider the key points presented here as a checklist for outlining as well as for revising the Introduction. By doing so, chances of your work being accepted increase, while the opportunities for reviewers to question your line of reasoning through the "why" questions diminish.

findings are consistent with the prediction, the theory is supported and new predictions may lead to new research. If the findings are inconsistent with the prediction, the theory may be modified, also leading to new predictions. By asking new questions based on theory, knowledge accumulates in a relatively orderly fashion.

In sport and exercise sciences, the motor schema is a well-known theory developed to explain movement control processes and factors that affect motor skill learning (Schmidt, 1975). One of the predictions made by schema theory is that variable practice (providing different types of practice when learning a skill) will result in more effective learning and transfer of motor skills than will constant practice (providing only one type of practice). Subsequent research found evidence supporting the prediction (McCracken and Stelmach, 1977) and thereby supported schema theory. Subjects, who were trained to make a 200 millisecond movement, were assigned to either a constant practice condition where only one movement distance (15, 35, 60, or 65 centimeters) was practiced, or a variable practice group where all four distances were practiced. Following the training sessions, subjects in each group were tested on an unpracticed 50 centimeter movement. The findings showed that during training, the constant practice group performed better than the variable practice group. However, for the novel 50 centimeter movement, the variable practice group performed better. These findings showed that for this skill, variable practice was more effective for transfer than constant practice. Figure 2.1 is a figure from this study.

Note that the findings from a single study do not constitute proof that one form of practice is superior to another form of practice—the findings from a given study are regarded as evidence. When assessing the overall strength of a theory, a researcher considers the weight of all the evidence. Subsequent to the study discussed above, many other studies were conducted to further test schema theory and variable practice effects.

Previous Research

Research investigations are normally designed to address a single specific question. However, a common by-product of an

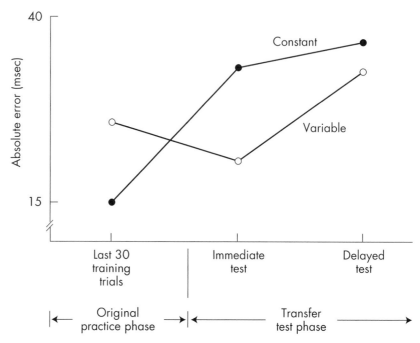

FIGURE 2.1 Performance in a ballistic timing task as a function of variability in practice conditions. (From McCraken and Stelmach: Journal of Motor Behavior 9:197, 1977.)

investigation is the uncovering of several new questions. For example, most studies are relatively limited in scope. New questions can be asked by broadening the scope of the original research by studying different populations under the same conditions, or by studying the same population under different conditions. Laboratory findings may be tested in the field, the findings from descriptive research might be tested experimentally, and so on.

Inconsistent findings from previous research provide another good source for research questions. It is not uncommon for the results of one study to support one theory or argument, and the findings from a different study to support a competing point of view. When this is the case, the Introduction to the report will contain a discussion of these conflicting or inconsistent findings and a description of how the present research will attempt to resolve the inconsistencies.

Practical Problems

Many studies are designed to address practical problems that are not necessarily based in theory. The goal of this research is usually to solve immediate problems rather than to test theoretical predictions. Practical problems provide a good source for research questions in sport and exercise sciences, as well as in other disciplines.

For example, understanding the factors affecting exercise adherence is a topic that has been extensively explored. In a study investigating exercise habits of college upperclassmen and recent college graduates, Calfas, Sallis, Lovato, and Campbell (1994) found that almost 50% of the recent graduates reported engaging in less physical activity than when they were in college. Both groups of subjects also reported becoming generally less active over time. Incentives such as enrollment in a fitness course, reduced membership fees to health clubs, and free physical activity instruction were reported to be important incentives in maintaining acceptable activity levels. Based on these findings, exercise programs could be developed and targeted toward these populations to help them remain physically active. The researchers in this study were not testing theoretical predictions. Rather, they investigated a practical problem with the goal of gaining information that could be used to better understand factors that affect exercise adherence and to develop effective programs.

The Discussion section of a research report is a good place to find new questions. Authors will commonly suggest new lines of research based on the findings presented in the report. By reading the most recent literature on a topic, you may be able to gain a sense of the most timely questions.

TYPES OF RESEARCH

When reading a report, you should try to classify the report into one of the types of research discussed next. By developing a sense of the types of research, it will help you appreciate the general goals, methods, and philosophy underlying a report.

Research in sport and exercise sciences, as well as in many other disciplines, can be categorized into several broad groups. These groups include basic and applied research, qualitative and quantitative research, descriptive and experimental research, longitudinal and cross-sectional research, and human and animal research. **Basic research** addresses fundamental questions; **applied research** examines practical problems. **Qualitative research** relies on observations of natural situations; **quantitative research** relies on strict experimental control and uses numerical information to describe behavior. **Descriptive research** describes behaviors and events as they naturally occur; **experimental research** examines cause-and-effect relationships. **Longitudinal research** tracks a specific group of individuals over time; **cross-sectional research** compares separate groups of individuals at the same point in time. **Human** and **animal research** rely on humans or animals as the subjects for the investigation.

Note, however, that these categories are not necessarily mutually exclusive. For instance, experimental research can be either basic or applied, longitudinal research can be qualitative or quantitative, and human research can be experimental or descriptive. The reasons why a researcher may use one type of research over another depend on the nature and goals of the investigation. For example, biomechanical research is usually experimental whereas historical research is usually descriptive. By the same token, biomechanical research can be basic or applied. In addition, an investigator might use a combination of these types of research so a question can be examined from more than one angle.

Basic and Applied Research

Two of the most common types of research are basic and applied. Applied research is designed to solve practical problems that are not necessarily theoretically based. The goal of basic research, on the other hand, is to explore fundamental principles that are normally theoretical in nature.

For example, a researcher in basic exercise physiology might study various biochemical adaptations to exercise while a researcher in applied exercise physiology might study the most effective methods for training middle distance runners. The findings from the biochemical studies may or may not result in the direct application of the information. The goal of this research is to further our understanding of physiological adaptations to exercise, and the findings will increase our depth of understanding of biological processes. Conversely, the training findings might have immediate application for runners. Both types of researchers are interested in how exercise affects behavior; the differences can be found in the underlying goals of the research.

Qualitative and Quantitative Research

It may be useful to think of the types of research as existing along a scale with gradations and overlap between methods. At one extreme, there is research that relies on observations of natural situations. This type of research is termed qualitative or *ethnographic* in nature. At the opposite extreme is research that depends on control over all aspects of the situation. Quantitative is the general term for this research. The terms qualitative and quantitative do not refer to any one specific research method. The terms are generic in nature and divide the range of research methods into two broad categories with shades of gray connecting the two. The two types of research can be used to complement each other within a single research study.

Qualitative research includes any research method that relies mainly on observations of behavior in natural settings. The goal of qualitative research is not only to describe what happened, but also *qualify* the description with language that clearly illustrates what happened. Qualitative research may take the form of a case study of an individual, a small group, or an event. Qualitative research is not conducted under as tightly controlled conditions and does not rely as much on numerical information as quantitative research does. Qualitative research also does not rely on the manipulation of independent variables or the administration of treatment conditions that are the cornerstone of quantitative research. Qualitative research affords flexibility in the way knowledge is pursued and developed. A qualitative researcher may begin a study based on a few observations and then evolve or change depending on what emerges. In qualitative research the researcher is the main tool for obtaining data and as such must be very skilled and careful.

A 1993 study titled, *Coping strategies used by national champion figure skaters* is a good example of qualitative research (Gould, Finch, and Jackson, 1993). They investigated how champion figure skaters develop coping strategies depending on their perception of sources of competitive stresses (see the box below). The researchers used interviews with the skaters as their method of gathering data. Based on the interviews, they concluded that figure skaters rely primarily on various aids such as self-talk, positive focus and orientation, and social support to cope with competitive stress.

Quantitative research lies at the opposite end of the spectrum. The term *quantitative* symbolizes the numerical nature of the data representing quantities of whatever is measured. The primary tools for the collection of information are tests and procedures that are examined for their reliability, validity, and objectivity. Extensive planning and laboratory environments characterize quantitative methods.

A sports nutrition study titled, *Prevalence of eating disorders in elite female athletes* is an example of quantitative

Coping Strategies Used by National Champion Figure Skaters

Daniel Gould, Laura M. Finch, and Susan A. Jackson

This investigation had two purposes: (a) to identify and describe the coping strategies used by national champion figure skaters and (b) to examine the relationship between coping strategies and particular stress sources. Participants were 17 of 20 (85%) Senior U.S. National Champion figure skaters who won titles between 1985 and 1990. All skaters were interviewed, and the interview transcripts were content analyzed. General coping dimensions reported by at least 40% of the skaters included (a) rational thinking and self-talk, (b) positive focus and orientation, (c) social support (for example, receiving support from coach, talking with friends and family), (d) time management and prioritization, (e) precompetitive mental preparation and anxiety management (for example, relaxation, visualization), (f) training hard and smart, (g) isolation and deflection (such as, not letting things get to me, avoiding/screening media), and (h) ignoring the stressor(s). It was also found that the skaters implemented different coping strategies depending on the specific stressors encountered.

From Gould D, Finch LM, and Jackson SA: Research Quarterly for Exercise and Sport 64(4):453-468, 1993.

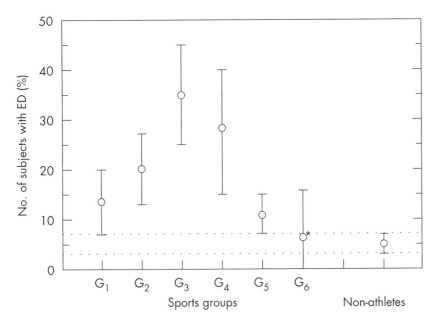

FIGURE 2.2 Frequency of all athletes in different sport-groups and nonathletes who met the criteria for anorexia nervosa, bulimia nervosa, or anorexia athletica. Results are shown as frequencies with 95% confidence intervals. The star indicates an upper one-sided 95% confidence interval. (From Sundgot-Borgen J: International Journal of Sport Nutrition 3[1]:35, 1993.)

research (Sundgot-Borgen, 1993). The investigator used a variety of measures to estimate eating disorder rates in Norwegian female athletes and nonathletic controls. The results showed that athletes suffered from higher rates of eating disorders than nonathletes. This is particularly true for athletes competing in sports where leanness or certain body weights are considered important attributes (see Figure 2.2).

Descriptive and Experimental Research

Two of the most common research categories are descriptive and experimental. Descriptive research attempts to describe and record naturally occurring events, while the premise underlying experimental research is the manipulation of variables to learn how these manipulations affect events or behaviors. As discussed in Chapter 1, descriptive research commonly precedes experimental research.

Descriptive researchers employ a wide variety of methods including surveys, observational techniques, historical investigations, and correlational measurements (see the box below). For example, wildlife biologists use sensitive microphones to record the sounds birds make as they complete their yearly migratory travels. The researchers are able to gauge the health of the populations by comparing the recordings from year to year. This type of research is descriptive because the

Stacking and "Stoppers": A Test of the Outcome Control Hypothesis

Brett D. Johnson and Norris R. Johnson

One explanation for stacking in sports is that minorities are excluded from positions with the greatest opportunity for determining the outcome of the competition, with the place kicker in football cited as an example. This paper postulated that the short relief pitcher in baseball also has high outcome control, and it hypothesized that minorities would be underrepresented in that position as well. We classified major league pitchers from the 1992 and 1993 seasons as starters, stoppers, or others and tested whether race or ethnicity was a factor in assignment to these positions. The hypothesis was not supported for either African American or Latin American pitchers. Minority group members were equally underrepresented in all categories of the pitcher position.

Major League Pitchers, by Race/Nationality and Role (as Starter, Stopper, or Other), for Combined 1992-93 Seasons

| | Starters | | Stoppers | | [Starters2*] | | Others | | Total | |
	%	N	%	N	%	N	%	N	%	N
White	82	121	87	28	[87	53]	86	227	85	376
Latin	12	18	6	2	[7	4]	9	23	10	43
Black	5	8	6	2	[7	4]	6	15	6	25
Unknown†		2						19		21
Totals	99	147	99	32	[101	61]	101	265	101	444
		149						284		465

*Values in this column are based on a looser definition that permits categorization of more than one stopper per team; these values are not included in row totals.
†Those categorized as Unknown are not included in calculating percentages.

From Johnson BD and Johnson NR: Sociology of Sport Journal 12(1):105, 109, 1995.

investigators are gathering information about naturally occurring events.

The goal of experimental research is to explore and understand cause and effect relationships and is based on the manipulation and measurement of variables (see the box below). For example, we might manipulate the mode of strength training (free-weights and weight machines) and measure strength gains to determine if one type of weight training is more effective than another. The causal factor is the mode of strength training, the effect is the change in levels of strength. This type of research is experimental because the investigators actively create two different situations or environments and then determine if the measured variable exhibits any changes.

Longitudinal and Cross-Sectional Research

One area of study in sport and exercise science focuses on changes in individuals caused by growth and maturation. As we progress from infancy through childhood, adolescence, adulthood, and old age, any number of physiological and

---

Baseball Bat Inertial and Vibrational Characteristics and Discomfort Following Ball–Bat Impacts

Larry Noble and Hugh Walker

This study examined the relationship between selected mechanical characteristics of aluminum baseball bats and sensations on the hands resulting from impacts. Sixteen skilled male Little League baseball players held each of two bats while they were impacted at the following locations by baseballs at speeds of approximately 27 m/s; near barrel end, center of percussion (COP), distal node of the fundamental mode, and 4 in. toward the hands from the COP. Results of a questionnaire regarding annoyance and discomfort were correlated with selected bat characteristics and vibrational characteristics associated with each impact condition. Results indicated that perceptions of annoyance and discomfort were related to the level of excitation of the fundamental mode and first overtone mode and that annoyance and discomfort were less with impacts on the COP and fundamental vibrational node.

Continued.

From Noble L and Walker H: Journal of Applied Biomechanics 10(2):132, 134, 1992.

Baseball Bat Inertial and Vibrational Characteristics and Discomfort Following Ball–Bat Impacts—cont'd

Mechanical Characteristics of Bats

Variable	Bat 1	Bat 2
Mass (kg)	0.797	0.644
Length (m)	0.765	0.760
Moment of inertia (kg · m²)	0.093	0.090
COP location (m)*	0.597	0.625
Fundamental frequency (Hz)	300	253
Proximal node location (m)	0.144	0.127
Distal node location (m)*	0.577	0.598
First harmonic frequency (Hz)	945	830
Proximal node location (m)	0.067	0.060
Middle node location (m)	0.337	0.304
Distal node location (m)	0.642	0.645
Distal impact point (m)*	0.686	0.682
Proximal impact point (m)*	0.507	0.533

Note. Moment of inertia and COP were measured about a point 0.15 m from knob end. All locations are given in distance from knob end.
*Indicates impact location.

behavioral changes occur. Researchers have traditionally used two types of designs for conducting this research: cross-sectional designs and longitudinal designs.

In cross-sectional designs, individuals of different ages are studied at the same point in time (see the box on p. 45). For instance, suppose we are interested in measuring the percent of body fat in elementary school children as a function of age. We could obtain a sample of first- through sixth-grade children by year (referred to as cohorts), and measure their body fat. We could then compare the findings among age groups to determine if there exists any differences in body fat in children as they mature. The main advantage of the cross-sectional method is that it is efficient in terms of time and resources—it yields results in a relatively short time period. A disadvantage of cross-sectional methods is that dividing children by class standing may result in groups of subjects that vary in age rather significantly within a given

Talent Identification in Swimming

Wendy L. Poppleton and Alan W. Salmoni

Summary
Much has been written about talent identification in sport from a theoretical perspective, while far less has been done at the sport research level. The present research focused on skill analysis in swimming. Female swimmers and controls from four age groups (8-10, 11-12, 13-14, and 15-17 years) were administered a battery of psychosocial and physical tests. In addition, the swimmers reported their best times for the 100 meter breaststroke, butterfly, freestyle, and backstroke. Although swimmers in all four age groups were superior to non-athletes in terms of the physical measures taken, they did not differ from other athletes of their own age, except for ankle and shoulder flexibility. From a questionnaire filled out by the parents, it was found that swimmers' parents had higher parental interest and encouragement scores than the parents of other children (both athletic and non-athletes). Swimmers scored higher in both athletic and swim competence than other children tested. Using multiple regression analysis (holding age constant), the only variables to be predictive of swim speed were shoulder and ankle flexibility, as well as athletic and swim competence. The results were interpreted to mean that parental interest and encouragement are important in determining a child's entry into sport, whereas variables such as flexibility are of importance in determining successful sport performance.

From Poppleton WL and Salmoni AW: Journal of Human Movement Studies 20:85-100, 1991.

group. The actual age of the sample of children in the sixth-grade, for example, can vary by as much as twelve months or more. In addition, the researcher cannot directly observe developmental changes since comparisons are made among different groups of individuals. Because we are comparing different groups of subjects, it can be difficult to determine if any observed differences are due solely to maturational factors.

For longitudinal designs, the same subjects are observed or measured repeatedly over a period of months or years (see the box on p. 46). In our body fat example, we would identify a sample of children, all in the first-grade, and then measure their body fat several times each year through the sixth-grade. The primary advantage of the longitudinal design is that developmental changes can be assessed more precisely over time. The main disadvantage of this design may

Performance Changes in Champion Swimmers Aged 30-84 Years

Alan A. Hartley and Joellen T. Hartley

Performance changes in champion swimmers aged 30 to 84 years were examined using both longitudinal and repeated cross section designs. When single cross sectional slices of the data were analyzed, decrements in performance with advancing age were found, similar to those reported in older track athletes. When the same individuals or cohorts were followed over time, the changes were found to be substantially smaller. The results also showed greater age changes in short, anaerobically-swum races than in longer, aerobically-swum races.

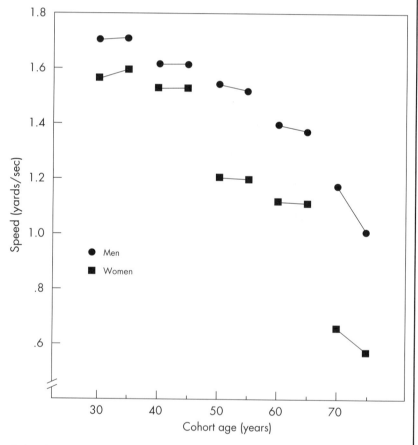

Swimming speed in United States championships as a function of cohort age. Lines connect performance by the same individuals in 1976 and 1981.

From Hartley AA and Hartley JT: Experimental Aging Research 10(3):142, 1984.

be apparent to you—it is time consuming and complicated to conduct a longitudinal study spanning several years. Losing subjects is a concern because some may be forced to drop out or become unavailable for many reasons as the study progresses.

Human and Animal Research

Conducting research with animals substituting for human subjects has a long history in many disciplines. The psychologist B.F. Skinner developed the principles of operant conditioning from his research conducted with pigeons and rats. Although Skinner used animals in his research, the findings are used to describe many types of behavior, including human behavior. Biomedical research often uses animals in research to study the effects of drugs or other medical procedures before they are applied to humans.

Sport and exercise sciences, by definition, have traditionally focused on human adaptations to exercise and activity. Yet conducting research with human subjects is limited by many factors. Investigations that include risks of either physical, psychological, or emotional harm to subjects are restricted for ethical reasons. In addition, researchers are constrained by the demands that can be imposed on subjects such as time commitments, effort, and limitations placed on subjects' daily activities. In some cases researchers also must provide incentives or compensation to motivate subjects to participate in a study.

Sport and exercise science researchers, and exercise physiologists in particular, are increasingly using animals in their research. Animals, such as laboratory rats, provide a good means of investigating acute adaptations to exercise in situations where using human subjects is not appropriate or convenient (see the box on p. 48).

An important advantage of using animal subjects is that research can be conducted under tightly controlled conditions. For example, animals of known ancestry, age, and other characteristics can serve as subjects. In exercise physiology research, factors such as exercise intensity, duration, mode, diet and rest can easily be controlled. Thus any effects identified in well controlled animal research can be perceived as generally valid. When using human subjects, it is more

Cocaine and Exercise: Physiological Responses of Cocaine–Conditioned Rats

K. Patrick Kelly, Dong H. Han, Gilbert W. Fellingham, William W. Winder, and Robert K. Conlee

Abstract

To compare the physiological response to a cocaine-exercise challenge in cocaine-conditioned animals with that of acute-cocaine animals, rats were injected i.p. with either cocaine ($20 \, mg \cdot kg^{-1}$) or saline, twice daily for 14 consecutive days. On the 15th day (test day) cocaine-conditioned rats received an i.v., injection of cocaine ($5 \, mg \cdot kg^{-1}$) (chronic group). One-half of the chronic saline rats also received the cocaine injection (acute group), while the other half received saline (saline group). Immediately after injection, all rats were either rested or exercised ($22m \cdot min^{-1}$, 10% grade) for 30 min. For most parameters there was no difference between the responses of the chronic and acute cocaine groups at rest or to the cocaine-exercise challenge. During exercise, both cocaine groups had similarly higher lactate values than the saline animals ($P < 0.05$). Both groups had similarly greater reductions in glycogen content of the white and red vastus muscles than occurred in the saline group; and both groups had similar increases in corticosterone. In contrast, cocaine-conditioned animals had greater rise in norepinephrine ($P < 0.059$) and epinephrine ($P < 0.001$) in response to cocaine-exercise than did the acute group. The mechanism responsible for the exaggerated catecholamine response in the chronic cocaine animals is unknown.

From Kelly KP, et al.: Medicine and Science in Sports and Exercise 27(1):65, 1995.

difficult to control factors such as these, as well as other factors like motivation, cooperation, and involvement in outside activities.

One disadvantage of animal research is the ability to make valid generalizations from animals to humans. The validity of these generalizations depends on the nature and goals of the research. For example, mammals have similar physiology; physiological adaptations to exercise observed in animals are expected to reflect adaptations that would be seen in humans under similar conditions. However, many variables (for example, drug dosage, intensity of exercise, exercise tolerance, etc.) are difficult to translate from the animal model to human.

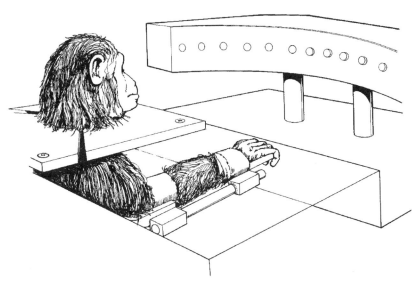

FIGURE 2.3   Experiment testing movement control in a primate. (From Polit A and Bizzi E: Journal of Neurophysiology 42:184, 1979.)

Animals have been used in studies other than exercise physiology. In researching motor control, studies have been conducted using primates to investigate how the nervous system controls voluntary movement skills. It is generally assumed that many of the same principles that describe animal movement and learning can be applied to humans (see Figure 2.3 for an example).

SUMMARY

The first section of a research report consists of the Introduction and Literature Review. The purpose of this section is to describe the research question and to present a review of the related literature. References are one important aspect of the research report that differentiate a report from other less formal forms of writing. The references make it possible to trace the origins of a body of knowledge and also to help distinguish between facts and speculation.

The research question is crucial to the development of knowledge. New research questions emerge from a variety of sources, but the best questions are usually the product of a keen interest and an understanding of the state of knowledge in a field. When reading your textbooks or studying class notes, try to think of new questions. As you become increasingly familiar with a body of knowledge, you will begin to ask even better questions.

EXERCISES

1 Describe the main differences between:
   Basic and applied research
   Qualitative and quantitative research
   Descriptive and experimental research
   Longitudinal and cross-sectional research
   Human and animal research

2 Look at the table of contents in three or four issues of *Medicine and Science in Sports and Exercise* and try to determine how reports describe animal research.

3 Read the discussion section from two or three research reports and try to find suggestions for future research.

4 Examine two or three issues of *Medicine and Science in Sports and Exercise* and *The Research Quarterly in Exercise and Sport* and try to determine how many reports can be classified as basic or applied research, descriptive or experimental research, and longitudinal or cross-sectional research.

5 From the box Editor's Viewpoint: Why ask "Why?" (on pp. 33-34), list and describe five important shortcomings or common errors present in many research reports.

Disseminating Knowledge

LEARNING GOALS

After reading this chapter you will be able to:

1 Describe the three main ways researchers disseminate information.

2 Differentiate among the four main sections of a research report.

3 Describe the purpose of the Abstract and References sections of a research report.

4 Understand the style requirements of research reports.

5 Explain how a research manuscript is organized.

6 Prepare references for a report in APA style and CBE style.

7 Understand how citations are written in a research report.

8 Describe the advantages and disadvantages of presentations, research reports, and posters.

9 Explain the difference between a primary and a secondary source.

TERMS

Poster
Introduction and Literature Review
Methods
Results
Discussion
Abstract
References
Author's Notes
Appendix
Footnotes
Table
Figure
APA
CBE
Primary sources
Secondary sources

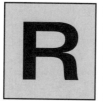esearch, reduced to its simplest form, is a two-step process. The first step is the development of new knowledge to further our understanding of events and behaviors. The second step is the process of disseminating the new knowledge. Our purpose in Chapter 3 is to discuss the information dissemination process. In the next chapter we will discuss the literature review process and where to look for information. As a student of sport and exercise science, it will be valuable for you to learn how new knowledge is made available, and more importantly, how to search for information.

Researchers disseminate the findings of work primarily in two ways: by giving presentations at professional meetings and through written reports. In this section we will discuss the most common methods of presenting and writing research reports.

PRESENTATIONS

Professional associations such as the American College of Sports Medicine (ACSM), North American Society for Psychology of Sport and Physical Activity (NASPSPA), and the American Alliance for Health, Physical Education, Recreation and Dance (AAHPERD) conduct national, regional, and local meetings on a regular basis that provide a forum for presentations. Presentations are regarded as an important aspect of the research process because they often represent the leading edge of knowledge. Researchers can present the findings from recently completed projects or discuss studies in progress. Presentations provide the researcher with an opportunity to receive feedback from colleagues and to address issues at a time when suggestions or modifications may be incorporated into current work. The main disadvantages of presentations are a limited audience and permanence. Limited audience refers to the fact that only a limited number of people can attend a presentation and the presentation typically only takes place once. Therefore, the information reaches only a limited number of people. The permanence limitation refers to the fact that most presentations do not result in a permanent and detailed record of the research. Although many professional associations such as AAHPERD publish abstracts of presentations

Fear of Personal Fatness and Discrimination Towards Obesity

Denise A. Monroe

In recent years, research studies have indicated that discrimination toward obesity in our society is very widespread, and that this bias may even become the next major battle of a civil rights nature. One variable that has not been associated with one's bias toward obesity is one's personal fear of becoming fat him/herself. The purpose of this study was to examine the relationship of fear of one's fatness and personal attitudes toward obesity. Students from introductory health and wellness courses and nutrition courses at a midwestern university served as the sample in this study. Students (N = 452) were administred the Fear of Fat Scale, the Bray Attitudes Toward Obesity Scale, items addressing their perception of their body weight and basic demographic information in a classroom setting. Pearson's coefficient analyses indicated a high relationship between Fear of Fat scores and Attitude Toward Obesity scores in both men and women. Preliminary ANOVA analyses indicated a significant difference in individuals fear of fat scores when perception of body weight (under weight vs. healthy weight vs. over weight) was held as the independent variable. Results suggest that individuals possessing a stronger negative bias against obesity are most fearful of their own personal fatness. Results also propose that individuals who perceive themselves as normal weight or underweight possess stronger fears of their personal fatness than those perceiving themselves as overweight. The study offers implications for health educators for dispelling bias toward obesity.

From Monroe DA: Research Quarterly for Exercise and Sport 66(1):A-41, 1995.

given at national meetings, many less formal meetings or seminars do not. Such abstracts are limited in length, and by definition, do not provide a comprehensive description of the research (see the box above).

POSTER PRESENTATIONS

Poster presentations at professional meetings are becoming an increasingly popular way to present the findings from recent research. A **poster** represents the middle ground between a presentation and a written report. During a poster presentation session, several researchers simultaneously display a brief written account of their work in a poster format. Usually the posters at a particular session are related in some way in terms of topic. For example, one poster session might be on exercise physiology, and a different session may be devoted to research on biomechanics. Individuals attending the session can circulate among the presenters, ask questions, and discuss the work with the presenter. Perhaps you have been to a science fair where different people display projects and demonstrations. If you have the opportunity to attend a poster session you'll see that they are modeled on this type of forum. Poster sessions are attractive because they are an efficient way for many researchers with similar interests to present their findings, and the sessions provide an opportunity for casual interaction among researchers that is generally not available during more formal presentations. Take a look around the building where your sport and exercise department is located and you may find a couple of posters on display.

Poster presentation formats vary from author to author, but most include approximately a dozen "pages." Common headings include abstract, purpose, methods, results, graphs, tables, photographs, discussion, conclusion, and references. A key ingredient for a good poster is a clear visual presentation that can be quickly and easily read by the viewer.

WRITTEN REPORTS

Written research reports provide a third forum for disseminating research findings. Written reports take a variety of forms, including journal articles, books, dissertations, technical reports, reviews, and abstracts. Research reports written for a school, department, industry, or the government are also common. Graduate students usually write a thesis or dissertation based on their research as part of the requirements for a graduate degree. These reports are located both in the library and in the department in which the student has studied. Some undergraduates write an honors thesis or a baccalaureate essay that is also kept by their school. Research reports are not always placed in the public domain. Reports written for business and industry may be protected for commercial reasons. Government and military reports may be classified for national security reasons.

With the growth of electronic mail and bulletin boards such as Internet, computer-based forums are becoming a popular medium for research discussions. Electronic methods allow individuals to post information and receive feedback from interested parties more quickly than traditional methods.

The primary advantage of written reports is they provide a permanent and detailed record of the research and the findings. These findings are housed in the libraries of colleges, universities, and other institutions. Students, faculty, and other interested individuals can gain access to this information as needed. No single library collects all written reports because of the costs involved in doing so. Rather, most colleges or universities normally maintain collections of the essential journals and books in all primary disciplines and other materials specifically related to the academic disciplines available at that institution. For example, medical school libraries subscribe to a wide range of medical journals that most schools without such a program would not. When researching a topic, you feel frustrated when you discover that your library does not subscribe to a particular journal or does not have a given book. However, the interlibrary loan service can usually acquire books or articles that your library does not have. Check with the interlibrary loan office at your school if you fail to find a specific article or book.

The main disadvantage of written reports, including journal articles, is the lag-time between the completion of the research and the appearance of the report in the literature. The time that elapses between the completion of a study and the appearance of the report can sometimes be measured in years. Factors contributing to this lag-time include how long it takes the researcher to write the report, the time needed to review the report, the time needed to complete revisions, and the production, printing, and distribution time. At a minimum, the lag-time is usually 6 months, but more commonly as much as 1 or 2 years. The longest known publication delay for a journal article to appear in the literature is 26 years! The obvious consequence of the publication lag-time is that even the most current journals or books are possibly behind the current state of knowledge.

Because of the advantages and disadvantages of presentations and written reports, most researchers use a combination of methods to disseminate information about their work: presentations and posters at professional meetings for recent work followed by the written report appearing in a book or journal sometime thereafter.

When walking through the journals and books maintained by a large research library, it is easy to form the impression that just about every research report ever written is eventually published. Because of the limited space in most journals and the numbers of manuscripts received, journal editors actually decline many reports. Some journals have an acceptance rate of less than 10% of the articles submitted. The general rule of thumb followed by journals is to publish only those reports that advance the body of knowledge in a meaningful way. Of course this is a subjective judgment, so standards vary from journal to journal or book to book.

Specific journals represent every academic discipline. In psychology, for example, there are dozens of journals each specializing in one or two specific psychology subdisciplines. More than three dozen journals publish research in sport and exercise sciences. Additionally, journals in psychology, physiology, sports medicine, nutrition, and history publish sport and exercise science research. A list of journals that publish sport and exercise science research is included in Chapter 4. As you read through the titles, you may see some titles that you recognize and many that may be new to you. The library at your school will have many, but probably not all, of these titles. It is very expensive to subscribe to the large number of journals, magazines, and newspapers, and to purchase the books needed by a comprehensive research institution (for example, the University of Colorado-Boulder spends about 2.5 million annually for its journal, magazine, and newspaper subscriptions). Multiply that by the other state-supported institutions in Colorado, such as Colorado State University and the University of Northern Colorado, and you can see that a great deal of money is invested in these collections.

CONTENT OF A RESEARCH REPORT

In this section we will discuss the content of a typical research report that you would find in a journal such as the *Research Quarterly for Exercise and Sport* and most other journals that publish research in sport and exercise sciences. As we described in Chapter 1, reports are divided into four main sections: the **Introduction and Literature Review** defining the question, the underlying theory and research hypotheses, and a discussion of the present knowledge in the area; the **Methods** detailing the procedures used in the study; the **Results** presenting the outcomes of the data analysis; and the **Discussion** where the findings are discussed and interpreted. In addition to the four main sections, two other sections are included: the **Abstract** summarizing the full report, and the **References** listing the citations in the report. Finally, in some reports, sections such as the **Author's Notes, Appendix,** and/or **Footnotes** may also be included. In this section we will briefly discuss the content of these sections and describe what the author is trying to convey to the reader.

Abstract

The Abstract provides the reader with a condensed description of the study and typically includes a few sentences from each of the main sections of the report. This helps the reader get a feel for the research question, the methodology employed, the results generated, and the conclusions drawn. The Abstract is normally about 100 to 200 words in length. Although the Abstract appears first in a report, it is usually written last because it must summarize the entire report.

Introduction and Literature Review

When writing the Introduction and Literature Review the researcher has several goals: introduce the research problem, discuss why the problem was investigated, outline the current state of knowledge and provide relevant references, discuss theoretical aspects of the projects, and present the research hypotheses tested in the study. It is a challenging task to create a well-written Introduction and Literature Review because of the need to incorporate the findings from other reports in an accurate yet concise way.

When reading the Introduction and Literature Review, several questions should be kept in mind. Was the research problem clearly introduced? Did information given from previous work accurately and adequately summarize the present state of knowledge in the area? Was there a clear distinction between fact and speculation? Did the authors cite a reference for all statements of fact?

Methods

The Methods section is intended to provide the reader with a detailed description of how the study was conducted. The goal in writing the Methods section is to provide enough detail so that the study can be reasonably replicated by someone else. The Methods section is usually the easiest section to write because it consists of descriptions of procedures, equipment, materials, subjects, and the experimental design.

The information in the Methods section is usually organized by subheadings. *Subheadings* help both the author and the reader present and locate important information in an efficient and organized manner. Examples of common subheadings include:

- *Subjects*—This subheading includes information about the number of subjects, how they were selected, and specific relevant characteristics (for example, age, gender, and fitness level). Descriptive statistics are often used to summarize this information.
- *Equipment or materials*—This includes information on the make and model numbers of equipment and the source for tests or surveys, or any other important materials. Because of space limitations, reports describing survey research ordinarily do not include the questionnaire. The address where someone can obtain a copy of it is usually provided.
- *Procedures*—The steps involved in the data acquisition process are described in the procedures section. For example, any information given to the subjects, how they were assigned to different conditions, and the activities the subjects completed are detailed here.
- *Experimental design*—This section consists of a description of the variables used in the study and their operational definitions. Experimental design information and statistical methods information is also provided here.

A given article may include any combination of the common subheadings or others not mentioned here. There are no strict guidelines authors are required to follow when organizing the subsections of the Methods section. Each research project is unique; therefore the methods presentation will be suited to the particular project described.

As with the Introduction, several questions should be kept in mind when reading the Methods section. Was it clear who the subjects were, the number of subjects tested, and how they were selected? Was the equipment well-described, including manufacturer names and model numbers? Were diagrams used to help describe complex laboratory set-ups? Were the specific procedures employed in the data gathering process clearly described? Is the experimental design clearly presented and is it appropriate for the experiment described? Would it be possible to replicate the study based on the information presented?

Results

The Results section contains the presentation of the findings. In quantitative research the Methods section consists of the summary of the statistical analysis of the data. In qualitative research, the "data" usually consist of text or descriptive information. The statistical analysis of data commonly takes two forms: *descriptive statistics* used to summarize the data, and *inferential statistics* used as evidence to support conclusions. Most authors use a combination of text, inferential and descriptive statistics, and Tables and Figures to present the results. The Results section is usually the most exciting section of a research report to write. Here the researcher presents the findings from the study and shows how the hard work led to an answer for the question.

Tables

Tables are used most often to present a concise summary of the descriptive and sometimes the inferential statistics discussed in the Results section. When preparing a manuscript for publication, each journal usually specifies how Tables should be prepared. However, there are certain features common to most journals. Tables are often limited to one per sheet of paper and must be "camera ready." The title should be centered at the top of each Table and should be complete enough to make clear what is presented in the Table even if it was not explained in the text. The units of measure for each variable should be clear. Both mean and variability statistics should be included and the number of subjects should be indicated. Even though a well-prepared Table will be able to stand by itself, Tables are referred to and discussed specifically in the text of the Results section.

Figures

Figures are any illustrations presented in the report. They include photographs, diagrams, maps, drawings, and most commonly, graphs. Graphs are particularly effective when a variable is measured over time or when the graph can effectively illustrate the results. As with Tables, all Figures are referred to in the text of the Results.

When reading the Results section ask yourself if the descriptive and inferential statistics were appropriate for the design of the study and the scale of measurement for the variables. As a student or novice researcher, this may be a difficult question to answer. As you gain experience, you will be better able to assess this issue.

Discussion

The purpose of the Discussion section is to answer the question posed in the Introduction and Literature Review. Similar to the Introduction, the Discussion can be difficult to write. Here the researcher has to use creativity, insight, and background to show how the present findings contribute to our knowledge in the field. In addition to this, it is also necessary for the researcher to describe the *limitations* and *delimitations* of the study. Few studies are perfect and some unanticipated event may occur or the researcher may lack control over certain conditions (for example, a study conducted at 5000 ft. above sea level). These factors or events are referred to as limitations. Delimitations are boundaries set by the researcher on the scope of the study (for example, a decision to use only female subjects).

Researchers will also discuss any similarities or differences between the results of the present study and the results of other related studies. Findings from a given study might support previous research while others may not. The Discussion section is often devoted to arguments supporting one set of findings or another based on the present research and previous studies. Besides describing the findings of the study, researchers often discuss the theoretical or practical importance of the findings. Finally, many researchers will offer suggestions for future investigations based on the findings of the present study.

When reading the Discussion you should keep several questions in mind. Were the major results clearly summarized and emphasized at the beginning of the Discussion? Were the similarities and differences of the results of the present study and previous studies discussed? Were the perceived limitations of the present study described and their consequences considered? Were suggestions for future research based on the findings of the present study described? Finally, did the report come to a conclusion with a summary or concluding paragraph?

References

The References begin on a new page following the Discussion and must contain a complete and accurate listing of each article cited in the paper. Only those articles cited in the paper should be included in the references. The citations that appear in the References section are commonly compiled gradually as the researcher writes the report. It is important for researchers to carefully check the references because it is easy to make typographical errors on page numbers, dates, or journal volume numbers. These errors can be very frustrating to those interested in locating a particular reference.

The issue of reference accuracy was examined in an article by Stull, Christina, and Quinn (1991). The authors examined the accuracy of references in a sample of articles from the *Research Quarterly for Exercise and Sport,* a popular journal in sport and exercise sciences. They found that out of 973 citations examined, 457 contained one or more errors. In other words, 47% of the citations contained at least one substantive error. The authors of the article noted that such high error rates have also been found in other journals such as the *British Journal of Surgery* and the *Journal of the American Medical Association.* However, much lower rates have been reported for other journals such as the *New England Journal of Medicine.*

Their recommendation was that authors need to carefully prepare a reference list to ensure that all citations are accurate.

Appendix

An Appendix is more commonly found in a student research project, thesis, or dissertation than in a journal article. The Appendix contains important details of the study that did not appear in the text of the paper. Listings for computer programs, mathematical proofs, survey questions, data, informed consent forms, or committee approval forms are examples of the kinds of information often placed in the Appendix.

Author's Notes

Authors occasionally wish to acknowledge the assistance or participation of individuals in conducting a research project or writing the report. Author's Notes are not necessarily required but often allow for a personal statement of appreciation from the authors. Author's Notes are also used, if relevant, to provide information concerning the funding source for a research project including the name of the funding agency and the project designation or account number.

Footnotes

Footnotes are not used extensively because they can be distracting to the reader. Footnotes usually contain supplemental information that does not fit well with the rest of the report. This information is placed in a footnote so the reader is not "interrupted" while reading the report.

PREPARING WRITTEN REPORTS

When a researcher writes a report for a book or journal, the report is expected to conform to a particular format. The format prescribes, for example, how to indicate the citations in the text of the report, how to organize and write the reference list, and how to prepare tables and figures. There are several commonly used formats that an author could follow with the differences between some formats relatively minor, while the differences between other formats are quite noticeable. Formats also evolve; editors are always looking for better and more effective ways to communicate information. It is important for researchers to keep abreast of format requirements. Journals follow a specific format so that all reports appear the same format in print.

Since journals often require a particular format they normally publish a Notes to the Contributor section describing the guidelines for a manuscript. Before preparing a report, researchers usually review the Notes to the Contributor and then write and organize the manuscript accordingly. Some journals provide relatively limited guidelines but then give a reference for a more detailed guide such as the *Publication Manual of the American Psychological Association* (APA). Other journals, such as *Medicine in Sport and Exercise,* provide very detailed guidelines. Next time you are in the library, glance through a few journals such as *Nature, Science,* the *Research Quarterly for Exercise and Sport,* and *Medicine and Science in Sports and Exercise* and try to identify some of the format differences.

In particular, notice how citations in the text of the article are given and how the reference list is presented. You will see, for example, that *Nature* and *Science* use very different formats than the *Research Quarterly for Exercise and Sport* or *Medicine and Science in Sports and Exercise.* There are also some obvious differences between the *Research Quarterly for Exercise and Sport* and *Medicine and Science in Sports and Exercise,* particularly in the appearance of the reference list (see the box on p. 64).

The APA Publication Manual (1994) gives detailed manuscript standards that many journals in the social sciences follow. Later in this chapter we provide examples of references and citations in APA style used by the *Research Quarterly for Exercise and Sport,* and in the Council of Biology Editors style (CBE), the basis for the format used by *Medicine and Science in Sports and Exercise.*

WRITING FORMATS

In writing a research report, the writer's main goal is to present all pertinent aspects of the research as precisely and

---

Examples of Various Styles Used for Writing References in a Research Report

Clinics in Sports Medicine

54. Deuster PA, Kyle SB, Moser PB et al: Nutritional survey of highly trained women runners. AM J Clin Nutr 44:954, 1986.

International Journal of Sport Nutrition

30. Fogelholm, G.M., and P.K. Lahtinen. Nutritonal evaluation of a sailing crew during a transatlantic race. *Scand. J. Med. Sci Sports.* 1:99-103, 1991.

Journal of Applied Sport Science Research

46. Steen, S.N. and S. McKinney. Nutrition assessment of college wrestlers. **Phys. Sportsmed.** 14:100-116. 1986.

Journal of Sport & Exercise Psychology

Borgen, J.S., and Corbin, C.B. (1987). Eating disorders among female athletes. *Physician and Sportsmedicine,* 15(5), 775-86.

Sport Medicine

Rosen LW, McKeag DB, Hough DO, and Curley V. Pathogenic weight-control behavior in female athletes. Physician and Sportsmedicine 14:79-86, 1986.

---

yet as concisely as possible. The writing style found in most reports consists of a straightforward description of the research.

Three aspects of written reports (and class assignments) should be kept in mind. First, most research reports are written in the past tense. Reports describe a completed study; the author explains the procedures, gives results, and presents conclusions, all of which have occurred in the past.

Second, research reports are usually written in third person. Phrases such "I think" or "we believe" should be written "it is believed" or "evidence suggests that." When written in third person, the information presented in research reports is perceived as more objective than when written in first person. First person gives the impression that the researcher is presenting personal opinion rather than relating objective information. An exception to this is a qualitative research report (see Chapter 8) in which first person is often used.

Third, research reports provide references for all sources of factual information cited in the paper. The presence of references can make reports distracting for the novice reader. However, references are essential information in a research report. They allow knowledge to accumulate in a structured fashion so future researchers can trace information to its source.

Next, we will discuss in more detail how research reports are written and in particular, how to write citations and references. You can use this information when writing reports for many of your classes.

ORGANIZING A MANUSCRIPT

Journals require that researchers organize the elements of a manuscript in a certain order (Figure 3.1). The outline below shows a common example.

1. Title page with the title, author(s) name(s) and affiliation(s)—page 1
2. Abstract—page 2
3. Text—starting on page 3, continuing without breaks, and including:
   Introduction and Literature Review
   Methods
   Results
   Discussion
4. References starting on a new page
5. Appendix starting on new page, if included
6. Author's Notes starting on new page, if included
7. Footnotes starting on new page, if included
8. Tables, with captions each on a separate page
9. Figure captions all together on a separate page
10. Figures each on a separate page

The first page of a research paper is the title page. It lists the title of the article, the name(s) of the author(s), and the name of the institution with which the author(s) is (are) affiliated. The title of a research paper should be kept as short

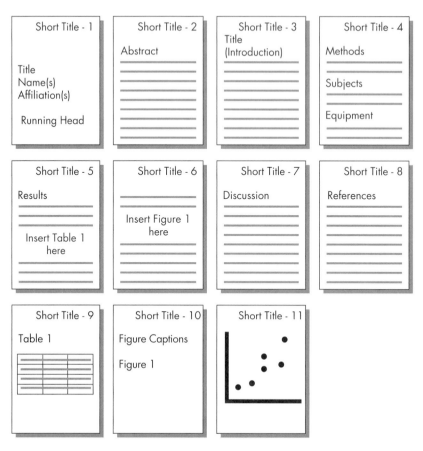

FIGURE 3.1 Organization of a manuscript.

as possible while at the same time providing information about the nature of the study. For example:

Cardiovascular fitness and maximal heart rate differences among three ethnic groups.

The effect of age and athletic training on the maximal heart rate during muscular training.

A simplified method for determination of residual lung volume.

Children and fitness: A pedagogical perspective.

A *short title* and the *running head* also usually appear on the title page. The running head appears centered at the bottom in upper case letters. The short title appears in the upper right-hand corner just above the page number and continues on each page of the manuscript. This information is used by the reviewer during manuscript evaluation and by the publisher to help keep the manuscript organized during the production of the report.

Although a research report is prepared and submitted to a publisher following the above organization, during the production process the manuscript is reorganized so each section appears properly in the final report. For example, Tables and Figures are photographically reduced and then placed in the body of the article at the proper location. Table and Figure captions are also placed and formatted according to the style followed by a given journal.

WRITING REFERENCES AND CITATIONS

The references that appear at the end of a research report are written following a specific format. The format specifies the placement of various elements of the reference, such as the date, the punctuation, the journal title, and so on. We will present examples from two reference formats used by many journals that publish sport and exercise sciences research: The American Psychological Association style **(APA)** and Council of Biology Editors **(CBE)** style.

Format for Journal Articles

When writing references, the author should follow the format requirements of the particular journal to which the report is being submitted. Even so, the way that the references in the original manuscript are written and how they appear in the published report may not necessarily be the same. For example, in APA style the title and volume information in the original manuscript are underlined, yet in a published article they are commonly printed in italics. Therefore, you cannot always follow a published report for format guidelines. When in doubt, it is best to check in the Notes to the Contributor.

Journal article with one author and no issue number in APA:
>Henry, M. F. (1952). Force-time characteristics of the sprint start. <u>Research Quarterly, 21</u>, 301-312.

Journal article with one author and no issue number in CBE:
> 4. Henry, M. F. Force-time characteristics of the sprint start. Research Quarterly 21:301-312; 1952.

Journal article with two authors and issue number in APA:
> Mero, A., Luthtanen, P., & Komi, P. V. (1983). A biomechanical study of the sprint start. <u>Scandinavian Journal of Sports Sciences, 5(1)</u>, 20-28.

Journal article with two authors and issue number in CBE:
> 7. Mero, A.; Luthtanen, P.; Komi, P. V. A biomechanical study of the sprint start. Scandinavian Journal of Sports Sciences 5(1):20-28; 1983.

Note that the main differences between APA and CBE are the location of the date, some punctuation differences, if the second and third line are indented and the number preceding the authors' names. In CBE style, references are alphabetized and in numerical order (in our examples the numbers are arbitrary).

Format for Books

The title of a referenced book is underlined and only the first word, proper nouns, and words following colons are capitalized. The city of publication and the publishing company follow the title. Notice the differences in the placement of the date between APA and CBE.

One author in APA:
> Berger, B. G. (1984). <u>Free weights for women.</u> New York: Simon & Schuster.

One author in CBE:
> 11. Berger, B. G. Free weights for women. New York: Simon & Schuster; 1984.

One author, second or later edition in APA:
> Sharkey, B. (1984). <u>Physiology of fitness.</u> 2nd ed. Champaign, IL: Human Kinetics.

One author, second or later edition in CBE:
> 12. Sharkey, B. Physiology of fitness. 2nd ed. Champaign, IL: Human Kinetics; 1984.

Edited books in APA:
> Haskell, W. Scala, J. & Whittam, J. (Ed.). (1982). <u>Nutrition and athletic performance.</u> Palo Alto: Bull Publishing.

Edited books in CBE

19. Haskell, W.; Scala, J.; Whittam, J.; editors. Nutrition and athletic performance. Palo Alto: Bull Publishing; 1982.

Format for Chapters in Edited Books

For edited books, the reference begins with the authors of the specific chapter cited, not the book. Only the title of the book is underlined.

One author in APA:

Schmidt, R. A. (1976). The schema theory as a solution to some persistent problems in motor-learning theory. In G. E. Stelmach (Ed.), <u>Motor control: Issues and trends.</u> (pp. 41-65). New York: Academic Press.

One author in CBE:

21. Schmidt, R. A. The schema theory as a solution to some persistent problems in motor-learning theory. In: Stelmach, G. E., ed. Motor control: issues and trends. New York: Academic Press; 1976: p. 41-65.

Other types of references include those from a presentation at a professional meeting, a dissertation, a magazine or newspaper article, or a personal communication between the author and someone else. Refer to a guide such as the *APA Manual* for the proper format for these less common references.

Citations in the Text of the Article

Research reports are based on previously published factual information. Researchers must cite their sources of this information so readers can refer to the original source. APA style journals use the author-date citation style in journal articles. The author(s) name(s) and year of publication are included in the text of the article for each citation and then listed in the reference section. Many CBE style journals use a number that corresponds to a number in the reference list. Use the following guidelines when writing a paper and note how citations in the text appear in journal articles.

In APA when the author's name is part of the narrative, the date of publication follows the name and is placed in parentheses. In CBE, a number is placed in parentheses and corresponds to a specific reference listed in the reference list (the numbers used in our examples are for illustrative purposes and do not correspond to any particular report):

In APA:

The various attempts to estimate the energy expenditure in soccer have been reviewed by Rielly (1979).

In CBE:

The various attempts to estimate the energy expenditure in soccer have been reviewed by Rielly (12).

In APA, when the author's name is not part of the narrative, both the name and date are placed in parentheses. In CBE, a number is given:

In APA:

Percent body fat was computed from body density measured by the underwater weighing procedure with correction for residual lung volume measured twice in succession by oxygen dilution (Wilmore, 1969).

In CBE:

Percent body fat was computed from body density measured by the underwater weighing procedure with correction for residual lung volume measured twice in succession by oxygen dilution (15).

In APA, when two authors collaborate on a paper, both names are cited. When the authors' names are part of the narrative they are joined by the word "and." When the citation is placed in parentheses the names are joined by the "&" symbol. In CBE, as in the examples above, a number or numbers are given:

In APA:

Ariel and Saville (1972) reported in six male weightlifters shorter total patellar reflex times during administration of an anabolic steroid compared to previous levels.

Cycle ergometry has long been a popular mode of exercise for researchers in exercise physiology (Astrand & Rodahl, 1977).

In CBE:

> Ariel and Saville (17) reported in six male weightlifters shorter total patellar reflex times during administration of an anabolic steroid compared to previous levels.
> Cycle ergometry has long been a popular mode of exercise for researchers in exercise physiology (21).

In APA, when three to five authors contribute to a paper, all names and the year are listed at the first citation. In all following citations only the first author's name followed by the abbreviation et al. (and others) and the date are given:

First citation in APA:

> Soviet investigators (Medvedev, Masalgin, Frolov, & Herrera, 1981) have studied characteristics of elite performers and have identified optimal kinematic and temporal parameters for each of these periods.

Following citations from the same article in APA:

> Medvedev et al. (1981) cite Cuban data which point to a high incidence of errors in the jerk by athletes of all skill levels.

In a paper with six or more authors the et al. abbreviation is given following the first author's name for every citation followed by the year. When two or more citations are given within one set of parentheses, the citations are given in alphabetical order by the first author and separated by a semicolon:

In APA:

> The dominance of the visual sense has been noted in protocols involving reaction time (Jordon, 1972; Kien & Posner, 1974), spatial localization and image perception (Kinney & Luria, 1970; Page & Locke, 1977), and balance (Dickenson, 1986).

In CBE:

> The dominance of the visual sense has been noted in protocols involving reaction time (6, 19), spatial localization and image perception (20, 24), and balance (7).

VOLUME AND ISSUE NUMBERS

Some journals are compiled annually by a *volume number* and a *journal issue number* while other journals only use a volume number. When the page numbers of a journal run consecutively for an entire year, only a volume number is used. When each issue of a publication begins with page 1, then an issue number is also included.

PRIMARY AND SECONDARY SOURCES

One unique characteristic of research reports compared to other forms of writing is the reliance on references and citations. References are categorized as either primary or secondary. **Primary sources** are research reports, books, or other sources prepared by the original author. **Secondary sources** are descriptions of primary references where someone else summarizes or interprets the words of the original author or source. Research reports that you find in scientific journals are normally a combination of primary and secondary resources. The primary resource is the original research reported by the authors in the report. The secondary resource is the author's descriptions of past research presented in the literature review.

It is important to review primary resources (original reports) before you write a summary rather than rely on the interpretations made by someone else. It is usually assumed that when a researcher cites, summarizes, or interprets a research article, they have actually read the article themselves.

SUMMARY

Researchers have several options when they wish to present their findings to their colleagues. The three common methods are presentations at meetings, written reports, and posters. Many researchers disseminate information using a combination of the three. In this section we focused on the research report as one method of disseminating information. As a student, you should become familiar with the organization of research reports; this will not only help you better understand reports, but will also help you organize and write reports for your classes.

EXERCISES

1 Check in the main office of your department to see if they have student membership information for professional organizations such as the American College of Sports Medicine or the American Alliance for Health, Physical Education, Recreation, and Dance.

2 Select an issue of *Medicine and Science in Sports and Exercise* and an issue of *The Research Quarterly in Exercise and Sport* and compare the writing and reference styles in the two journals. How many similarities and differences are you able to identify?

3 List the main questions that the critical reader should be able to answer after reading each section of a research report.

4 Explain why the Introduction and Literature Review section and the Discussion section are usually the most difficult parts of a research report to write.

5 List the names of the main sections of a research report. Describe the purpose of each section and outline the type of information found in these sections.

Literature Review

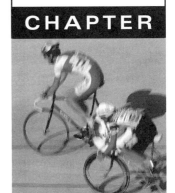

CHAPTER 4

LEARNING GOALS

After reading this chapter you will be able to:

1 Explain the difference between an abstract, an index and a review.

2 Explain why CD-ROMs have made the process of searching for information more effective.

3 Identify other disciplines associated with sport and exercise sciences where you can find related research.

4 Define the term *Internet.*

5 Describe some of the emerging information resources associated with the Internet.

6 Explain how to read an IP address.

7 Explain the terms *E-mail, Telnet,* and *FTP.*

8 Describe the World Wide Web.

TERMS

Abstract
Index
Internet
IP address
http
html
Telnet
FTP
World Wide Web

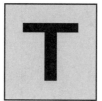he term *literature review* refers to the process of searching for information on a topic and then presenting a summary of the current state of knowledge. This presentation is an integral part of the Introduction section and Literature Review of journal articles, books, and research presentations. The purpose of the literature review is to present a summary of findings from previously published research relevant to the question under investigation. A crucial skill for any researcher is the ability to effectively and efficiently find and evaluate information on a topic.

Research results are published in many formats, and the most common and accessible is the journal article. However, when searching for information on a topic unfamiliar to you, journal articles may be the least effective place to start. Therefore, when beginning a search, it is best to start with one of the several sources that compile, summarize, and organize research articles in a systematic way.

SEARCHING FOR INFORMATION

Suppose your professor gives you an assignment to conduct a literature review on a topic in sport and exercise sciences such as the effects of exercise on arthritis. Your first step should be to look up the Library of Congress subject matter headings for exercise. These subject headings can be found in the *Library of Congress Subject Headings* book in the reference section of the library. If you consult with books such as this before starting an assignment, you will be able to identify the exact subject headings that will help you locate information. Subject headings are arranged alphabetically by topic. Always start with the most specific heading you can identify—for example, human locomotion, motor ability, running, and so on. It is important to remember that most card catalogs or computer catalogs use only those headings found in the *Library of Congress Subject Headings* book. If you are using a different heading, you could miss important information on your topic.

Next, using subject headings, search the subject card catalog or computer catalog to identify the holdings for your topic. If you want to find research reports on a topic, rather than looking for books, you can use an index or CD-ROM to locate recent reports. A good place to start is the *Physical Education Index.* The information found in the *Physical Education Index* will give specific reference information (for example, authors, journal or book title, volume, year, and page numbers) in other publications. If you want additional information without searching a specific article, you can use abstracts such as *Sport Search* or *Psychological Abstracts.* In addition to reference information, an abstract provides a summary of an article.

If available at your school, you should learn to use the CD-ROM resources. CD-ROMs are very effecient because they have powerful searching capabilities. When using a CD-ROM resource such as *Medline, PsyLIT* or *SPORT Discus*, make sure you are using the most appropriate subject headings to search for reports. Some of the CD-ROM resources use somewhat different headings than given in the *Library of Congress Subject Headings* reference book.

For instance, *Medline* uses *MeSH* subject heading terms to organize research reports; for example, *Exercise* and *Exertion* are two MeSH headings that you might find useful. Reports related to exercise, physical fitness, fatigue, and other related areas would be found under these headings. Before searching for information with a CD-ROM resource, ask the reference librarian of the index of subject headings for that resource.

In addition to using appropriate subject headings, it is also important to understand Boolean operators when using a CD-ROM. A Boolean operator is a term that limits the scope of a search. The most often used operators are *and, or,* and *not.* For example, if you are searching for information on the effects of exercise on arthritis, Boolean operators would help limit the number of reports that meet the Boolean requirements. If you use the search string *exercise and arthritis,* the operator and would narrow the search to only those reports containing both terms. If you use the search string *exercise or arthritis,* the operator or would broaden the search to all articles containing either the term exercise or the term arthritis. Using the string *exercise not arthritis,* the operator would exclude reports on exercise containing the term arthritis. As you can see in Figure 4.1, each of these three search strings

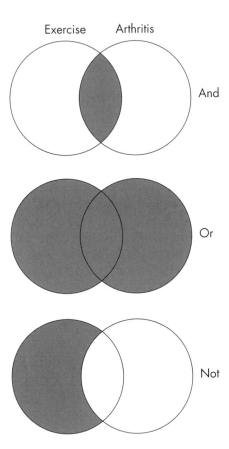

FIGURE 4.1 Search strings.

would return a different set of articles. In addition to operators, you can limit a CD-ROM search by using other qualifiers such as date, language, and author.

Once you have made a list of articles related to your topic, you can look for the articles in the library. The reports you locate will include a list of related references that will lead you to other reports. A good strategy is to look up recent reports first, and then look up related reports found in the reference list.

TRADITIONAL INFORMATION RESOURCES

Traditional information resources are those resources that researchers have relied on for many years, still rely on, and will rely on in the future. These include abstracts, indexes, CD-ROMs, and reviews. As a student, you should become familiar with how to use these, and in particular, how to use CD-ROMs.

Abstracts

Abstracts are reference books that give both reference information and a brief summary (an abstract) for research reports. Many academic disciplines have at least one abstract in that area. Here are some examples you may find useful:

Annual Meeting of the American College of Sports Medicine
Biological Abstracts
Completed Research in HPER
Dissertation Abstracts
Medical Abstracts
Psychological Abstracts
Sociological Abstracts
Sport Search

The box below is an example from the *Sport Search* abstract. Notice that the abstract contains the title of the article, the

---

Sample Sport Search Abstract

Kinematic Analysis of Male Olympic Cross-Country Skiers Using the Open Field Skating Technique

B.S. Heagy

The kinematic characteristics of 17 elite male cross-country skiers competing in the 50 km race of the 1992 Winter Olympic Games were determined. Each skier used the open field skating technique one of four skating techniques used in free technique cross-country ski races. Skiers were filmed by the use of three video cameras, placed at a filming site on a flat portion of the racing course. Digitized data from the video were used to determine selected kinematic parameters which included: cycle velocity; cycle length; cycle rate;

Continued.

From Heagy BS: Sport Search 11(3):20, 1995.

Sample Sport Search Abstract—cont'd

center of mass (CM) velocity vector angle; CM lateral displacement; CM lateral velocity; CM horizontal velocity; ski angles; ski edging angles; several types of pole angles; and hip, knee, and trunk angles. Temporal characteristics including strong side and weak side ski and pole phase times were also calculated. Cycle velocity and cycle length were found to be significantly related as were cycle velocity and the maximum strong side knee angle (r [greater than] .48, p [less than] .05). Cycle velocity and the CM velocity vector angle were found to have only a moderate non-significant relationship as did cycle velocity and the strong and weak side ski angles. For those skiers using the open field skating technique, CM lateral motion (as measured by the CM velocity vector angle and the ski angles) did not seem to be a distinguishing factor between faster and slower skiers, as hypothesized. However, cycle length and the maximum strong side knee angle did seem to distinguish faster from slower skiers. Skiers who covered more distance throughout a cycle tended to have faster cycle velocities. Contributing to this increased distance could have been the thrust to the strong side ski. Skiers with the most strong side knee extension tended to ski the fastest. Thus, it seems that greater leg extension results in greater propulsive forces and greater velocity.

name of the author, where it can be located, and a summary of the report.

Indexes

Indexes are reference books that give just article reference information, but no abstract. There are many indexes specializing in different subjects ranging from accounting, advertising, history, and music to physical education, sociology, and women's studies.

Indexes, as well as abstracts, are located in the Reference Department in the library. Each index has a "how to use" guide in the beginning of each volume. Though the information in indexes is usually organized alphabetically, there are differences in the notations or formats depending on the index. Your library will probably have all of the following indexes:

Abridged Index Medicus
Applied Science and Technology Index
Business Periodicals Index

Education Index
General Sciences Index
Health, Physical Education and Recreation
  Microform Publication
Index Medicus
Life Sciences Index
Physical Education Index
Physical Fitness/Sport Medicine
Sport Bibliography
Social Sciences Index

CD-ROM

Compact Disc Read Only Memory (CD-ROM) is a high storage capacity optical disk that can hold the equivalent of about 300,000 typewritten pages of text. CD-ROMs are ideal for storing and retrieving large quantities of reference information. Searching for information by CD-ROM takes far less time than a search in the printed versions of reference materials. As discussed previously, CD-ROM allows searches by subject, author, title, year of publication, place of publication, and key terms. Results of a search can usually be downloaded to a 3.5" diskette or printed. Most CD-ROM resources are more similar to a printed abstract and include summaries. Some full-text CD-ROMs are also available. Full-text CD-ROMs often contain information that would be difficult to access in other formats. An example is information from the U.S. Government census which is primarily available only on CD-ROM. If you are unfamiliar with how to use the CD-ROM at your school, ask the reference librarian for assistance. Some examples that you may find useful are given in the following list:

Biological Abstracts—Comprehensive coverage of the life
  sciences literature from 1985 through the present.
Cambridge Life Sciences—Comprehensive coverage of the
  biological sciences from 1982 through the present.
Census of Population and Housing, 1990—Contains a wealth
  of demographic information from the 1990 U.S. census.
Direct Access to Reference Information (DATRIX)—This is
  the CD-ROM version of *Dissertation Abstracts* from
  University Microfilms.

DISCLOSURE—Contains recent financial and management information on more than 10,000 public companies from their annual reports.

Economic Census, 1987—Contains results from the censuses of the U.S. commercial trade including retail trade, wholesale trade, service industries, transportation, and manufacturing.

Educational Resources Information Center (ERIC)—ERIC includes education journal articles, books, reports, conference proceedings, and audiovisual materials from 1966 to present. It corresponds to the print indexes *Resources in Education* and *Current Index to Journals* in Education.

GenBank—A computerized compilation of DNA sequence data gathered by a wide range of institutions. It began in 1982 and is updated three times a year. Contains more than 53,000 DNA fiber sequences.

General Science Index—This index covers 139 periodicals in areas such as food and nutrition, physiology, and biology from 1984 to present.

IMPACT—This is a database that indexes U.S. Government publications since 1976.

Life Sciences Index—Life Science Index covers more than 5000 journals, books, and conference precedings in 17 life science disciplines. Coverage is from 1982 to the present and abstracts are provided.

Medline—This is the CD-ROM version of *Index Medicus* and covers all areas of clinical medicine and biomedical research from 1966 to present. Medline is a composite resource of three printed indexes: *Index Medicus*, *Index to Dental Literature*, and the *International Nursing Index*.

PsyLIT—PsyLIT covers more than 1000 journals in psychology and behavioral sciences from 1974 to present, plus book chapters from 1987 to present. It is updated quarterly and has abstracts.

Sociofile—This is an index that contains abstracts of the literature in sociology from nearly 2000 journals that covers from 1974 to the present and is updated three times a year. It contains citations and abstracts from both *Sociological Abstracts*, and *Social Planning Policy and Development Abstracts*.

SPORT Discus—This CD-ROM provides a multidisciplinary coverage of sport- and fitness-related publications covering such subject areas as biomechanics, economics, executive fitness, sociology, sport law, stress management, sport administration, sport fitness for the disabled, sport history, nutrition, sport psychology, and training. It is updated quarterly.

The following box is a sample abstract from SPORT Discus. As you can see, the SPORT Discus abstract contains the article title, author's name, journal name, level of research, subject headings, and an abstract (see the box below).

SPORT Discus Abstract Sample

Title—	TI	TITLE: The effects of anabolic steroids on myocardial structure and cardio-vascular fitness.
Author—	AU	AUTHOR: Sachtleben,-T.-R.; Berg,-K.-E.; Elias,-B.-A.; Cheatham,-J.-P.; Felix,-G.-L. Hofschire,-P.-J.
Journal— Name	JN	JOURNAL: Medicine-and-science-in-sports-and-exercise-(Indianapolis,-Ind.); 25(11), Nov 1993, 1240-1245 Refs:29
	PY	PUBLICATION YEAR: 1993
	LA	LANGUAGE: English
	DT	DOCUMENT TYPE: Serial-Article
Level of — Research	LE	LEVEL: Advanced
	DE	DESCRIPTORS: anabolic-steroid; man-; weight-training; myocardium-echocardiography-; oxygen-consumption; body-consumption
Subject — Headings	SH	SUBJECT HEADINGS: (931030) DRUGS-AND-DOPING-DOPING-SUBSTANCES-ANABOLIC-STEROIDS-PHYSIOLOGICAL-EFFECTS
	SC	SUBJECT CODES: 931030, 931
Compre- — hensive Abstracts	AB	ABSTRACT: To determine the effects of anabolic steriods on myocardial structure, VO2max, and body composition, experienced age-matched male weight trainers (M age 26.5 yr) who either used (U) (N = 11) or did not use (NU) (N = 13) anabolic steriods were evaluated.

Continued.

From SPORT Discus, Sport Information Resource Center, Gloucester, Ontario.

SPORT Discus Abstract Sample—cont'd

Steroid users were tested while off cycle (U-OFF) for at least 8 wk, again at the peak (U-ON) of their subsequent cycle, and to the nonuser group of weight trainers. Echocardiographic measurements revealed significant differences in left ventricular (LV) mass (182.8 plus/minus 26.9 g vs 210.6 plus/minus 42 g; P less than 0.05) and interventricular septum thickness (IVS) (10.3 plus/minus 1.2 mm vs 11.1 plus/minus 1.2 mm: P less than 0.05) between U-OFF and U-ON, respectively. NU measurements were also significantly different than U-ON for LV mass and IVS (186.5 plus/minus 36.2 g; P less than 0.05 and 9.3 plus/minus 1.2 mm; P less than 0.05, respectively). LV diameter in diastole was significantly greater in U-ON (59.2 mm) than in NU (55.7 mm; P less than 0.05). In addition, LV posterior wall thickness in diastole was greater in U-ON compared with NU (11.2 mm vs 9.5 mm; P less than 0.05). VO2max values for both user groups were significantly lower than those for NU (U-OFF = 41.0 plus/minus 4.5 ml.kg-1.min-1, U-ON = 41.0 plus/minus 5.7 ml.kg-1.min-1, and NU = 50.2 plus/minus 6.4 ml.kg-1.min-1; P less than 0.05). Despite these morphological changes within the myocardium, there were no concomitant increases in shortening fraction.

CP   COUNTRY OF PUBLICATION: United-States (840)

SF   SUBFILE: SIRC

AN   ACCESSION NUMBER: 341277

UD   UPDATED CODE: 9404

Reviews

Reviews are bound collections of reports written to summarize a broad range of information on a specific topic. There are several reviews you might find useful in sport and exercise studies as well as in social sciences, education, and the biological sciences. Check with the reference librarian if you need help locating any of the following publications:

Annual Review of Physiology
Annual Review of Psychology
Athletic Performance Review

Encyclopedia of Education Research
Encyclopedia of Physical Education, Fitness and Sport
Exercise and Sport Science Reviews
Physical Fitness Digest
Science and Medicine of Exercise and Sport
What Research Tells the Coach

Journals and Books

Once you have identified specific research reports that you are interested in, the next task is to locate them in the library. The reports you are looking for will normally be found in either a book or a journal. *Books* consisting of research reports typically contain several related reports with a certain theme and are published only once. Some examples of book titles include *Coding processes in human memory* or *Enhancing human performance: Issues, theories and techniques. Journals*, similar to books, also normally focus on specific topics. Examples include the *Journal of Sport History* or the *Journal of Biomechanics.* Journals are published several times a year, usually quarterly, some monthly, and some less frequently. As you can see in the following list of journal titles, there is a considerable number of journals publishing sport and exercise science research. Additionally, journals in related fields such as psychology, physiology, or nutrition also publish relevant research. You may find that your library subscribes to some journals in paper form, and others in Microfiche. Microfiche is a microfilm version of a journal that you read on a special machine. If you fail to find a particular journal in your library, check with the librarian—they may have the Microfiche version.

Journals, as books, are usually organized by Call Numbers. The Call Numbers can vary from library to library for a given journal. For example, the Call Number for the *Sociology of Sport Journal* at the University of Wyoming is *GV706.5.S62*. At Arizona State University, the Call Number for the same journal is *GV706.5.S645*. Libraries normally use the same subject matter Call Number, here *GV706.5*, with the second element of the Call Number unique to the specific collection. See Table 4.1 for a list of journals that publish research in sport and exercise sciences.

TABLE 4.1 Scientific Journals

Sport and exercise research journals	Call number
Adapted Physical Activity Quarterly	GV445
Advances in Pediatric Sport Sciences	RC1218
Bulletin of Physical Education	GV201
British Journal of Sports History	GV561
Canadian Journal of History of Sport	GV571
Canadian Journal of Sport Sciences	RC1200
Clinical Kinesiology	RD795
Exercise and Sport Sciences Reviews	RC1200
Dance Research Journal	GV1580
Human Movement Sciences	QP301
International Journal of the History of Sport	GV561
International Journal of Physical Education	GV201
International Journal of Sport Biomechanics	RC1235
International Journal of Sport Psychology	GV706.4
International Review Sociology of Sport	GV706
Journal of Aging and Physical Activity	QP301
Journal of Biomechanics	QP303
Journal of Applied Biomechanics	RC1235
Journal of Applied Sport Psychology	GV706.4
Journal of Applied Sport Science Research	GV514
Journal of Biomechanics	QP303
Journal of Electromyography and Kinesiology	QP303
Journal of Human Movement Studies	QP303
Journal of Leisure Research	GV1
Journal of Motor Behavior	QP303
Journal of the Philosophy of Sport	GV706
Journal of Physical Education, Recreation and Dance	GV201
Journal of Sport Behavior	GV561
Journal of Sport and Exercise Psychology	GV706.4
Journal of Sport History	GV571
Journal of Sport Management	GV713
Journal of Sport and Social Issues	GV561
Journal of Sport Sciences	GV561
Journal of Swimming Research	GV836
Journal of Teaching in Physical Education	GV363
Pediatric Exercise Science	QP301
Perceptual and Motor Skills	BF311
Psychology and Sociology of Sport	GV706
Quest	GV201

TABLE 4.1 Scientific Journals—cont'd

Sport and exercise research journals	Call number
Research Quarterly for Exercise and Sport	GV201
Review of Sport and Leisure	GV561
Scandinavian Journal of Sports Sciences	RC1200
Sociology of Sport Journal	GV706.5
Soviet Sports Review	GV263
Sport Psychologist	GV706.4

Psychology journals	Call number
Behavioral and Brain Sciences	QP376
Canadian Journal of Psychology	BF1
Developmental Psychology	BF699
Human Development	QP86
Human Factors	T58
Human Performance	BF636
Journal of Experimental Psychology: General	BF1
Journal of Experimental Psychology: Learning, Memory and Cognition	BF1
Journal of Experimental Psychology: Human Perception and Performance	BF1
Learning and Motivation	BF683
Memory and Cognition	BF371
Psychological Bulletin	BF1
Psychological Review	BF1
Psychophysiology	QP351
The Psychological Record	BF1

Physiology journals	Call number
Annual Review of Physiology	QP1
American Journal of Physiology	QP121
Canadian Journal of Applied Physiology	GV561
Circulation	RC681
European Journal of Applied Physiology	QP1
Journal of Applied Physiology	QP1
Physiological Reviews	QP1
Respiration Physiology	QP121

Continued.

TABLE 4.1 Scientific Journals—cont'd

Sports medicine journals	Call number
American Journal of Sports Medicine	RC1200
Annals of Sports Medicine	RC1200
Australian Journal of Science and Medicine in Sport	RC1200
British Journal of Sports Medicine	RC1200
Clinical Journal in Sport Medicine	RC1210
Clinics in Sports Medicine	RC1200
Electromyography & Clinical Neurophysiology	RC77.5
International Journal of Sports Cardiology	RC1200
International Journal of Sports Medicine	RC1200
Journal of Sports Medicine and Physical Fitness	RC1200
Journal of Sport Rehabilitation	RC1200
Kinesiology and Medicine for Dance	GV1580
Medicine and Science in Sports and Exercise	RC1200
New Zealand Journal of Sports Medicine	RC1200
Physician and Sportsmedicine	RC1200
Sports Medicine	RC1210

Physical therapy/Rehabilitation journals	Call number
Archives of Physical Medicine and Rehabilitation	RM845
Journal of Cardiopulmonary Rehabilitation	RC682
Journal of Orthopaedic & Sports Physical Therapy	RD701
Physical Therapy	RM695

Nutrition journals	Call number
American Journal of Clinical Nutrition	RC584
Annual Review of Nutrition	QP141
Human Nutrition	TX341
International Journal of Obesity	TX553
International Journal of Sport Nutrition	RC1235
Journal of the American Dietetic Association	RM214
Journal of Nutrition	RM214
Journal of Nutrition Education	QP141
Nutrition Abstracts	RM214
Nutrition Reviews	TX341
Topics in Clinical Nutrition	QP 141

TABLE 4.1   Scientific Journals—cont'd

Health journals	Call number
Educational Gerontology	LC5201
Health Education	LB 3401
Journal of Environmental Health	RA565
Journal of Health Education	LB3401
Wellness Perspectives	RA733

EMERGING INFORMATION RESOURCES

This section is titled "emerging information resources" because many of these resources are relatively new and unfamiliar to many of us. Additionally, many of these resources are rapidly evolving and changing. The Internet is a prime example. How to access the Internet and the resources available electronically is literally changing every day. Until very recently, finding new information, locating specific journal articles, or just browsing with the hope of finding something new and interesting required going to the library. With the advent of personal computers, information services, and networks, the libraries are increasingly, and rapidly, coming to us. Many university libraries are joining consortiums that allow access to any library in the system. For example, the Regent's universities in the state of Kansas are electronically linked with *KARENET* (KAsas REgents NETwork) so students at one institution can search the holdings at another institution. Students at the University of Colorado can use networking programs to search the library holdings at the University of Wyoming, Arizona State University, University of Maryland, and many others. In return, students at each of these schools can search the University of Colorado library system. As more universities offer World Wide Web Home Pages, access to the library catalog will become widely available.

One fact that most students learn early on is that the library at their school may not have all of the books and journals they may be interested in. However, you can obtain many books and reports through the interlibrary loan system. Normally, you have to submit a form to the loan office and then wait a few days, at a minimum, for the item to be delivered. Many universities have an electronic interlibrary loan request system where loan requests can be made with electronic mail. The *Interlibrary Loan Memorandum* (ILLM) is an online interlibrary loan request system whereby the user can request an item and receive notification when it arrives, all electronically. In effect, the interlibrary loan system itself is a computer network which facilitates the sharing of resources by libraries worldwide. Thus it is possible to search the holdings of a library in a different state and place an interlibrary loan request, while never leaving the office or home.

Layered CD-ROMs

With the advent of CD-ROMs, we can now access information that is maintained in one form or another, but has not been readily available as a result of costs or other reasons. For example, the most recent U.S. Census is available in CD-ROM and contains extremely detailed census information down to a city-block by city-block level. The cost of printing this detailed information is prohibitive, and therefore not readily available. With CD-ROMs, not only is the information available, it is also much easier to search and locate specific information than is the hard-copy version.

Some textbooks and journals may soon be available in compact disk (CD) format. There is already a substantial number of titles available on CD including the complete works of Shakespeare, World Atlas, and First Aid instruction to mention just a few.

CD technology is also evolving. In a few years a new type of CD termed the layered disk may reach the market. The layered CD will have the capacity to hold about 6.5 billion bytes of data by storing information on up to 10 optical layers on a disk. With the increased storage capacity, the ability to store pictures and movies will be enhanced considerably beyond what is presently available. A single CD could store the equivalent of several thousand 200-page books.

Document Delivery Services

UnCover is an online periodical indexing and document delivery service and has more than 5 million items in its database and is growing continuously. UnCover was developed by the Colorado Association of Research Libraries (CARL) as a reference resource. Today, many universities have free access to UnCover and it can be searched with a personal computer or terminal. In the U.S., articles cost $8.50, plus copyright royalty fee, and can often be received in less than an hour if a FAX number is available. The World Wide Web address for CARL is *http://www.carl.org/carl.html* (no period at the end of the address).

INTERNET

Internet is the network or computer networks linking universities, government, businesses, and individuals worldwide. The current Internet originally began in 1969 with the experimental ARPANET system that connected computers at four institutions. Internet as it is used today began in the early 1980s and is fast becoming a valuable resource for information through discussion groups, bulletin boards, libraries, electronic mail, and many other resources. If you haven't already, you should request an electronic-mail address and password from the appropriate department at your school and enroll in a training course. Internet access is free at most colleges and universities for faculty and students.

Internet Addresses

Internet addresses come in two formats: a numeric address, or a name address. Each computer on the Internet has a unique address termed an **IP address**. In numeric form, the IP address contains a series of numbers connected by periods such as *192.231.192.1*, which is the address for the Big Sky Telegraph free-net. The number farthest to the left is the broadest identifying the largest network, then working to the right, increasingly more specific information until a specific computer is identified by the last number at the right. Because numeric addresses are inherently difficult to remember, most sites now use name addresses. For example, *stis.nsf.gov* is the name address for the National Science Foundation Science and Technology Information System. Name addresses are read in just the opposite direction as numeric addresses. The name address indicates the most specific information on the left and becomes increasingly general working to the right. In this case, *stis* is a specific computer operated by the National Science Foundation, *nsf* stands for the National Science Foundation, and *gov* stands for the U. S. Government. The final address symbol on the right, *gov* falls into a few general categories.

The symbol *com* indicates U.S. commercial domains, *edu* indicates educational sites, *net* refers to administrative organization for a network, and *org* stands for other types of organizations. Name addresses are more commonly used (any site can have either form of address) because they are obviously easier to interpret and remember than the numeric addresses.

A second type of Internet address is the *universal resource locator (URL) address*. These addresses are used for sites containing hypertext documents that are identified with the prefix *http://*. For example, the URL address for the Library of Congress Homepage is *http://lcweb.loc.gov/home-page/lchp.html* (no period). The address for Purdue University Writing Lab is *http://owl.trc.purdue.edu/* (no period). Some of these addresses can become quite long, but in general they are easy to decipher. **HTTP** stands for Hypertext Transfer Protocol and **HTML** stands for Hypertext Markup Language, which is a programming language used to create hypertext documents. Information on how to create Hypertext documents can be found at *http://home.mcom.com/assist/net_sites/index.html* (no period at the end of the address).

Basic Internet Applications

The Internet system has three basic applications that make it useful and popular. They are electronic mail, file transfer, and remote logon.

Electronic mail (E-mail)

Electronic mail is a very convenient way to communicate with others via the Internet. When ARPANET was first designed,

E-mail was added as an afterthought. Since then, the growth in the popularity of E-mail and amount of E-mail traffic has been tremendous. Researchers worldwide rely heavily on E-mail to discuss current projects with colleagues both nationally and internationally. With an E-mail address you can send messages to friends at other schools or perhaps communicate with your professors. You can even send E-mail to the U.S. President at *president@whitehouse.gov*.

E-mail has distinct advantages over other modes of long distance communication—mail and telephone. The obvious advantage of E-mail over standard mail (snail-mail) is the nearly instantaneous transmission of the message. When you become accustomed to communicating with E-mail, you begin to regret when you have to use "snail-mail" because of the delivery time. In addition, the computer stores your E-mail until you have the time to read it. Most systems allow you to maintain a permanent log file of your important messages. Some universities have electronic application forms for student admissions that you can submit with E-mail.

Remote login (Telnet)

Telnet provides the ability to log-on to a computer at a different location, either across town, in the next state, or overseas. Of course, for many systems you have to have a user's name and password. Other systems are designed to allow anyone access (at least to certain files) from any remote site. The great advantage of Telnet is you can either work with a computer that you have access to from anywhere else, or the owners can make available certain functions or files to anonymous users. For example, researchers who need access to super computers for their work often rely on Telnet. Other systems, such as library catalogs, are accessible from remote sites because of Telnet.

File transfer (FTP)

FTP stands for File Transfer Protocol and allows files of various types to be sent from one type of computer to another type of computer. Anonymous FTP is a means by which you can connect to another computer and gain access to files without having a users account. You usually enter "anonymous" as your user name and your E-mail address as your password.

DISCUSSION GROUPS

By using electronic mail, remote log-in, and file transfer capabilities, a wide range of services and discussion groups have evolved that take advantage of the Internet capabilities. Discussion groups provide a forum for people with common interests to exchange information and opinions.

USENET (User's Network)

USENET is a large collection of various newsgroups. A newsgroup is a collection of articles (E-mail message posting) about specific topics. USENET was one of the earliest features of the Internet and is still very popular. You can read messages, submit new messages, or reply to or comment on other messages. There are literally thousands of newsgroups from scientific to recreational topics. USENET topics are divided into several broad categories including *comp* for information of computer hardware, software, and many other computer-related topics; *sci* indicates groups related to scientific topics; *soc* is used to designate groups concerning social and cultural discussions; *talk* covers a wide range of topics; *rec* groups include discussions on sports, automobiles, movies, and TV to mention just a few; and *alt*, which is a broad category of topics such as cooking, books, ham radio, and many others.

BITNET (Because It's Time Network)

BITNET connects about 1500 organizations in more than 50 countries and is operated by the Corporation for Research and Education Networking. It was created in 1981 and was designed to connect universities to a network so faculty and researchers could easily communicate with one another. BITNET works like an E-mail system where information is automatically distributed to groups of people interested in specific topics rather than to individuals. Just as E-mail is commonly used as a one-to-one system, BITNET is a one-to-many system. There are dozens of topics available on BITNET. See Gilster (1993) for a complete discussion of USENET, BITNET.

SPORT AND EXERCISE SCIENCE DISCUSSION GROUPS

There are two discussion groups you may find interesting: BIOMCH-L and SPORTSCI. Each of these groups contain discussions in sport and exercise sciences.

BIOMCH-L

BIOMC-L is a BITNET-based electronic discussion group for researchers in biomechanics and related fields. BIOMCH-L is intended for the free exchange of information worldwide, complementing traditional means such as journal articles, conferences, and/or newsletters. BIOMCH-L includes discussions, reports, calls for information or help, calls for papers, announcements of new publications and other items. This would be a good place for you to start if you are interested in exploring BITNET and sport and exercise discussions related to biomechanics in particular.

To subscribe, send an E-mail message to: *listerv@nic. surfnet.nl* or *LISTSERV@HEARN.BITNET*. State in the message: *subscribe BIOMCH-L.* An archive of posted items can be retrieved with the command *SEND BIOMCH-L LOG9206.*

SPORTSCI

SPORTSCI is also related to sports and exercise sciences. Topics include field and physiological tests, nutrition, diet and supplementation, sport in extreme environments, technological developments and new equipment, training (specificity, periodization, overtraining), topics from biochemistry, biomechanics, biostatistics, motor learning, sport medicine, sport psychology or other disciplines if related directly to human performance. Anyone with an interest in sports and exercise science can subscribe and contribute to SPORTSCI. To subscribe, send an E-mail message to: *majordomo@stonebow. otago.ac.nz.* State in the message: *subscribe sportsci.*

World Wide Web

The **World Wide Web** (WWW) is a network of servers that allows you to access hypertext documents. *Hypertext* documents are linked to one another so that you can start with one resource and then access other resources linked to it. Most resources contain some combination of text files, sound files, picture files, and even movie files. If the file is an audio file, it can be played back through the speaker in the computer; if it's a video or movie file it can be displayed on the screen. Hypertext allows you to jump from the middle of one document to the same place in another document that has related information. For example, suppose you are researching the great art museums of the world. A section of an article about the National Gallery in Washington D.C. might be linked to another document about the National Gallery that contains picture files of the artwork. In effect, WWW is a universe of network accessible resources.

The best way to access the World Wide Web is with programs such as Mosaic or Netscape which are discussed below. With this software and a network connection, you can access an amazing range of resources such as U.S. Supreme Court decisions at *http://www.law.cornell.edu.* The U.S. Geological Survey server can be found at *http://info.er.usgs.gov* and is a great resource for a wide range of information in earth science fields. The NASA server is found at *http://www.nasa.uiuc.edu* and has a variety of images from the Hubble Space Telescope and space shuttle (see the box on pp. 97–98).

Web Access Software

Mosaic and Netscape are examples of programs that connect a computer to the World Wide Web. As mentioned earlier, these programs are appealing because they are easy to use and can handle text files, image files, sound files, and even movie files. Not only will they locate information in a variety of formats, but in most cases you can download all types of files to your own computer. Different versions of these programs are available for computers with different operating systems such as Macintosh, Microsoft Windows, or X Windows. The address for NCSA Mosaic is: *http://www.ncsa.uiuc.edu.* The address for Netscape is: *http://home.netscape.com/* (no period at the end of the address).

Interesting, Fun, and Useful World Wide Web Sites

Abstracts and Indexes
http://www.lib.iupui.edu/erefs/ab_in.html

Art History
http://rubens.anu.edu.au/

Biomechanics World Wide
http://gpu.srv.ualberta.CA/~ploaudin/biomch.htm

History of Medicine Division, NLM
http://www.nlm.nih.gov/hmd.dir/hmd.html

The Internet Movie Database
http://www.cm.cf.ac.uk/Movies/

The Internet White Pages
http://home.netscape.com/home/internet-white-pages.html

Library of Congress
http://lcweb.loc.gov/homepage/lchp.html

Macintosh Software
gopher://gopher.archive.merit.edu:7055/11/mac

Museums
http://www.comlab.ox.ac.uk/archive/other/museums.html

National Public Radio
http://www.npr.org/index.html

Pathfinder—Time Warner Electronic Publishing
http://www.timeinc.com/pathfinder/

Public Access United States Government
http://Thomas.loc.gov

Purdue University Writing Lab
http://owl.trc.purdue.edu/

San Francisco Exploratorium
http://www.exploratorium.edu/

Smithsonian Institution Servers
http://www.si.edu/

Sport and Recreation Information on the World Wide Web
http://amdahl1.cs.latrobe.edu.au:8080/SARA/moreSport.html

Views of the Solar System
http://www.c3.lanl.gov/~cjhamil/SolarSystem/homepage.html

Continued.

Interesting, Fun, and Useful World Wide Web Sites—cont'd

The Visible Human Project
http://www.nlm.nih.gov/extramural_research.dir/visible_human.html

Weather Information
http://ast1.spa.umn.edu/weatherinfo.html
http://www.atmos.uiuc.edu/

The White House
http://www.whitehouse.gov/

The Whole Internet Catalog
http://nearnet.gnn.com/wic/newrescat.toc.html

World Wide Web Home Page
http://info.cern.ch/

The WWW Virtual Library
http://www.w3.org/hypertext/DataSources/bySubject/Overview.html

Yahoo-A Guide to WWW
http://www.yahoo.com/

Information Search Engines

With the advent of the World Wide Web, powerful information search software became necessary. These search engines allow you to search for information in many different ways—some engines search titles or headers of documents on the net, others search the documents themselves, still others just search other indexes or directories (see the box on p. 99).

How successful your search is depends on many factors. These include your topic, the resource searched, the key words that you use, and your patience and skills. At this time, more information is available on the World Wide Web on some topics, such as computer, technology, commercial services, and recreational topics. If you are looking for specific information, such as the effects of exercise on arthritis, for example, you will probably be less successful finding useful information. The information you find also depends on the resource searched. Some resources only give you location of other Web sites, while others list specific documents and files. Different key words can result in very different findings. At

---

World Wide Web Search Engines

Centre Universitaire d'Informatique World Wide Web catalog (CUI)
http://cui_www.unige.ch/w3catalog
Search results on the term sports and exercise:
0 items found
Search results on the term sports:
more than 50 WWW resources found
Search results on the term exercise:
only a few resources found, mostly commercial products

The Lycos Home Page: Hunting WWW information
http://lycos.cs.cmu.edu/
Search results on the term sports and exercise:
11,338 items found

WebCrawler Searching
http://webcrawler.com
Search results on the term sports and exercise:
181 documents found

World Wide Web Worm (WWWW)
http://www.cs.colorado.edu/home/mcbryan/WWWW.html
Search results by title on the term sports and exercise:
0 items found
Search results by title on the term sports:
15 items found
Search results by title on the term exercise:
2 items found called **Exercise(medicine)**—Links from here to a long list of items with exercise as a key word. Many related to human exercise, many others not.

---

this point, information on the Web is not as systematically organized as it is in more traditional resources. Finally, your patience and experience plays a crucial role in how successfully you can search for and find information on the Internet. For most novices the process can be slow, confusing, and not very productive. However, with the right software (Mosaic in particular), searching the Internet and the World Wide Web can be enjoyable and useful. Electronic information resources will continue to expand rapidly. If you develop your skills now, it can only help you later.

Electronic Agents

World Wide Web is a *second generation graphical user interface* (GUI) computer that allows easy access to text, images, sound and movie files (Apple Macintosh and Microsoft Windows are GUI systems). Mosaic and Netscape, along with commercial servers such Prodigy, America Online and eWorld are all examples of second generation resources.

In both cases, the user must actively search for information. What you ultimately find depends on the type of service you use and your information search skills and knowledge. The next advancement in computer information search and retrieval will be with electronic or intelligent agents. Electronic agents are being designed to make networks smarter about people rather than requiring people to be smart about networks. *Electronic agents* are programs assigned to a specific individual or group that functions, in effect, as a personal servant. The owner will be able to instruct the agent to look for information, organize E-mail, "run errands," and even shop online while the owner is doing something else. The agent will "report back" to the owner if and when it has accomplished a certain task. Initial services such as PersonaLink from AT&T and Intelligent Communications from IBM will be oriented toward business and commercial users.

Academic agents will no doubt become available that will allow students and faculty to search for information and resources using this technology. Suppose for example that you are interested in the effects of exercise on arthritis. Your agent would monitor various information resources and let you know when some new information on the subject becomes available. The agent will automatically download the information, place it in a specific folder, and inform you that it is there.

INTERNET RESOURCES

A wide range of resources and materials are available over the Internet and the World Wide Web—computer software, university catalogs, and information on a wide range of topics, to mention a few.

University Home Pages

Many universities are developing World Wide Web Home Pages that are similar to the university catalog. Home Pages usually contain information about the university, programs of study, admission requirements, as well as links to other World Wide Web sites. In addition, many Home Pages have links to the local library. You can use your terminal to examine the library holdings at the university to which you are linked. One note of caution: Remote access is not necessarily universal. In some cases, access may be denied if you are not a student at that institution. For an extensive list of university Home Pages see *http://www.mit.edu:8001/people/cdemello/univ.html.* Figure 4.2 is a sample university home page, and the box on p. 102 lists a number of other university home page addresses.

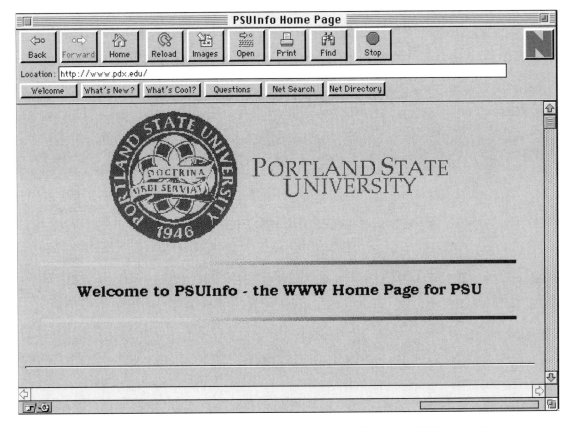

FIGURE 4.2 Portland State University home page. (From Portland State University, 1995, Portland, Ore.)

Sample University Home Page Addresses

Colorado State University
http://www.colostate.edu/

Hobart and William Smith Colleges
http://hws3.hws.edu:9000/

Idaho State University
http://www.isu.edu/welcome.html

Oregon State University
http://gopher.orst.edu/

University of Iowa
http://www.uiowa.edu/

University of Maryland
http://www.umd.edu/

University of Vermont
http://www.uvm.edu/

Electronic Journals and Newsstands

When you visit the periodicals room at your library you'll see dozens and dozens of printed journals covering all fields of study. Networks are now providing an alternative means of disseminating journals and information. The electronic journal (E-journal) is becoming an increasingly popular medium for journal publications. These E-journals range from peer reviewed journals to informal journals and newsstands.

Several sites on the World Wide Web offer a wide range of electronic magazines, texts, and journals. The number of offerings is growing rapidly. Experiment with the sites listed below, or try searching for sites with a program like Webcrawler in Netscape:

Electronic Newsstand
http://www.enews.com:2102/enews.html

Electronic Texts Journals Newsletters Magazines and
    Collections
http://www.lib.ncsu.edu:80/stacks/

Figure 4.3 shows the WebCrawler search pages and Figure 4.4 is the Biomechanics World Wide Web Site.

Project Gutenberg

Project Gutenberg is an on-going effort to make a wide range of books and other documents available electronically. You can download items in the Project Gutenberg library to your computer and save the information on disk. Project Gutenberg amounts to an electronic library accessible from anywhere in the world where Internet is available. Most of the books are either classics such as *Alice in Wonderland* or informational books such as the *CIA World Factbook*.

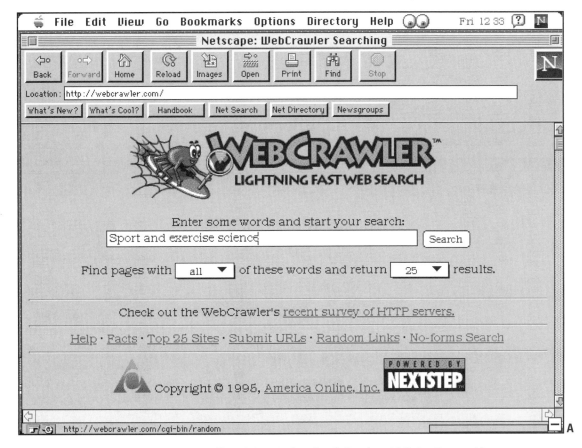

FIGURE 4.3 Sample WebCrawler pages. (Copyright 1995 America Online, Inc. All Rights Reserved.)

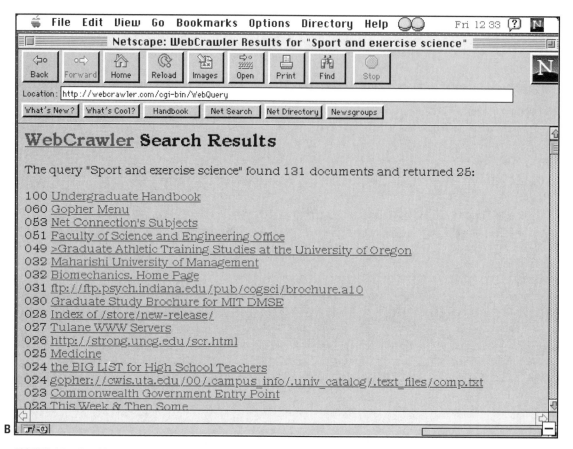

FIGURE 4.3 Cont'd

Project Gutenberg Home Page
http://jg.cso.uiuc.ed/PG/Welcome.html

THE VIRTUAL LIBRARY

The Library of Congress is planning to create a virtual library of digitized images of its collections of books, manuscripts, photos, and other materials for access over computer networks. A Digital Library Coordinating Committee is seeking donations in addition to appropriations from Congress to support the project. Their goal is to convert many of the documents by the year 2000. Any personal computer or terminal can become a *virtual library* in the sense that you can search, order, and/or download information

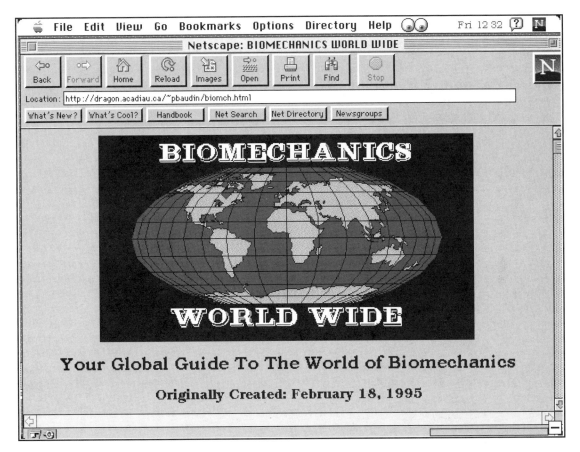

File Edit View Go Bookmarks Options Directory Help   Fri 12 32

Netscape: BIOMECHANICS WORLD WIDE

Back Forward Home Reload Images Open Print Find Stop

Location: http://dragon.acadiau.ca/~pbaudin/biomch.html

What's New? What's Cool? Handbook Net Search Net Directory Newsgroups

BIOMECHANICS

WORLD WIDE

Your Global Guide To The World of Biomechanics

Originally Created: February 18, 1995

FIGURE 4.4 Biomechanics home page. (From Baudin JP: Biomechanics World Wide, Acadia University, 1995, Wolfville, Nova Scotia.)

from literally anywhere in the world from one location. For example, you can use Internet to access library catalogs in Asia (Australia, New Zealand, Japan), the Western Hemisphere (the Americas), Europe and Africa from home, the office, or at campus terminals.

Figure 4.5 shows examples of the Virtual Library Home Pages on the World Wide Web that has links to a wide range of library resources. Virtual Library Home Page: *http://www.w3.org/hypertext/DataSources/bySubject/overview.html*

One limitation however, is that although you can examine the holding for many libraries, you cannot directly access the materials. The Center for Library Initiatives is a consortium of 12 universities: Indiana, Michigan State, Northwestern, Ohio

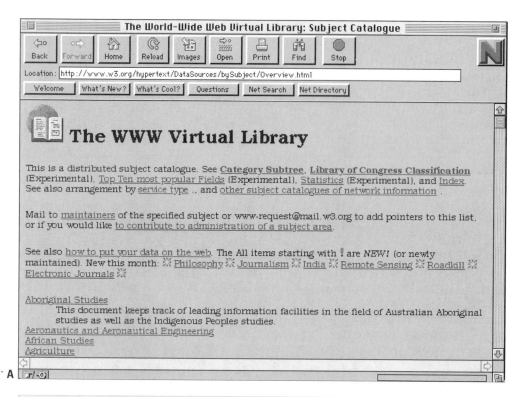

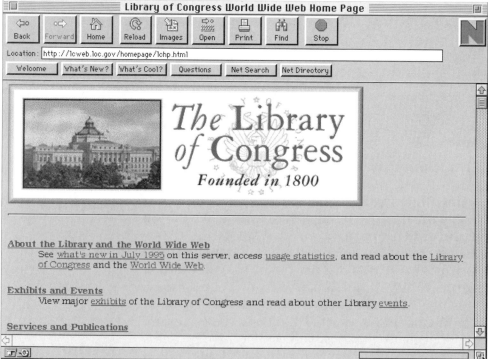

FIGURE 4.5 **A,** Virtual library home page (Courtesy Secret, A and Berners-Lee, T). **B,** The Library of Congress World Wide Web home page.

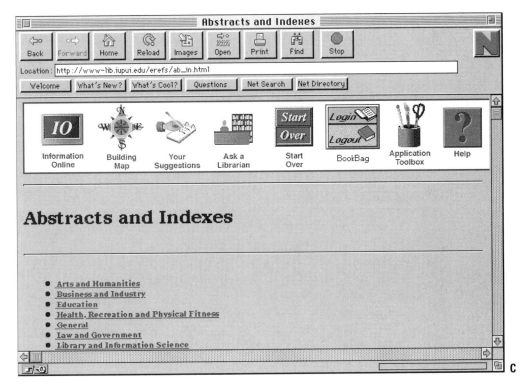

FIGURE 4.5 cont'd C, Abstracts and Indexes page at Indiana State University. (From University Library, Indiana University-Purdue University, 1995, Indianapolis, Ind.)

State, Pennsylvania State, Purdue, and the Universities of Michigan, Chicago, Illinois, Iowa, Minnesota, and Wisconsin. They have recently entered into a cooperative arrangement where the schools will pool library resources and make them available electronically. As a student at any of the participating institutions, you will be able to access information at any of the other institutions. As this type of cooperative sharing of resources expands, quick access to information will increase tremendously.

SUMMARY

There is no doubt that we live in the information age. For many of us the problem is not finding enough information, the problem is finding time to stay current with all of the new information. Efficient and effective information search skills are becoming more essential every day as the range of potential information resources expands and the volume of information grows. In this chapter we presented many of the information resources that researchers use to locate information. As a student, you should familiarize yourself with these resources. As you research topics for class projects, you will be more efficient and effective when searching for information.

EXERCISES

1 Request a user's name for your university computer system and learn to use the E-mail system.
2 Ask your advisor for their E-mail address so you can communicate with them when you have questions.
3 Exchange your E-mail address with friends at other schools.
4 Go to the library and find out which information sources they have available on CD-ROM and which resources are in book form.
5 Practice using the CD-ROM resources. In particular SPORT Discus, Medline, and PsyLIT.
6 Find out if the computer center has Mosaic software installed on the computers. If so, explore the World Wide Web.

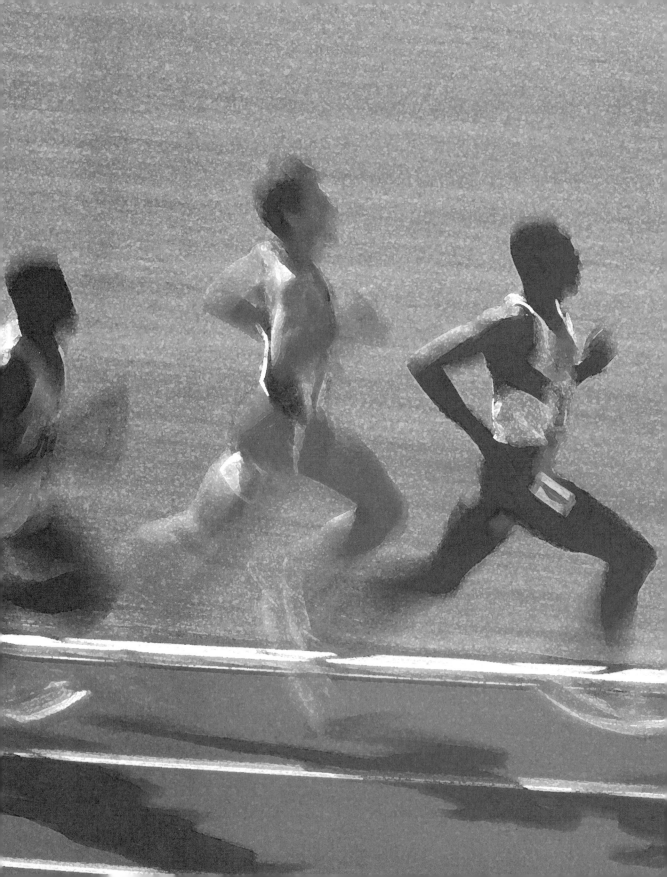

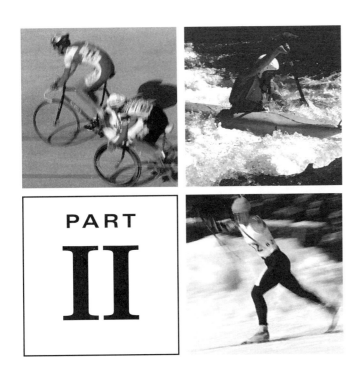

Methods

Experimental Research

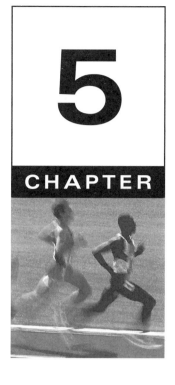

5

CHAPTER

LEARNING GOALS

After reading this chapter you will be able to:

1 Explain the difference between the terms *parameter* and *statistic.*

2 Discuss the qualities of proper sampling.

3 Describe the differences between a random sample, a stratified sample, and a cluster sample.

4 Explain the difference between an independent variable, a dependent variable, and a control variable.

5 Describe why independent variables have levels.

6 Identify some of the alternative terms for independent and dependent variables.

7 Explain how operational definitions define variables.

8 Understand the threat imposed by confounding variables on research findings.

9 Differentiate between primary variance, secondary variance, and error variance.

10 Explain how to maximize primary variance, control secondary variance, and eliminate error variance.

11 Differentiate between the terms *external validity* and *internal validity.*

TERMS

Parameter
Sample
Statistic
Population
Independent variable
Dependent variable
Operational definition
Control variable
Confounding variable
Primary variance
Secondary variance
Error variance
Internal validity
External validity

METHODS OVERVIEW

The purpose of the Methods section of a research report is to explain the details of how the investigation was conducted. The Methods section generally follows the Introduction and the Literature Review sections of the report. As you recall, the Introduction section contains an explanation of the particular problem the researcher is investigating and a description of the scope (or limits) of the investigation. Usually, hypotheses to be addressed at the conclusion of the report are also found in the Introduction.

The Literature Review (which is carried out before conducting the study) is then summarized to provide the background that leads to the development of the specific problem at hand. It is this backdrop that provides the context for the research described in the report. It is somewhat analogous to a sentence and the paragraph in which it is located. The paragraph (for example, the Literature Review in the analogy) provides meaning to the sentence (for example, the research project). Once the researcher has provided specifics of the research problem and how it fits into what is previously known in the area, the next task is to describe how the investigation will be conducted, and this is done in the Methods section.

A general rule of thumb for judging the quality of a Methods section is to ask whether or not sufficient detail is provided to allow another investigator to replicate the study. This would require enough detailed information about how the subjects involved in the study (if any) were selected and enough information about their relevant characteristics (for example, age, weight, social background, level of education, etc.) that a similar group of subjects could be identified at some other location and at some other time.

Additionally, pertinent information about facilities and equipment used in the study should be presented again with sufficient detail to permit replication. This often requires even model numbers to be reported when specific equipment is utilized.

In most cases the bulk of the Methods section will contain information about the procedures used by the investigator. Depending on the type of research involved, the description of the procedures will contain varying types of information. Examples of details located in the Methods section include length, duration, and types of treatments provided in an experimental study; development of criteria for variable selection in a meta analysis; explanation of validating techniques to determine if an item should be included on a questionnaire; or precautions taken to prevent bias from entering into the interview process in a qualitative study. Many other examples could have been given here to illustrate the variety of procedural details that might be found in the Methods section. These examples demonstrate that the methods used in a research project define the "type" of research conducted. This concept was illuminated in previous chapters.

It is very difficult to categorize research in sport and exercise sciences into neat, nonoverlapping compartments. Many concepts (for example, the need for reliable and valid measurements) are critical to any type of research and, conversely, other details apply only to one specific type of study.

The box on pp. 116-118 is an excellent editorial describing the importance of the Methods section of a research report.

Most research in sport and exercise sciences involves measuring characteristics of humans or animals. In the Methods section of a research report the investigator describes how the "subjects" were selected and also any relevant attributes so that another researcher could replicate the study. Because it is seldom true that all of the members of a population of interest can be measured, a subset of the population is selected and the measurements made in this subset (called a sample) are inferred to represent the population.

If it were possible to measure all members of a population (called a census) any resultant fact about the population is called a **parameter**. Usually Greek symbols are used to indicate parameters. For example, if a teacher was interested only in collecting information on a certain class and measured the height of each member of the class, the average of these measurements would be represented by μ (mean).

A **sample** is any subset of a population. Facts about a sample are called **statistics** and they represent estimates of parameters. If the teacher collected height measurements on some subset of the members of the class, the average of these measurements would be a statistic represented by $\overline{X}$ (mean)

Editor's Viewpoint: Who's on First, What's on Second?

Maureen R. Weiss

In the famous dialogue between Abbott and Costello, "Who's on First?" Lou Costello is thoroughly confused about the lineup of ballplayers that Bud Abbott has put together for a game. Abbott patiently tries to explain to Costello the players and their positions: Who is on first, What is on second, I Don't Know is on third, and so on. In exasperation Costello finally blurts out, "I don't give a darn," to which Abbott calmly replies, "Oh no, that's our shortstop!"

Grappling with the Method section of a research article is in many ways analogous to sorting out the lineup in this baseball skit. Like Costello, the reviewers and readers seek to learn about the "players" in the Method lineup. It is the author's responsibility to ensure that the least amount of confusion and as much relevant information as possible is communicated about the methodology. Therefore, I recommend that the methodology lineup include the first baseman (Who), second baseman (What), left fielder (Why), right fielder (How)[1], and center fielder (Because). I also suggest banishing the third baseman (I Don't Know) and, by all means, the shortstop (I Don't Give A Darn) to the minor leagues forever! The purpose of this Editor's Viewpoint is to illuminate what information should be provided in the Method section in order to score points with the fans (the readers) and umpires (the reviewers).

Let's start with Who, the first baseman. *Who* are the subjects? Describe your sample as thoroughly as possible, including characteristics relevant to your particular study, such as number and breakdown by age, gender, gender within age groups, ethnicity, and experience or skill level. Also state the reason for selecting these particular subjects. For example, explain why certain age groups or skill levels were chosen. Provide appropriate and clear operational definitions for criteria such as elite athlete or expert performer. Clarify why subjects were included or excluded; that is, what system was used to select or remove subjects from the available pool to meet specific requirements of the research question. These criteria should be mentioned in the discussion of the sample and either clarified here or in the design section.

The next player is What, the second baseman. *What* type of study design did you employ (for example, experimental, correlational, qualitative) to answer your research questions or hypotheses? Describe the groups of subjects selected for testing the proposed hypotheses and the protocol used to gather data about the subjects (for example, experimental manipulation, in-depth interview, participant observation). Identify the independent and dependent variables (if appropriate), distinguish the levels of the independent variable, and operationally define the dependent measures. In short, use the design section to give reviewers and readers the "big picture" of how the study was developed to answer the major research questions.

The next player in the methodology lineup is the big hitter and left fielder, Why—a review of measures and/or instrumentation. Describe the measures that were chosen to represent the constructs of interest, along with their validity and reliability characteristics. Explain *why* these forms of assessment were selected instead of possible alternatives. Provide information about the instrumentation used, such as the make and model of equipment and how key variables were derived (for example, physiological or biomechanical data

---

[1]In the Abbott and Costello skit, the only player not identified by name was the right fielder. I have taken the liberty of inserting How, the right fielder, into my methodology lineup.

From Weiss MR: Research Quarterly for Exercise and Sport 65(2):iii-iv, 1994.

Editor's Viewpoint: Who's on First, What's on Second?—cont'd

estimates). Describe any calibration steps and inter- or intrarater procedures used to ensure the reliability or consistency of subject responses. If questionnaires, fitness tests, or surveys were used, describe as much relevant data as possible: number of items (total and subscale), item response format (for example, 5-point Likert-type), and procedure for computing scale scores. Provide validity and reliability data from previous research that assessed constructs using the same type of sample (for example, children) or a reason why the measure should be valid with your sample (for example, pilot study data).

Social science researchers often develop a measure or several items to assess a construct central to answering the research question. In this case, it is essential to the integrity of the study that you provide the following: (a) information about how the instrument was developed (for example, derived from items used in previous research, pilot study), (b) a listing of the items or a sample of items, and (c) the psychometric characteristics available (for example, content, factorial, concurrent validity). It is not sufficient just to say, "the questionnaire is available from the first author," because reviewers need information to evaluate how accurately and reliably the research questions were answered in the study. With interpretive or ethnographic studies using qualitative methods, describe how behaviors are assessed using observational procedures, how participant conditions and affect are inferred using interview schedules, and the coding schemes used during participant observation or critical incident reporting.

The procedure section is covered nicely by the right fielder, How. Provide a step-by-step outline of *how* the study's purposes were carried out. The major objective is to maximize the readers' ability to "replay" the study if they had the resources to do it. Indicate how informed consent was obtained from subjects, as well as how subjects were recruited to participate in the study, what events transpired on entering the research setting, and the general procedures in collecting the data (for example, length of time, debriefing). In survey studies, describe the series of steps designed to maximize the return rate (for example, follow-up mailing after 2 weeks, postcard after 4 weeks) and report the final return rate. For qualitative studies, document procedures such as in-depth interviews and participant observation in enough detail that readers can follow the natural process of data collection and the eventual interpretation of that data.

Rounding out the batting order in the methodology lineup is the center fielder, Because, of the data analysis section. This section serves as a "road map" for how the data will be analyzed to answer the research questions and should provide the reasoning behind your choice of statistical techniques (for example, "A DM MANOVA was conducted *because* the sphericity assumption was violated."). In this section, specify the descriptive and correlational analyses that will be conducted, reliability assessments, and the major analyses to specifically address the research hypotheses. The Results section should naturally follow from the data analysis information; readers now know exactly the order of events in the forthcoming section.

In sum, as authors you can get the benefit of a "good call" by conscientiously putting together a strong lineup of players in the Method section. To do this, carefully consider the following points when writing and editing your papers prior to submission:

- *Who* is on first: provide a detailed account of subject characteristics, operational definitions (for example, inexperienced),

Continued.

Editor's Viewpoint: Who's on First, What's on Second?—cont'd

and criteria used to include or exclude subjects from the study.

- *What* is on second: elaborate upon the nature of the study design, how the design specifically addresses research hypotheses, and relevant independent and/or dependent variables.

- *Why* is in left field: identify the measures employed, discuss psychometric properties, and explain the derivation of scores as well as their interpretation.

- *How* is in right field: systematically account for the procedures employed to carry out the study so that they can be replicated by other researchers.

- *Because* is in center field: provide a road map specifying which data analyses were conducted to answer key research questions. Explain the reasoning behind the choice of your statistical techniques.

The Method section is a crucial place for authors to explain essential elements of their study. It is important to do a "crackerjack" job of highlighting the study sample, design, measures, procedure, and data analysis. Once you have convinced the "umpires" of a representative sample, sound design, adequate measures, systematic procedures, and logical statistical analyses, then "pitching" our results should not throw any curveballs to the readers. Remember Costello's confusion and frustration. Take complete control of your methodology lineup and clearly and coherently inform the readers.

and be an estimate of μ. The accuracy of this estimate would depend on several factors, the most important of which is how the sample was selected from the population. This "sampling" process is critical to the outcome of a research project.

To begin, the researcher must first clearly identify the population of interest. The definition must be precise enough to eliminate any ambiguity regarding who is and who is not included. The next step (which is often more difficult than it seems) is to identify *all* members of the population selected. If the population is to be sampled and all members of the population are not identified, it is possible that the resulting sample will not correctly represent the population. Such a sample is said to be *biased*.

Once the population is defined and its members identified, the researcher has two questions to answer: how large a sample should be selected and how exactly will the individuals be picked to be in the sample.

The decision about the number of individuals to include in a sample is a complex one and generally revolves around statistical considerations. Precision, reduction of error probability, and reliability are examples of some of the concepts involved. As a general rule, as the size of the sample increases the accuracy of research increases. However, there are two situations where increasing the sample size is not productive.

Some research involves costly procedures, either in terms of time, money, facilities, and/or personnel. There can exist a situation in which the increases in accuracy are not worth the additional costs of increasing the sample size. More serious, however, is using a flawed procedure to select the sample from the population. No matter how large a sample is, if it is biased and therefore does not accurately represent the population, it may lead to erroneous conclusions.

One of the most infamous cases of sampling error was the poll taken by *The Literary Digest* during the 1936 presidential election between Roosevelt and Landon. They commissioned a very ambitious poll of ten million voters (about one out of every four voters) and predicted, based on the results of the poll, that Landon would win the election. Much to their surprise and embarrassment, Roosevelt won. Gallup (1948) diagnosed why the results were in error:

> The reasons the *Digest* poll went wrong in 1936 are obvious to anyone who understands modern polling methods. *The Literary Digest* sent out its ballots by mail and, for the most part, to people whose names were listed in telephone directories or to lists of automobile owners. From the point of view of cross section this was a major error, because it limited the sample largely to the upper half of the voting population, as judged on an economic basis. Roughly 40 percent of all homes in the United States had telephones and some 55 percent of all families owned automobiles. These two groups, which largely overlap, constitute roughly the upper half or upper three-fifths, economically, of the voting population.
>
> *The Literary Digest* in previous straw polls had sent post card ballots to the same group, but the *Digest* did not reckon for two factors in 1936—the decision of votes along income lines which began with Roosevelt's

administration in 1932, and the substantial increase in the voting population which took place between 1932 and 1936. These new voters came predominately from the poorest levels—from income groups which favored Roosevelt.

The *Digest* not only failed to select a proper cross section, but the means by which the magazine reached voters—mail ballots—also helped to introduce error into the findings.

Persons most likely to return mail ballots are those in the higher income and educational levels, and, conversely, those least likely to return their ballots represent the lowest income and educational levels. So, even if the *Literary Digest* had actually used lists of voters throughout the country as they did in a few cities, instead of names selected from telephone books and automobile lists, post card ballots would still have been responsible for a substantial error in the *Digest's* findings (Gallup, 1948, 73-75).

As you can see, it was improper sampling techniques that were the source of the error, not the size of the sample. The *Digest* was interested in the voting preferences of the eligible voters (the **population**) but sampled in such a way that not everyone in the defined population had the possibility of being included in the sample. A second error was that a large sample was necessary and that it would necessarily be representative of the population. Many nationwide surveys conducted today use samples ranging from about 600 to 2400 respondents. Statisticians have shown that if a sample is representative, samples of this size can describe the population with an acceptable margin of error.

What then is the proper way to select individuals to ensure a nonbiased sample? The answer is to use a simple random process to select the subjects from the population. However, two conditions must be met. Every member of the population must have an equal probability of being selected, and the probability of an individual being selected must be independent of the selection of any other individual.

The reason for the requirement of being able to identify every member of the population mentioned earlier now becomes clear. If some members of the population are not identified, they don't have an equally likely chance of being selected. An example of violation of the independent condition would be including a second individual in the sample because he or she was a sibling of someone already selected to be in the sample. Such a procedure would not lead to a random sample.

Once these two conditions are met then any process that uses random selection of individuals will produce a nonbiased sample. Using a table of random numbers or a random number generator computer program, drawing names from a hat, or any other nonsystematic process may be used. Although this seemingly simple process is usually the best way to proceed, there are other ways to select a sample as well. Some of these are satisfactory under certain conditions while others are not satisfactory but still used. Other sampling techniques are explained next.

SYSTEMATIC SAMPLING

If a complete list of the individuals comprising the population of interest is available but it is arranged in some systematic fashion (for example, alphabetical) every nth name could be selected to arrive at a sample. For example, if the list contained 1000 names and it was decided to have a sample of 50 subjects (5%) then every twentieth person could be selected. Through a random process a member between 1 and 20 would be selected (for example, 7) and then this individual and every twentieth name thereafter (27, 47, . . . 987) would comprise the sample. In most situations this procedure would lead to a random sample as long as the list contained all members of the population.

STRATIFIED RANDOM SAMPLING

The population is first divided into relevant subgroups and then random sampling techniques are applied to each subgroup. For example, suppose that 20% of the students at a college are seniors, 20% are juniors, 25% are sophomores, and 35% are freshmen and your goal is to select 100 students for your sample. To arrive at a stratified sample you would randomly select 20 seniors, 20 juniors, 25 sophomores, and 35 freshmen from a list containing the names of all students organized by class standing. With this method, you can be certain that the sample represents the population precisely in terms of student level and have confidence that the entire student population is adequately represented in every other characteristic.

Stratification may be done on more than one variable but normally is done only on variables that are relevant to the dependent variable. Using the United States census data, professional polling organizations use stratified sampling techniques to ensure their relatively small samples are representative of the entire population in ways that are important to whatever they are investigating.

QUOTA SAMPLING

This technique is like stratified sampling but does not involve random selection from the various levels identified. As an example, suppose you are conducting a survey on the exercise habits of the students at a university, and you want to compare the habits of the students at each level of class standing. You learn from the admissions office that the undergraduate population is 20% seniors, 20% juniors, 25% sophomores, and 35% freshman. You can afford to print 100 copies of the survey, so your goal is to survey the first 20 seniors, first 20 juniors, first 25 sophomores, and first 35 freshman that you can recruit at the student union.

As you can see, the results may not necessarily represent the true habits of the entire student body. The quota method would exclude those students who, for example, were not at the student union at the time you conducted the survey, or those students who do not often go to the student union. Although this sampling method is convenient and does not require you to have a complete list of all students by class standing at the university, it would not be possible to defend any conclusions obtained as being representative of the entire student population.

CLUSTER SAMPLING

Another sampling technique designed for surveying large populations where it is impractical or impossible to obtain lists of all members of the population is called cluster sampling. For example, suppose you decide to conduct a survey on the exercise habits of the elementary school children in your state. In most states, it would be impractical to randomly select subjects from all elementary school children. As an alternative to simple random selection, you might use a random cluster sample. Cluster samples consist of groups of subjects selected from the population. Suppose your state is divided into 100 counties. The first step would be to randomly select, say, five counties. Next, you would randomly select five school districts from each of the five counties. Finally, you would randomly select five schools from each of the school districts. All the students in the selected schools would become subjects in the survey. As you can imagine, it is much more efficient for the researcher to survey all the students at a specific school rather than survey few students at many schools all over the state.

Although this may be the only sampling method available to you and it is certainly preferred over simply locating a few elementary school children in the state to survey, it does not lead to a random sample and therefore conclusions derived from the survey cannot be claimed to represent the desired population. Even though the schools eventually selected were obtained by a random process, the "independence" rule has been violated using cluster sampling. All the students in a particular school are included in the sample and thus they are "connected" to each in some ways and cannot be considered to be chosen independently. If conducted carefully and a sufficient number of clusters are included, this type of sampling is less problematic than accidental sampling in which the "equally likely to be chosen" principle is violated.

ACCIDENTAL SAMPLING

This technique involves the use of a self-selected sample and is commonly seen in many magazine surveys, street-corner surveys, and television surveys. The respondents, in self-selected samples, tend to be particularly interested in an issue and are therefore willing to take the actions necessary to become involved. For example, suppose your local television station asks its viewers to express their opinion on the legality of abortion by telephoning one number to register support for the current laws and a different number to register opposition. Those people who choose to call will probably be those with strong opinions on the issue, pro and con, and may not equally reflect moderate views of the public. In addition, the survey would, of course, exclude anyone who was not aware of it. This method of obtaining a sample is totally unacceptable for a research project.

In summary, the only absolutely appropriate sampling technique for a research project is simple random sampling. However, for a variety of reasons, mostly involving practical considerations, it may not be possible to use this process. Does this mean that any research project that does not utilize random sampling is invalid? Probably in the strictest sense the answer to this question is yes. However, if a researcher can show that the sample used does not differ in any important way from the population of interest, it may be possible to regard the sample as representative of the population. While it is true that strict adherence to sampling rules would probably slow down our research efforts, it is equally true that results of research not using these methods must be accepted with some degree of caution.

Just as nearly all research projects involve some type of sampling procedures to select the individuals to be studied, research projects also involve measurement of some characteristic of these individuals. The act of measurement implies it is possible to quantify these characteristics and that these characteristics have the potential to change. Characteristics that have the ability to change are termed *variables* and a general discussion of variables in research follows.

THE ROLE OF VARIABLES IN RESEARCH

Imagine a class assignment where your professor asks you to design and conduct a small experiment on any one of several physiological responses to exercise. You decide to investigate the effect of bicycling on body weight. Your plan is to cycle 10 miles per day at an average intensity of 40% of maximum heart rate, 3 days a week for 6 weeks. You weigh yourself on the first day, conscientiously follow the cycling program, and then weigh yourself at the end of the sixth week. The questions is: Will your professor detect any flaws in your experiment? To answer this question, we need to examine the factors that contribute to a well-designed experiment.

VARIABLES

At the simplest level, a variable is a characteristic (an attribute or dimension) that will exhibit different values under different conditions. For example, heart rate can be thought of as a variable because it will vary under different conditions. Exercise intensity, emotional state, temperature, and other factors cause heart rate to vary. In your bicycling experiment, body weight is a variable. The assumption underlying the design of your experiment is that body weight will change (or vary) as a consequence of the cycle training. The goal of the experiment is to determine how much and in what direction weight will change. However, weight is only one of the variables in your experiment; other variables include the type of exercise (bicycling), the intensity (40% of maximum heart rate), the frequency (3 days a week), the duration (10 miles), and the length of the program (6 weeks).

A fundamental goal of research is to understand how variables behave or react to different conditions in the environment. Exercise physiologists explore how physiological or biochemical variables change or adapt to different levels or types of exercise. Motor behaviorists study how learning variables influence the acquisition of motor skills. Biomechanists examine how variables such as force, torque, or acceleration change with variations in movement.

Independent Variables

Independent variables are those variables that are manipulated by the investigator. The term *manipulation* refers to the active process of selecting a variable, and then deciding on the different levels of the variable to be investigated. The process of identifying a variable, and then manipulating it (setting it at different levels) is the central feature of experimental research. The term *cause-and-effect* relationship refers to the ability to describe changes in the value of an affected variable when a first variable (the independent variable) is manipulated. At the conclusion of your bicycling experiment, you might conclude that the exercise program (the cause) resulted in a reduction in body weight (the effect).

Research projects may have one independent variable, or several independent variables. To study the behavior of tennis racquets when hitting a tennis ball, Knudson (1991) strung different racquets at one of three tensions with one of two types of string. The first independent variable manipulated by Knudson was *string tension*, set at three levels: 50, 60, and 70 lbs. The second independent variable, *string type* was set at two levels: synthetic gut and natural gut string. To study the effect of the menstrual cycle on athletic performance in young women, Quadagno et al. (1991) utilized one independent variable, *cycle phase*, set at three levels: premenstrual, menstrual, and postmenstrual. Shank and Haywood (1989) manipulated three independent variables in their study of visual responses of college baseball players. The first independent variable, *skill level*, had two levels: expert and novice. The second independent variable, *delivery type*, had two levels: wind-up and stretch. The third independent variable, *pitch type*, also had two levels: fastball and curveball.

In each of these examples, the researchers identified variables that they believed would affect the behavior of a ball rebounding from the face of a tennis racquet, athletic performance in women, and perceptual responses in baseball players in important, but at the time, unknown ways. See Table 5.1.

It is important for you to recognize that in each example there is at least one independent variable, and each independent variable has two or more levels. The simplest experiment has one independent variable at two levels, and one dependent variable (discussed next). The Quadagno et al. experiment was slightly more complex than the simplest experiment—it had one independent variable with three levels. The Knudson experiment was more complex with two

TABLE 5.1 Independent Variables

Knudson (1991)	**String tension:** 3 levels	**String type:** 2 levels		
Quadagno et al. (1991)	**Cycle phase:** 3 levels			
Shank and Haywood (1989)	**Skill:** 2 levels	**Delivery:** 2 levels	**Pitch:** 2 levels	

independent variables, the first with three levels, and the second with two levels. The Shank and Haywood experiment was the most complex of these three examples having three independent variables each with two levels.

Dependent Variables

The **dependent variable** is the variable measured in an experiment, sometimes called the outcome variable. Knudson measured two dependent variables: the rebound accuracy and velocity following a tennis ball impact. Quadagno et al. measured four dependent variables: two measures of strength, bench press and leg press, and two measures of swimming speed, 100 and 200 meter freestyle times. Shank and Haywood also measured two dependent variables: number of correct responses and eye movement reaction time. Table 5.2 shows the dependent variables from the Knudson, Quadagno et al., and Shank and Haywood studies.

Independent and dependent variables are the foundation of the research process. Selection, manipulation, and measurement of these variables allow researchers to explore the relationships between and among them. Knudson found greater rebound accuracy at low tension (50 lbs.) than at high tension (70 lbs.). Quadagno et al. determined that cycle phase had no effect on strength or swimming speed. Shank and Haywood found that expert baseball players were more accurate at identifying pitches than novices but found no difference in eye movement time between the two skill level groups.

Remembering the distinctions between independent variables and dependent variables can initially seem difficult because the definitions are not very intuitive. Table 5.3

TABLE 5.2   Dependent Variables

Knudson (1991)	Accuracy ratio	Velocity ratio		
Quadagno et al. (1991)	Bench press	Leg press	100 meter swim time	200 meter swim time
Shank and Haywood (1989)	Correct responses	Eye reaction time		

TABLE 5.3 Independent and Dependent Variables	
"One researcher's independent variable is another researcher's dependent variable"	
Independent variables	**Dependent variables**
• Manipulated variables	• Outcome variables
• Experimental variables	• Measured variables
• Treatment variables	• Estimated variables
• X-variables	• Y-variables
• Factors	• Criterion variables
• Predictors	• Response variables

provides some alternative terms that may help you understand and remember the difference between these two terms.

Operational Definitions

An **operational definition** formally defines the characteristics of a variable (independent or dependent). For example, *endurance athlete* can be an independent variable, but from a research perspective the term endurance athlete alone is not specific enough to be useful. Swimmers, runners, cross-country skiers, or cyclists all might be considered endurance athletes. Within any group there can be several categories: runners can specialize in 5k, 10k, marathon, or ultra-marathon events; swimmers, skiers, and cyclists also have similar specializations. In the Quadagno et al. study, menstrual cycle was operationally defined as: premenstrual, 3 to 5 days before menses; menstrual, days one through three of menses; and postmenstrual, ten to twelve days after the onset of menses. Operational definitions are important so other researchers can completely understand the details of the research.

As an example of how some variables can be considered an independent and a dependent variable in different studies, consider body weight. In a study to determine various training regiments on strength development, a researcher could include body weight as an independent variable with three levels—subjects weighing 100-120 lbs., subjects weighing 130-150 lbs., and subjects weighing 160-180 lbs. In another study investigating the effectiveness of three types of diets, body weight might be the dependent variable.

Control Variables

In experimental research it is important to pay attention to any factor that might possibly cause changes in the dependent variable other than those that are manipulated (the independent variables). If these factors are not attended to the researcher cannot be certain that it was the manipulation of the independent variable(s) that caused changes in the dependent variable. This issue is addressed through the use of control variables and control groups. A **control variable** is a variable that is held constant (for example, only one level is present) during an experiment. Control variables fall into two categories: experimental and statistical.

Experimental control variables

In most experiments the number of control variables is greater than the number of independent and dependent variables. In the Knudson study there were five control variables: the type of racquet (Prince CTS 90), size of the racquet head (90 sq. inch), the position of the racquet (clamped), the speed of the ball (19 m/s), and the angle of incidence (25.6°) were all control variables and held at one value throughout the experiment. The Quadagno et al. study also had five control variables, and the Shank and Haywood study had at least three controls. The control variables for these experiments are shown in Table 5.4.

TABLE 5.4 Control Variables					
Knudson (1991)	Frame size	Frame type	Impact velocity	Frame position	Impact angle
Quadagno et al. (1991)	Normal cycle	No oral contraceptives	Measurement methods	Strength training methods	Subject qualifications
Shank and Haywood (1989)	Videotape stimulus events	Viewing environment	Feedback information		

You may recognize that these control variables could have been independent variables if the investigators had been interested in determining their influence on the dependent variables. For example, in the Knudson study, frame size (90 sq. inch, 110 sq. inch, and 125 sq. inch) could have been an independent variable and string tension could have been a control variable held constant at 60 lbs. A crucial aspect in designing experiments is to identify and fix as many control variables as possible so the effect of the independent variable on the dependent variable can be isolated. Notice, however, that the selection of a control variable also limits the eventual discussion of results to the level of the control variable picked. For example, Knudson cannot assume his findings are accurate for any other type or size of racquet, position, ball speed, or angle.

Statistical control variables

Some statistical techniques are available in specific experimental situations to provide control over variables that might impact the results of an experiment. For example, suppose an investigator is interested in examining the effect of three different training protocols on muscular strength development. Even though the investigator has the ability to randomly assign subjects to the three treatment groups, it is known that body weight is correlated with muscular strength and the investigator wants to ensure any differences in body weight are not responsible for any changes detected in muscular strength. Through the use of a statistical technique called *Analysis of Covariance* (ANCOVA) the final muscular strength scores (dependent variable) are mathematically adjusted as if the groups were equal in body weight. This procedure "controls" the variable, body weight.

Why, you might wonder, isn't this technique used all the time? "There is no free lunch," is the answer. This procedure "costs" something in terms of other statistical concerns. More importantly, as noted above, this procedure is applicable only in certain situations and the issues involved will be explained in more detail later in a section on quasi-experimental methods.

Control groups

As will be explained in more detail later in the Experimental Design chapter, another method of controlling the variables

TABLE 5.5 Types of Variables	
Independent variable	The manipulated variable
Dependent variable	The measured variable
Control variable	The constant variable

other than the independent variables is the use of control groups. The procedure in theoretically simple. An additional level is included in the independent variable and this group is, as nearly as possible, exposed to everything the treatment groups are except the specific treatments. This, in effect, isolates the treatment as the only possible cause of any detected differences.

Table 5.5 summarizes the types of variables.

Confounding Variables

A **confounding variable** is a variable that is unintentionally allowed to vary. Suppose, for example, that unknown to the researcher in the Knudson study, the racquet strung at 50 lbs. was positioned at a 90° angle to the path of the incoming ball and the racquets strung at 60 and 70 lbs. were accidentally positioned at a 93° angle. Racquet angle was intended to be a control variable and set at 90° throughout the experiment. Because two racquets were unintentionally positioned differently than the other racquet, the effect on rebound accuracy, if any, could be the result of differences in string tension (the independent variable), or caused by the angle of the racquet (the confounding variable). If this had happened one could say that the *effect of string tension* on rebound *was confounded* by the difference in racquet angle. The researchers may argue that tension causes differences in rebound accuracy, but in this case, one could also argue that the racquet angle was the main causal factor. Either explanation is equally plausible.

When researchers plan or evaluate experiments they pay special attention to identifying potential confounding variables. Confounding variables can negate the results of an experiment by providing alternate explanations for the findings. The failure of investigators to account adequately for all relevant control variables leads to one of the most common criticisms of research.

We have defined a variable as a characteristic (attribute or dimension) that exhibits different values under different conditions. Of primary interest in most research is this quality of differing values and what causes differences to exist. To address this we will look at a construct called variance.

VARIANCE

Measurements obtained from one observation to the next, from one subject to the next, or from one condition to the next can, and do vary. The construct *variance* quantifies the variable nature of measurement and it is made up of several parts (see Table 5.6).

Primary Variance

Primary variance (or systematic variance) is the expected or desired variance in the measurement of the dependent variable and is caused (in part) by the effect of the independent variable. Primary variance is the *wanted* and *consistent* variation in the measurement of the dependent variable. The Knudson study on tennis racquets showed that rebound accuracy and velocity *varied* (or differed) as a result of string tension and string type.

TABLE 5.6 Types of Variance	
Primary Variance (systematic variance)	*Consistent* and *wanted* variation on measures of the dependent variable.
Secondary Variance (extraneous variance)	*Consistent* and *unwanted* variation on measures of the dependent variable.
Error Variance	*Inconsistent* and *unwanted* variation on measures of the dependent variable.

Secondary Variance

Secondary variance (or extraneous variance) is the *consistent* but *unwanted* variation in the measurement of the dependent variable. An example would be an inaccurately calibrated scale that added two pounds to every weight measurement. Although weight would be measured consistently, it would always be two pounds above true weight. If sources of secondary variance are present in the measurement methods, then results will consistently overestimate or underestimate the true value of the dependent variable.

Error Variance

Error variance is the *inconsistent* and *unwanted* variation in the measurements of the dependent variable. Some variability in measurement is present for unknown or unexplained reasons. People differ on characteristics and we don't always know precisely why. For example, people differ in body weight. Gender, heredity, diet, and age are some variables that we could use to explain some of the variability among body weights but they would not account for all the differences. This "left over" variance is called error variance. The experimentalist can also introduce error variance through imprecise measurement. For example, when making skinfold measurements, you need to carefully identify the correct measurement site and then use proper measurement techniques or error variance will affect the scores. The effect of error variance is unpredictable and reduces the accuracy of the measurement of the dependent variable. Research instruments and procedures are developed and tested with the intent of reducing error variance.

Maximizing Primary Variance

One goal of research is to show the effect of different levels of an independent variable on the dependent variable(s). To do this, the researcher needs to fix the independent variables at levels far enough apart that an effect may be observed. In the tennis racquet study, string tension was set at 50, 60, and 70 lbs. If string tension affects rebound, then a 10 pound difference between racquet frames should show the effect. Although the effect might be observed at 51, 52, and 53 lbs., it is less likely. Second, the levels of the independent variables should be set at realistic levels. The three levels of string tension selected for the tennis racquets were within the normal range of tensions used by tennis players. If the researcher selected 10, 15, and 20 lbs., an effect may have been observed, but the findings would be of little value because these tensions are outside the normal range for stringing tennis racquets. By fixing the independent variable string tension at 50, 60, and 70 lbs., the researcher hoped to maximize the effect of tension on rebound in ways that would apply to the real world.

Finding the optimal values for the levels of the independent variable is crucial in any experiment. Researchers will often adopt levels similar to those used in other related studies. This increases the comparability among studies and improves the chances that the researcher will find consistent relationships if they exist.

Controlling Secondary Variance

Careful control of sources of secondary variance improves the value of research findings. One way secondary variance can be reduced is by careful selection and assignment of subjects to experimental groups. Randomization or matching are two methods of controlling unwanted consistent differences between subjects. Blind experimental design procedures will help reduce experimenter bias or expectancy influences. This means the experimenter does not know which subjects are receiving which treatments, the subjects do not know which treatments they are receiving, or both. When both are unknown, it is called a double blind procedure. Properly calibrated equipment is another way to control sources of secondary variance.

Minimizing Error Variance

Inconsistent measurements are controlled by using care and precision when gathering data. Individual differences between subjects can be controlled by using samples that are representative of the population. Appropriate and careful measurement procedures for the dependent variable will help avoid inconsistent variations in obtained values. Finally, careful and proper data analysis techniques can also help reduce error variance.

RESEARCH VALIDITY

Careful selection and measurement of the independent and dependent variables does not guarantee a good experiment. Issues related to the validity of the overall experiment are important. Experimental validity issues are broadly classified into internal and external validity concerns.

　　Internal validity—Refers to the technical quality of a study. It involves the certainty with which the results of an experiment can be attributed to the effect of the independent variable rather than some confounding variable(s). If internal validity is high, then the effects on the dependent variable can be attributed to the independent variable. If internal validity is low, then the observed effect of the independent variable on the dependent variable is less convincing. The internal validity of any given study will range along a scale from very high to very low, although the exact level may not be readily apparent. Assessing internal validity is a subjective process because there is no definitive way to measure this construct.

　　External validity—Refers to the level with which the findings of a study can be generalized to other situations, people, or environments. In other words, how well can the findings describe, explain, or predict the behaviors of individuals other than those in the study. The term *generalize* (or generalizable) is also used for the same concept. If external validity is high, then the results apply to a wide range of situations or populations. If external validity is low, then findings only apply to a narrowly defined situation. As with internal validity, the external validity of any given study also ranges along a scale from very high to very low. Like internal validity, assessment of external validity is also subjective because there is no exact way to measure it.

　　Researchers balance the benefits of internal and external validity when designing an experiment because they tend to be inversely related. An experiment can be designed to have very high internal validity by using very strict experimental control, but can have low external validity (for example, generalizability) because the experiment may bear little resemblance to the situation to which you desire to generalize the results. It is also possible to design a very generalizable experiment that suffers from low internal validity. If the internal validity is too weak, the overall value of the findings is questionable.

Factors Threatening Internal Validity

Uncontrolled variables are the single largest threat to the internal validity of a study. Internal validity is reduced by factors such as the loss of subjects during the course of the experiment, uncontrolled events that occur during the experiment, and other factors detailed below. Threats to internal validity generally fall into two categories: threats concerning subjects and their behavior or treatment during the experiment, and threats related to experimental procedures or instrumentation.

Local history is defined as any unanticipated event occurring during the study that may have altered the subjects' behavior in an uncontrolled and unaccountable way. Because experimental treatments often take place over an extended time period it is possible that a local event may occur and affect treatment groups differentially. For example, many of the subjects in one treatment group may decide to sign up for and play in an intramural basketball league. If the dependent variable in the study is impacted by this experience the internal validity of the experiment could be reduced. One way to eliminate local history threats is to remove affected subjects from the study, if they can be identified. However, eliminating affected subjects decreases sample size and reduces statistical power so this should only occur with good reason. Local history threats are also controlled by using control groups and by maintaining equal conditions among groups.

Maturation of subjects is a threat to internal validity when this change affects the subjects' behavior in unaccounted ways. For example, did the junior high school students get stronger because of the weight training class or because they matured physically over the semester? Random and/or matched random subject assignment procedures are the best ways to control for subject maturation by distributing it equally among groups. Matched random subject assignment occurs when subjects are matched on some important control variable (for example, body weight) and then the subjects who have been matched with one another are randomly assigned to treatment groups. A second technique is using norms to compare changes in the subjects to normal maturation effects. The main problem is that norms for the behaviors being studied may not be available. Statistical control using covariables is another technique for controlling maturation effects.

Pretesting is a threat to internal validity because subjects may "learn" how to take the posttest and this experience causes the subsequent improvement rather than the treatment. For example the VO2max test is used to asses physical fitness by measuring oxygen consumption during exercise. One problem with the VO2max test is it can be intimidating to the subjects because of the procedures and equipment used. Therefore, investigators often include a "learning" trial in their design. Yet pretesting a VO2max test could by itself produce superior posttest results simply because one learns how the test works and subjects' apprehension is reduced because they have been through it before. The main trade-off in not using a pretest is the loss of group equivalence information.

Instrumentation refers to the effect of human or equipment measurement errors during the data collection and/or data analysis phase of a study. Suppose, for example, that during a study measuring body composition, the skinfold calipers were dropped and damaged. Continued use of those calipers could result in inaccurate measurements. Carefully training research assistants and calibrating equipment are the two best methods of controlling instrumentation threats. Another way to control for instrumentation threats is to conduct a pilot study so that testing procedures and equipment calibrating can be evaluated. The main drawback to pilot studies is they can be time consuming and use resources such as supplies, time, and/or subjects.

Statistical regression is the statistical tendency for extreme scores to move toward the group mean when measured a second time. It is also referred to as regression to the mean. For example, if subjects are selected for participation in a study because they scored either very low or very high on a test of physical fitness and were then measured a second time, the unfit group would tend to score higher and the fit group would tend to score lower even though their fitness level did not change. The effect of statistical regression is controlled by using the most reliable measure available, double testing subjects, and using statistical techniques that make allowances for its presence.

Differential selection of subjects is present when the subjects in the different treatment conditions are not equal on relevant characteristics as a result of improper or unavoidable selection and/or assignment procedures. For example, volunteers, because they are willing to join the experiment, may be different than those who choose not to join. Thus an experiment that relies on volunteer subjects may be exposed to this threat. Another example is the use of "intact groups." Two different intact fifth grade classrooms may differ in important but unknown ways. Random subject selection and/or assignment to groups, matching subjects so that treatment groups are known to be equivalent on relevant control variables and/or using a statistical procedure called blocking are all good methods for eliminating differential subject selection threats. Statistical blocking, in effect, removes from the error variance, variability caused by the presence of a control variable.

Experimental mortality refers to the uneven loss of subjects from the various treatment categories during the course of the study. If one condition in an experiment is physically more demanding and thus leads to injuries or stress, more subjects may be lost in this group than are lost in a less physically demanding group. This is only a problem if there is differential mortality or if subjects are lost from one group and not from another for a certain reason. If the loss of subjects is random, then the problem becomes a loss of data leading to a reduction in statistical power caused by reduced sample size.

The effect of experimental mortality can be limited by any one of several methods including: (1) providing incentive for subjects to complete the study, (2) determining the types of subjects that tend to drop out and removing similar subjects from other groups, (3) using random assignments methods, and (4) beginning the study with more subjects than you need.

Increasing Internal Validity

Researchers attempt to address internal validity issues by controlling several basic aspects of studies. For example, selecting an appropriate experimental design is important. The use of a two group design rather than a single group with a pretest and posttest is an example of selecting an appropriate design. Reasons for this will be explained in the next chapters. Carefully conducting the experiment increases internal validity by reducing threats such as instrumentation errors, local history events, differential selection of subjects, and others.

The systematic elimination of potential confounding variables may be the most important factor in protecting the internal validity of a study. Although not all confounding variables are equally threatening to the validity of a study, the presence of any confounding variable always reduces the internal validity of a study. Perhaps the best recommendations to maintain strong internal validity are: (1) randomly assign subjects to groups, (2) use control groups, and (3) be as careful as possible in making measurements.

Factors Threatening External Validity

Recall that external validity refers to how well the findings of a study generalize to other people and to other situations. Threats to this category of validity include the following.

Subjects—Most behavioral research, including research in sport and exercise sciences, relies on college students as subjects. Sears (1986) and Smart (1966) found that college students served as subjects in psychological research in more than 70% of the studies reported in selected psychology journals. Besides the question of how well one set of college students represent all college students, the larger external validity issue is how well college students represent other members of society.

Pretest Sensitization—Pretesting is a commonly used method of assessing group equivalence before the initiation of treatment trials. However, because pretesting is uncommon in real life, this procedure may result in limiting one's ability to generalize to the population. A pretest may sensitize the subjects to the nature of the study and may influence their behavior during the treatments or on the posttest. This is a good example of the tradeoffs confronting the researcher when considering the internal and external validity issues in designing a study. Pretesting serves to improve internal validity by assuring that groups are equivalent at the inception of a study, but can reduce external validity because the subjects in the study differ from the general population to which the researcher would like to generalize the results—the subjects have been pretested but the population has not. One way to deal with the problems posed by a pretest is to design the study so that half of the subjects are pretested and half are not. Specific statistical designs have been developed for this purpose. A second method is to replicate the study but without a pretest. In either case, the number of subjects required is increased and additional time and resources are invested in the study. If possible, it is better to rely on proper random sampling procedures rather than a pretest to ensure initial group equivalence.

Expectancy—This refers to the unintentional effects on the study caused by the researcher's prior beliefs of the outcome of the study. This is also referred to as "the self-fulfilling prophecy." Methods to control expectancy effects are using double blind or automated procedures whenever possible. Perhaps the best control for expectancy effects is awareness of this issue and guarding against it. This is an important issue in qualitative research.

Hawthorne Effect—The Hawthorne effect comes from a study involving the Hawthorne Electric Company where people were shown to be more productive simply because they knew they were subjects in an experiment. A control group and unobtrusive measures are the two best means of limiting the Hawthorne effect.

Overgeneralizing—Experiments are based on a limited number of independent and dependent variables. An external validity issue is the problem of generalizing experimental findings beyond the conditions of the original experiment. The Quadagno et al. (1991) study on menstrual cycle and athletic performance investigated two measures of swimming speed and two weight lifting exercises during three stages of the menstrual cycle in college-age women. They found there was no reduction in athletic performance during menses. Can these finding be generalized to performance in other sports or to different populations? It would not be possible to generalize this way until further experiments are devised to examine a larger range of activities in a larger range of women. See the box below for a summary of the issues affecting research validity.

Improving External Validity

Subject selection is an important factor when considering external validity. Defining the population of interest as completely as possible and then sampling this population properly are the two keys involved in improving external validity.

   Replication is the best method for demonstrating external validity. Replication, either exactly or conceptually, with different subjects, in a different environment, or under modified experimental conditions helps establish the level of external validity. Conceptual replication is more common than exact replication. Conceptual replication occurs when a study

---

Internal and External Validity Threats

Internal validity (True effects of experiment)
- Local history (a hidden effect)
- Pretesting (practice effects)
- Maturation (changes over time)
- Instrumentation (changes in measurements)
- Differential subject selection (preexisting subject differences)
- Statistical regression (unreliable measures—toward the group mean)
- Mortality (nonrandom mortality is a type of differential subject selection)

External validity (Generalization)
- Population (people) and ecological (setting)
- Subjects (who do they represent?)
- Pretesting sensitization ("That's interesting.")
- Hawthorne effect ("I'm a guinea pig.")
- Expectancy (self-fulfilling prophecy)
- Overgeneralizing (different operational definitions)

is modified by changing the independent variables or measuring the dependent variable differently. The goal is to demonstrate similar results under a broader range of conditions than the original research. For example, in the Quadagno et al. study a replication with running or bicycling rather than swimming could serve to examine the external validity of the original findings.

Relationship between Internal and External Validity

Judgments about the external validity of a study are dependent to some extent on judgments of internal validity. If an experiment is found lacking in internal validity, examination of its external validity is not important since the results of the study are in doubt and thus its generalizability becomes a moot point.

Example from sport and exercise sciences

Whitehurst and Menendez (1991) investigated the effect of endurance training on blood lipids in older women (mean age 69.5 years). The limited number of published reports on the effect of exercise on blood lipids in older women motivated the researchers to conduct the study. One of their desired outcomes was to determine if similar previous research on younger women was generalizable to older women (external validity). Whitehurst and Menendez were not motivated by questions of the soundness of previous research, but rather by knowledge that only certain types of subjects had been used in previous experiments. They were interested in determining if knowledge obtained with 20- and 30-year-old subjects also applied to individuals in their 60s. One way to determine this is to study older people following procedures similar to those used with gathering data on younger subjects.

Examples of studies that add to the generalizability of a research question are found in the works of Gabbard, Kirby, and Patterson (1979), Cotten (1990), Engleman and Morrow (1991), Nelson, Yoon, and Nelson (1991), and Kollath, Safrit, Zhu, and Gao (1991). There has been considerable research interest in the use of an upper body strength measure in physical fitness testing. Each of the above studies was designed to estimate the reliability of upper body strength tests. The investigators used a variety of upper body strength tests and they all used subjects having a wide range of ages. A summary of their results indicate that upper body strength tests are quite reliable, regardless of the particular upper body test used and the ages of the individual subjects involved.

SUMMARY

To understand a research report, presentation, or poster it is essential to develop a "researcher's vocabulary." Understanding terms such as parameter and statistic, sample and population, independent and dependent variable, internal and external validity is essential for not only researchers, but also for students. In this chapter, we described these terms in detail, why they are important, and how they are used in research.

EXERCISES

1 Identify the independent and dependent variable(s) for each of the following:

   a A researcher wants to examine cardiovascular adjustments (heart rate, blood pressure) to exercise (low intensity, moderate intensity, high intensity) and thermal stress (temperature: 70°, 80°, 90° and humidity: 50%, 70%, 90%).

   b A teacher wants to determine whether the method of instruction (small group discussion or large group lecture) affects department majors differently than non-majors. The teacher plans on measuring attendance and final exam scores.

   c In a research study on the effects of carbohydrates on exercise recovery, rats were injected with either a zero-dose, 1-dose, or 2-dose level of either a sucrose or a fructose solution. Time spent resting following 60 minutes of moderate intensity exercise was measured.

d A researcher correlated actual movement error and subjective estimates of error in novice and trained subjects when provided with knowledge of results information after every trial, or after every other trial, or after every five trials.

e A researcher examined if the mode of sensory feedback (visual, auditory, proprioceptive) differentially affected the acquisition, retention, and transfer of simple versus complex novel motor skills.

2 Describe the independent, dependent, and control variables that could be used in each of the following investigations:

a Research into the effects of exercise on the average amount of sleep.

b An examination of possible differences in basic motor abilities between athletes and nonathletes.

c A comparison of body composition and exercise patterns during growth and development (ages 5 through 10).

d The role of physical activity on the rate of aging.

e The effects of oxygen inhalation as an aid to recover from exercise.

ANSWERS

1 a Independent variable(s): Exercise, temperature, humidity.
Dependent variable(s): Heart rate, blood pressure.

b Independent variable(s): Method of instruction, type of major.
Dependent variable(s): Attendance, final exam scores.

c Independent variable(s): Level of the dose, type of sugar.
Dependent variable(s): Time resting.

d Independent variable(s): Skill level, frequency of feedback information.
Dependent variable(s): Correlated movement error scores.

e Independent variable(s): Sensory feedback mode.
Dependent variable(s): Skill acquisition, retention, transfer.

Experimental Designs

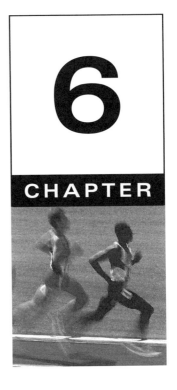

6

CHAPTER

LEARNING GOALS

After reading this chapter you will be able to:

1 Describe the components of good experimental design.

2 Discuss the advantages of conducting experiments to gain new knowledge.

3 Explain why some experiments use two or more independent variables.

4 Explain the difference between an independent group and repeated measures experimental design.

5 Compare the simple random assignment procedure with a matched random assignment procedure.

6 Explain why repeated measures design experiments require counterbalancing.

7 Descibe why a Latin Square is used to counterbalance.

8 Explain the advantages and disadvantages of using a posttest only experimental design versus a pretest-posttest experimental design.

9 Describe the features of a quasi-experimental design.

TERMS

Independent groups
Repeated measures
Carry-over effects
Order effects
Counterbalancing
Latin Square
Demand characteristics
Quasi-experimental design

WHAT IS AN EXPERIMENT?

Now let us evaluate our hypothetical experiment posed at the beginning of the last chapter. You had decided to investigate the effect of bicycling on weight loss. Your plan was to weigh yourself on the first day, then carefully complete the 6-week bicycling exercise program and weigh yourself after 6 weeks. The question is: Does this qualify as a "good" experiment for determining the effect of bicycling on body weight? The dependent (outcome) variable is body weight as measured on a standard scale. The independent variable is the exercise program. The experiment as currently designed would be identified as a one-group pretest-posttest design where a single subject (or it could be a group of subjects) is given a pretest, a treatment, and then a posttest.

Although this design appears reasonable, it has several potential problems. A crucial missing feature is a second level of the independent variable. To better assess the effect of bicycling on weight loss, the exercise program needs at least a second level. The second level could take many forms: A control group that does not cycle, or perhaps a group that rides 15 miles a day rather than 10 miles a day. The point is, the original design lacks a condition against which you can compare the results of the bicycling program.

You should also consider the need to identify important control variables. For example, would it be important to control diet and participation in other forms of aerobic training (for example, running or swimming) during the experiment? If these factors are not controlled, then any change in body weight could not be attributed to the cycling program alone.

Figure 6.1 shows the original study on the left with one independent variable having one level and one dependent variable. The design on the right shows the independent variable with two levels. The second design is better suited to generate meaningful cause-and-effect information about the effects of bicycling on body weight. The two-level design is better because subjects can be randomly assigned to a group and differences between the groups can be attributed to the bicycling program (if this was the only behavioral difference between the two groups).

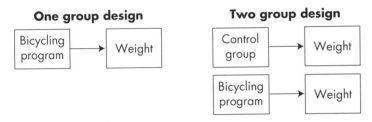

FIGURE 6.1 One and two group designs.

ADVANTAGES OF EXPERIMENTS

Experiments provide important advantages over simple observation for developing knowledge. *Experimental control* means that sources of extraneous variation that may affect the results are controlled or eliminated. Control can occur statistically or experimentally. By identifying as many control variables as possible and fixing each of these variables at a single level throughout the experiment, causal factors can be examined. For example, Knudson found that as string tension and string type were varied, rebound accuracy and velocity changed. This knowledge was gained through careful manipulation of independent variables, measurement of dependent variables, and control of related variables.

MORE THAN ONE INDEPENDENT VARIABLE

Experiments in sport and exercise sciences frequently involve two or more independent variables. Examples of such studies were presented in the previous chapter. The Knudson study on tennis racquets used two independent variables— string tension and string type. The Shank and Haywood baseball study involved three independent variables: skill level, delivery type, and pitch type. These researchers conducted experiments with two or three independent variables for several reasons. It is more efficient to conduct one experiment with two or three independent variables than to conduct a series of experiments each with a single independent variable. The efficient use of resources such as time, money, subjects, and equipment is increased in "complex" experiments.

Experiments with multiple independent variables also simulate the real world better than experiments with a single independent variable. For example, heart rate is influenced not only by exercise intensity, but also by exercise duration, fitness level, drugs, and several other factors. To study the effect of exercise on resting heart rate, you might design an experiment with three independent variables: exercise duration (15 minutes and 30 minutes), exercise intensity (25% of maximum and 75% of maximum), and age (20-29 years and 30-39 years) and then use other means to control as many other potential confounding variables as possible. Knudson considered the string tension and string type together because they are naturally related to one another.

The most important reason experiments with two or more independent variables are conducted is to allow researchers to examine how independent variables act in combination. How independent variables combine their effects on the dependent variable is termed *interaction* and will be discussed in detail later in Chapter 8.

Adding independent variables to an experiment also has disadvantages. As the number of independent variables increases, the complexity of the experiment increases. As the experiment becomes increasingly complex, the interpretation of the results also becomes increasingly difficult. Researchers try to balance the benefits of additionally complex experiments with the side effect of complicated results to obtain the most meaningful findings. You will discover that the majority of experiments in sport and exercise sciences use two or three independent variables (often with several levels of each), and in the very complex experiments, up to four or five independent variables.

MORE THAN ONE DEPENDENT VARIABLE

Often researchers will also measure several dependent variables in a single experiment. In the study on the effects of menstrual phase on athletic performance, the researchers measured four dependent variables: two measures of strength and two measures of swimming speed. In your hypothetical bicycling experiment, any number of factors might be affected by a cycling program. In addition to body weight, percent body fat, resting heart rate, lactic acid levels, or anaerobic threshold could also be dependent variables.

Similar to independent variables, the principal advantage of measuring more than one dependent variable is the efficient use of time and resources. The primary disadvantages of adding dependent variables is the increased complexity of the statistical data analysis and the additional demands placed on the subjects.

However, the inclusion of multiple dependent variables is more like "real life." The effects of a particular experiment are generally not isolated on a single variable (for example, life is "multidimensional in nature"). Thus research should be conducted that attempts to reflect the magnitude and scope of the effect of the independent variables on the dependent variables.

EXPERIMENTAL DESIGN

Experimental design is to a researcher what a blueprint is to a builder—it helps organize, conduct, and complete projects. Blueprints provide the builder with a formal set of plans to ensure that the finished building is in the proper location, built to specifications, and structurally sound. Experimental designs provide the detail and explanations of the various methodologies used by researchers to formally answer research questions.

Although experimental design appears to be a complex and confusing process to the novice, it is essential to have knowledge of the basics of this process to be able to interpret scientific research. Like a blueprint, which is concerned with site elevations, building dimensions, and construction materials, experimental design focuses primarily on four ingredients integral to research: devising subject selection and assignment procedures, writing operational definitions for the independent and dependent variables, selecting appropriate statistical analysis tests, and planning the experimental procedures used to gather the data.

SUBJECT SELECTION AND ASSIGNMENT

Three basic experimental designs are defined by the manner in which subjects are assigned to groups in an experiment:

TABLE 6.1 Methods of Assigning Subjects to Groups	
Independent Groups	Separate subjects serve in each condition.
Repeated Measures	The same subjects serve in each condition.
Mixed Group	Combines independent group and repeated measures methods.

independent groups design, repeated measures design, and mixed groups design. Independent groups and repeated measures approaches can be used in designs with one or more independent variables. Mixed designs can only be used in complex experiments with two or more independent variables. See Table 6.1 for a summary of these groups.

INDEPENDENT GROUPS DESIGN

Independent groups (also termed between-groups or between-subjects design) is an experimental design in which each treatment condition is administered to a separate group of subjects. Independent groups designs are used in situations where participation in one treatment condition necessarily excludes that subject from serving in a second treatment condition. For example, in a study on the effects of aspirin in preventing heart disease, one group of doctors took a small dose of aspirin while a second group of doctors took a placebo. This is an independent groups design because any one subject could not serve in both the aspirin and the placebo group at the same time.

It seems logical that all experiments could or should be conducted using independent groups designs. In fact, however, independent groups designs do have some disadvantages. The single biggest disadvantage is the potential for groups that are not equivalent on some important variables at the beginning of the study. For example, in the aspirin study, one must assume that the doctors in the two groups have basically equal levels of risk for heart disease at the inception of the study. As explained in the last chapter, the most commonly used and effective method for establishing group equivalence is random or matched random subject assignment methods. Researchers know that when random assignment methods are properly used, with a sufficient number of subjects, individual differences will average out among the groups and any differences that do exist are only caused by chance.

Simple Random Assignment

Simple random assignment is the most common method of assigning subjects to independent groups. A variety of techniques are available for assigning subjects to groups randomly. These include simply drawing names from a hat, using specially designed computer programs, and using tables of random numbers found in most statistics and research methods books. The important features are that group determination is equally likely and independent for each member of the defined population. This means that every member of the defined population has exactly the same chance of being selected to be in any group in the experiment and the selection of one subject from the population has no connection with the selection of any other subject.

Matched Random Assignment

Matched random assignment has the same goal as simple random assignment, but utilizes more involved assignment methods. This method is used when the researcher wants to ensure initial group equivalence on the dependent variable or a variable highly correlated with the dependent variable. Matched random assignment is most often used when limited numbers of subjects are available or when there is a reason to question the effectiveness of simple random assignment.

The first step is to select a variable that is related to the dependent variable. For example, if percent body fat is the dependent variable, then body weight could be the matching variable. The subjects are then measured on the matching variable (body weight) and the scores are listed from the highest to the lowest. If the subjects are to be divided into two groups, the subject with the highest score is paired (or matched) with the subject with the second highest score, and so on. Finally, the subjects in each pair are randomly assigned to the two groups.

Thus matched random assignment ensures that the groups are equivalent on some variable prior to the experiment commencing. Of course, this procedure does not ensure the groups are equal on any other variable.

REPEATED MEASURES DESIGN

Repeated measures (also termed within-subjects or within-groups design) is an experimental design in which two or more treatment conditions are administered to the same groups of subjects. Reasons for choosing a repeated measures design over an independent groups design depend on the nature of the experiment and the demands placed on the subjects. The Quadagno et al. study on the effects of the menstrual cycle on athletic performance utilized a repeated measures design. The subjects were tested on three occasions during different phases of the menstrual cycle for strength and swimming speed (see Table 6.2). The researchers could have used an independent groups design and recruited separate groups of women for each of the three tests. In this study however, a repeated measures design had definite advantages over an independent groups design.

TABLE 6.2	Study on the Effects of Menstrual Cycle on Athletic Performance: A Repeated Measures Design			
Subjects	**Independent variable**	**Level 1**	**Level 2**	**Level 3**
12 recreational weight lifters and 15 university swim team members	Cycle phase	3 to 5 days prior to menses	Days 1 through 3 of menses	10 to 12 days after menses onset
	Dependent variables			
	Strength and swim speed	First tests	Second tests	Third tests

The first advantage is that fewer subjects are needed than with independent groups. Quadagno et al. used 12 subjects in the strength portion of the experiment. Those same 12 women were tested during each of the three phases of the menstrual cycle. If the researchers wanted to maintain 12 measurements in each condition, but used independent groups with 12 women in each group, 36 subjects would have been needed (3 conditions × 12 subjects = 36 subjects). A second advantage of repeated measures designs is that it is more sensitive than an independent groups design to dependent variable differences between treatment groups. Because the same subjects serve in all treatment conditions, they are identical in every other respect (since they are the same subjects). This reduces between-subjects variability and improves the chances of detecting any effects caused by the independent variable. In later chapters this increased sensitivity to finding differences; if they exist, will be called statistical power. It is important to use a "powerful" research design when it is appropriate to the hypotheses under investigation.

Repeated measures designs also have disadvantages that researchers consider when designing an experiment. The main drawback is the chance of **carry-over effects** from one treatment condition to another. Carry-over effects are present when exposure to a previous treatment or condition interferes with a subject's behavior in a subsequent treatment. For example, the women in the Quadango et al. study could have experienced a "training effect" as a result of repeated strength and swimming tests. If, for example, strength was found to be the greatest in the postmenstrual cycle, the difference could be caused by the testing and training effect achieved during the premenstrual and menstrual tests, or as a result of some effect of the menstrual cycle on strength, or both. This possibility must be considered and controlled if it presents a problem.

Carry-Over Effects

If subjects are tested on several occasions, the previous treatment conditions or testing sessions may affect their behavior in ways more closely linked to the repeated testing than to the treatment itself. The possible effects of repeated testing are divided into several categories.

Order Effects

Order effects occur when the result of one treatment condition is still present when the second treatment is administered. There are two categories of order effects, practice effects and fatigue effects. A *practice effect* results in an improved performance on the second of two measures as a result of becoming "test wise" and learning how to take the test rather than to improvement in the characteristic resulting from exposure to the treatment itself. *Fatigue effects* are the opposite of practice effects, and are present when performance deteriorates as a consequence of repeated measurements. Fatigue effects have several sources, including actual physical fatigue, boredom, or loss of interest on the part of the subject. Order effects can be mitigated by counterbalancing.

Counterbalancing

Controlling for order effects in a repeated measures design is accomplished primarily by counterbalancing the order in which treatments are presented. **Counterbalancing** neutralizes the potential order effects in a repeated measures design by exposing the subjects to different treatment orders or testing conditions either systematically or randomly. For example, in the Quadango et al. study, for the test of swimming speed, half of the subjects completed the 100 meter swim, followed by the 200 meter swim. The other half of the subjects swam the two distances in the opposite order.

With *complete counterbalancing*, all possible orders of presentation are included in the design of the study. However, complete counterbalancing quickly becomes complicated when the number of treatment conditions increases beyond three or four. In general, there are $k!$ possible treatment orders where k is the number of treatment conditions (! exclamation point is the notation for the factorial operation). In a study with two treatment conditions there are two possible treatment or testing orders ($2! = 2 \times 1 = 2$). If a third condition is added the number of possible orders grows to six ($3! = 3 \times 2 \times 1 = 6$). If there are five treatment conditions, the

TABLE 6.3 Complete Counterbalancing of Orders for Three Treatment Conditions ($k = 3$)	
Order number	Treatment sequence
1	A-B-C
2	A-C-B
3	B-A-C
4	B-C-A
5	C-A-B
6	C-B-A

number of possible orders is 120 ($5! = 5 \times 4 \times 3 \times 2 \times 1 = 120$). For such a study as found in Table 6.3, the number of subjects required would be a multiple of six. For example, if 30 subjects were involved, by random procedures five subjects would be assigned to each of the six possible treatment sequences.

LATIN SQUARES

A **Latin Square** is a matrix of k rows and columns that contains a subset of all possible treatment orders. A Latin Square is used to control for order effects without the need for complete counterbalancing. As with complete counterbalancing, a Latin Square designates the treatment order for a given set of subjects. The use of a Latin Square for a repeated measures design having 4 levels of an independent variable is illustrated in Table 6.4. With 12 subjects, each would be randomly assigned to one of the four treatment sequences with three subjects in each sequence. The key feature of a Latin Square is that each treatment condition (1, 2, 3, and 4) appears only once at each position in the matrix. For example, the subjects in order A, would experience treatments 1, 2, 3, and 4 in that order. Subjects in order B would experience the same treatments, but in a 2, 3, 1, and 4 order. In addition, each treatment follows each of the other treatments only once, and each treatment precedes each of the other treatments only once. In this way, potential order effects are controlled and the counterbalancing

TABLE 6.4	Latin Square Counterbalance for an Independent Variable with Four Levels (1, 2, 3, and 4)			
Orders	**Treatment sequence**			
A	1	2	3	4
B	2	3	1	4
C	3	4	2	1
D	4	1	3	2

is more concise than setting up all possible orders of treatment administrations. Notice that only four of the possible 24 (4! = 4 × 3 × 2 × 1 = 24) treatment sequences occur in this particular Latin Square.

Demand Characteristics

Another problem with repeated measures designs is that subjects are exposed to all treatment conditions and thus may gain unintended insight into the nature of the experiment. If subjects figure out the true nature of the experiment, they may behave differently than they would if they were experimentally naive. This chance of subjects altering their behavior as a result of experimental knowledge is referred to as **demand characteristics**.

Researchers are concerned with carry-over effects and demand characteristics because both are potential threats to the validity of a study. Both of these issues impact internal validity, and demand characteristics also affect external validity. Repeated measures designs with greater than two levels of the repeated factor have an additional statistical assumption (for example, sphericity) which should be acknowledged and addressed by the researcher. Sphericity has to do with an assumption underlying repeated measures designs and specifically requires that the variance of the differences for all pairs of repeated measures be equal.

Nonetheless, repeated measures designs are very common and very effective designs when these potential threats are acknowledged and controlled.

REPEATED MEASURES AND LEARNING EXPERIMENTS

Repeated measures designs are used in many learning experiments and thus are very common in motor learning and motor control research. Many motor learning studies are designed to investigate factors that influence skills acquisition and movement. Subjects commonly practice a skill or skills for a certain number of trials. The practice trials are divided into blocks to measure the rate of skills acquisition. These blocks of trials are not counterbalanced. All subjects practice block 1 first, block 2 second, and so on.

WELL-DESIGNED EXPERIMENTS

Recall that experimental design is the action plan for how the research will be conducted. Well-designed experiments can be very simple: one independent variable at two levels, one dependent variable, and two groups of subjects—a control group and a treatment group (and as many control variables as necessary). Well-designed experiments can also be very complex: two or more independent variables each at two or more levels, several dependent variables, and several groups of subjects—a control group and the different treatment groups (and as many control variables as necessary).

The amount of information generated in a study is limited by the experimental design. Complex experiments can yield more information than simple experiments, but simple experiments are easier to manage, complete, and interpret. Even though the complexity of experiments varies widely, well-designed experiments have two basic features in common: (1) random subject selection and/or assignment, and (2) a control group. We will now examine some research designs you may encounter in the literature and explain the advantages and disadvantages of each.

INDEPENDENT RANDOM GROUPS POSTTEST-ONLY DESIGN

The independent random groups posttest-only design is an uncomplicated yet effective design that forms the basis for more complex designs that will be described later. The design

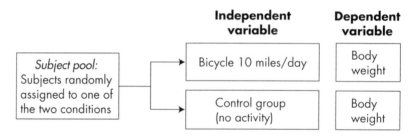

FIGURE 6.2 Independent random groups posttest-only design.

achieves control over extraneous variables by setting control variables and by assigning subjects to groups randomly.

The first step is to randomly select a group of subjects from the defined population and assign them randomly to the treatment condition or to the control group. Of course additional levels of the independent variable are possible. For example, in Figure 6.2 it would be possible to have other distances (for example, 15 miles/day) or other types of activities (for example, swimming). Nevertheless, the subjects would be randomly assigned to however many groups are involved. The goal is to achieve groups that are equivalent on relevant variables at the onset of the experiment. Of course, no groups of subjects are ever *exactly* equal, but random assignment methods average subject characteristics among groups so that any actual differences will be minor and caused only by chance. This assumption is particularly true if the number of subjects is relatively large and if random assignment procedures are properly executed.

Next, the subjects experience the treatment condition(s) (or in the case of the control group, no treatment). Finally, the dependent variable is measured and the results for groups are compared. If the groups were equivalent at the onset, and extraneous variables were controlled, any differences in the dependent variable can be attributed to the effect of the independent variable.

INDEPENDENT RANDOM GROUPS PRETEST-POSTTEST DESIGN

Initial group equivalence is assumed in posttest designs because of the random subject assignment methods. This assumption is particularly true when "large" numbers of subjects are involved. In some cases, however, the number of subjects is limited. In other cases, the researcher wants to measure changes over the course of the experiment in each treatment group. In these cases, a pretest is added to the design of the experiment. This design makes it possible to ascertain initial group equivalence or to detect any changes that may occur during the experiment. Each design has some advantages and disadvantages. A disadvantage in this design is the extra time required to make pretest measurements. In addition, there is the chance that subjects will become sensitized to the nature of the experiment, which could affect their behavior during the posttest. As explained in the previous chapter, pretesting also introduces external validity problems. The pretest-posttest design is the simplest repeated measured design.

Let's see what your bicycling experiment would look like if you used a pretest-posttest design (Figure 6.3). In this case the independent variable, bicycling, has two levels: a control group that does not exercise beyond normal daily levels, and the bicycling group. An independent groups design would be best since the same subjects could not realistically serve in both the control group and the bicycling group. In this experiment, it would make sense to weigh the subjects before starting the cycling program and then, of course, weigh them at the conclusion of the program. The pretest would provide group equivalence information prior to the bicycling program; the posttest would allow calculation of the changes in body weight among the groups following the program.

Both the posttest-only and the pretest-posttest designs may appear rather simple, but when used well, they are effective experimental designs. Many more complex experiments

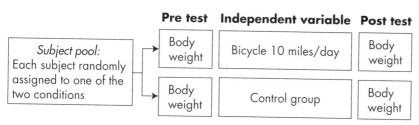

FIGURE 6.3 Bicycling experiment.

just extend the basic elements of these designs by adding additional independent and dependent variables.

POORLY DESIGNED EXPERIMENTS

Well-designed experiments have as a minimum an independent variable with at least two levels—a dependent variable, and a control group. When any of these elements is missing, then the design of the experiment is not strong. Recall the original bicycling program proposed in the previous chapter. Your plan was to cycle 10 miles per day at an average intensity of 40% of maximum heart rate, three days a week, for 6 weeks. You planned to weigh yourself on the first day, complete the program, and then weigh yourself at the end of the sixth week. The question was, will your professor detect any flaws in your experiment? The answer is yes, your professor probably will find a few flaws.

Your original design would be classified as a *one-group pretest-posttest design*, and it lacks an important element—a comparison or control group. Your hypothesis was, all other factors being equal, that a bicycling program should result in a loss in body weight. Using the one-group (actually, one subject) pretest-posttest design, you weighed yourself at the start of the experiment, completed the bicycling program, and weighed yourself at the conclusion. The question is, can any changes in body weight be attributed solely to the effects of the bicycling program? Without a control group it is not possible to claim that the treatment (bicycle program) was responsible for any body weight loss. Figure 6.4 illustrates the pretest-posttest design.

QUASI-EXPERIMENTAL DESIGNS

Technically, to qualify as an experimental design, random assignment of the subjects to treatment groups must occur.

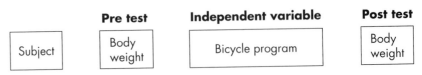

FIGURE 6.4 One-group pretest-posttest design.

Although random assignment does not guarantee that treatment groups are absolutely equal on all variables of interest, it is the best method available to approximate this condition. Differences that do exist can only be attributed to chance, and statistical techniques can account for chance.

When planning an experiment it is quite simple to indicate that random assignment of subjects will occur. It is another matter to actually accomplish this objective. For example, subjects may object to being in the control group because they don't get the "neat stuff" the treatment group does.

Another potential problem is the financial or time cost of the treatment and measurements required (for example, treadmill assessment of VO2max) may severely limit the size of the possible sample. Even with random assignment, the equivalence of treatment groups becomes less probable with a very small sample.

A third concern can be in actually selecting from the population the sample to be used in the study. The procedures to do this (drawing names from a hat, using random number generators, etc.) all assume it is possible to identify and locate every individual in the population. History is replete with descriptions of experiments that went bad because the original selection of subjects was biased in some way. An example is randomly selecting subjects from a phone book and forgetting the fact that not all individuals have a phone or a listed number.

All these issues are troublesome and researchers must address them for experiments to be valid. There are times, however, when random assignment of subjects is not possible and yet experiments are still conducted.

Quasi-experimental designs usually result when practical reasons prevent the possibility of random assignment to treatment groups. A common example of this situation is the use of intact groups. This might occur when a group of subjects who are already together for some reason (for example, they are enrolled in a particular section of a course) is exposed to one level of the independent variable and another group (for example, a different section of the course) is exposed to another level. The major problem that arises with quasi-experimental designs is in the area of internal validity. If differences are found between the treatments, the investigator cannot be certain whether the differences are caused by the treatments or some initial differences present in the intact groups.

Attempts to "correct" for the inability to randomly assign subjects to groups (for example, pretesting or using statistical procedures such as Analysis of Covariance) help but they introduce new concerns with external validity and interpretation of results. The random assignment of subjects to treatment groups is by far the best procedure to use in an experimental design. It should only be abandoned when for practical reasons it is not possible.

SUMMARY

When reading a research report, try to identify the design of the experiment and the justification for the selection of a particular design. In some reports you may find that the design is clearly described; in other reports it may be more difficult to determine the nature of the design. As you gain experience and knowledge, identifying designs will become easier for you.

In this chapter we introduced the basics of experimental design. When designing an experiment, an important question the researcher has to consider is how to best use the subjects in the study. Three of the basic methods are independent groups design, repeated measures design, and mixed group design. Each design has advantages and disadvantages including factors such as the total number of subjects needed, the effects of repeated measurements on the subjects, and the demands placed on the subjects' time.

In this chapter, we have examined some independent groups and repeated measures designs. In the next chapter, some examples of mixed group designs will be introduced. In some situations the researcher is not able to use a true experimental design and may have to rely on a quasi-experimental design instead. This is particularly true when intact subject assignment procedures are used.

EXERCISES

1 What is the primary difference between an independent groups design and a repeated measures design?

2 Suppose you conducted an experiment on three types of weight training (free weights, isokinetic machines, isotonic machines) on strength gains. Why would an independent groups design be a better choice than a repeated measures design? Why?

3 If you investigated taste preferences for three brands of power bars, why would a repeated measures design be a good choice? Why?

4 If you used a repeated measures design in the power bar example, why would it be important to counterbalance the order of the samples? Explain.

Complex Experimental Designs

LEARNING GOALS

After reading this chapter you will be able to:

1 Describe the two main methods of increasing the complexity of an experiment.

2 Explain the advantages and disadvantages of an experiment with two or more independent variables.

3 Understand how to interpret the shorthand description of an experimental design (for example, $2 \times 2 \times 2$).

4 Define and explain the terms *main effects* and *interaction*.

5 Discuss the importance of interaction information.

6 Explain how a graph can show the presence of an interaction between two variables.

7 Describe the difference between a manipulated independent variable and a categorical independent variable.

TERMS

Factorial design
Main effect
Interaction
Categorical variable

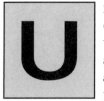ntil now we have only discussed simple experimental designs with one independent variable at two levels and one dependent variable. You will find that most research in sport and exercise sciences is actually more complex than this. Although high quality studies are conducted with simple designs, many questions are better answered with more complex designs. The labeling of experimental designs as "simple" or "complex" is largely arbitrary—no rating system exists to classify design complexity. For our purposes we will consider designs involving one independent variable with two levels as simple designs. As levels are added to the first independent variable, or as additional independent variables are added to the design, complexity increases. Following this progression, the next most complicated design would have one independent variable with three levels.

INCREASING THE NUMBER OF LEVELS OF THE INDEPENDENT VARIABLE

The main shortcoming of simple designs with one independent variable at two levels is that only simple linear relationships can be shown. By adding a third or fourth level to the independent variable, more complex relationships, if they exist, can be examined. The figure on p. 167 shows a simple design with the levels being a control group and a 10-mile-per-day bicycling group. The 10-mile bicycling group showed an average 5-pound loss of body weight, and on average the members of the control group gained a couple of pounds (see Figure 7.1).

You can argue, based on these results, that bicycling affects body weight. An example of one thing these results cannot tell us is what would happen if the subjects rode distances other than 10 miles each day. Suppose the subjects rode 15 or 20 miles daily. Would they lose weight at the same rate as the 10-mile group? Would weight loss level out? With the simple design there is no way to answer these more complex questions.

The easiest way to increase the information yield from an experiment is to increase the number of levels of the independent variable. In the bicycling experiment, a third level of the independent variable could be added, say a

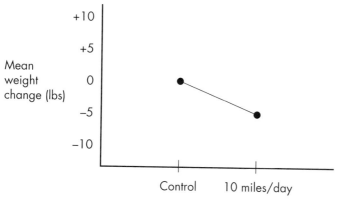

FIGURE 7.1 Simple design with one independent variable.

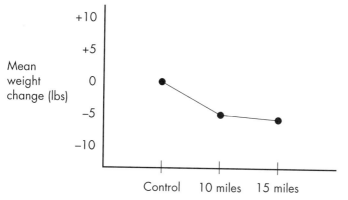

FIGURE 7.2 Hypothetical findings from a three level design.

15-mile-per-day group, without increasing the complexity of the design.

Figure 7.2 shows a hypothetical finding from a three level design. In this case, the riders in the 15-mile group lost about the same amount of weight as did the riders in the 10-mile group. This finding changes our understanding of the effects of bicycling on body weight and leads to some new questions. Although there was no appreciable increase in the loss of scale weight in the 15-mile group, other changes may have occurred. Perhaps the 15-mile group lost more body fat, but also gained more muscle mass than the 10-mile group.

This speculation could lead to a hypothesis to be tested through further experimentation. We might also have decided to go the other way. Is it necessary to ride 10-miles per day to achieve this weight loss? Perhaps a 5-mile-per-day group could be examined. This is a common occurrence in research—attempting to answer one relatively simple question often results in more questions than answers.

EXPERIMENTS WITH TWO OR MORE INDEPENDENT VARIABLES: FACTORIAL DESIGNS

A second and more important way to increase the complexity of an experiment is to include additional independent variables in the design. Because the words "factor" and "independent variable" are synonymous, an experiment that has two or more independent variables often is said to have a **factorial design**. The goal of factorial designs is to explore how two or more independent variables act alone and in concert.

Factorial designs have several advantages over experiments with only one independent variable. Factorial designs reflect real life conditions better than experiments with one independent variable. Almost always more than a single factor affects behavior. Factorial experiments are also more efficient than single factor experiments. It is less time consuming and more efficient to conduct one experiment with two independent variables than it is to conduct two separate experiments with one independent variable in each. Perhaps the best reason for using factorial designs is the availability of information termed interaction. This has to do with how independent variables combine to affect the dependent variable. Interaction information is only available in designs with two or more independent variables.

The simplest factorial design would consist of one dependent variable and two independent variables, each with two levels. This would be referred to as a 2 × 2 (two by two) design. A 2 × 2 design has four treatment *conditions*. That is, there are four combinations of the levels of the independent variables. A 3 × 3 design has two independent variables, each with three levels, with a total of nine treatment conditions. Any factorial design can be described using this general format:

[Number of levels of first independent variable] ×
[Number of levels of second independent variable] × . . .
[Number of levels of nth independent variable]

To find the total number of treatment conditions, you multiply the number of levels of each independent variable: $2 \times 2 = 4$ conditions; $2 \times 2 \times 3 = 12$ conditions.

FACTORIAL DESIGNS

Suppose your exercise physiology professor assigns an in-class experiment. This assignment is to conduct experiments on the effects of exercise on the aging process. The basic question your professor wants you to investigate is how does exercise affect age-related variables? Rather than using human subjects, the class is given access to the animal laboratory and the experiments will be conducted using lab rats as subjects. Each student is given 12 rats and the rest of the experiment is left up to you.

An Experiment with the Age Factor Alone

Based on feedback from your professor on the bicycling experiment, you realize that each independent variable needs at least two levels, subjects must be randomly assigned to groups, and as many extraneous factors as possible need to be controlled. The independent variables are age and exercise intensity, the dependent variable is exercising time to exhaustion. You decide to investigate the effects of each independent variable separately and begin with the independent variable *age*. You divided the rats into two age groups: young (12 to 14 months), and old (48 to 50 months).

Independent Variable Age

Young	Old

The rats are identical in all other respects: they all come from the same type of laboratory rats, their diets are the same, their living environments are the same, and so on.

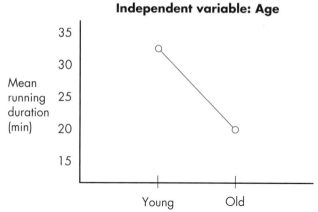

FIGURE 7.3 Results of the hypothetical experiment.

The treatment condition is the exercise training program. All the rats run on a treadmill 3 times each day at 50% of maximum capacity, for 15 minutes each session, for a duration of 6 weeks. The dependent variable is the total time the rats can run on the treadmill until exhaustion (defined as when they stop running) at the conclusion of the training program. Figure 7.3 shows the results for this hypothetical experiment. Following the training program, which was identical for both groups, the young rats were able to run for an average of about 34 minutes while the old rats were able to run for about 20 minutes. Therefore, with the same amount and type of training, younger rats are more resistant to fatigue than older rats.

An Experiment with the Exercise Intensity Factor Alone

In the second experiment the independent variable is exercise intensity. One group of rats is trained at 25% of maximum capacity (low), while

Independent Variable Exercise Intensity

Low	High

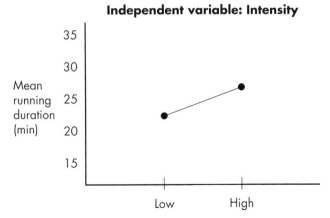

FIGURE 7.4   Results of the second hypothetical experiment.

the second group is trained at 75% of maximum capacity (high). In this experiment, the rats are randomly assigned to one of the two exercise intensity conditions irrespective of age. All other control variables remain the same. Figure 7.4 shows that following the training program, the rats that trained at low intensity (25% of maximum) were able to run for a mean of about 23 minutes while the rats that trained at high intensity (75% of maximum) were able to run for about 27 minutes.

You now have two sets of findings: The first experiment showed that as age increased, exercise duration capacity decreased. In the second experiment, increases in exercise intensity led to greater exercise duration capacity. One problem with the second experiment is that the professor asked you to study the relationship between age and exercise and this experiment did not address the age issue. The problem with the first experiment was that it was limited to just the age factor, and didn't address the exercise intensity issue. Can you simultaneously investigate both age and the exercise intensity? The answer is to conduct one experiment with two independent variables—a factorial design.

An Experiment with the Age and Exercise Intensity Factors Combined

Instead of researching the effects of training intensity and age on exercise duration in separate experiments, it is possible to study both factors is a single experiment. The combined form of the experiment is described as a 2 × 2 factorial design. There are two independent variables (age and exercise intensity) each having two levels (young and old; low and high). With a 2 × 2 factorial design there are four separate treatment conditions or cells: (1) low intensity with young rats, (2) low intensity with old rats, (3) high intensity with young rats, and (4) high intensity with old rats.

In our hypothetical experiment, each student is given 12 rats, so you can randomly assign three old and three young rats to each exercise intensity. Following the assignment of the rats to treatment conditions, the experiment is run, and the data are analyzed. Let's assume that the same results were obtained in the factorial experiment that were obtained in the two separate experiments. Figure 7.5 shows a breakdown of the factors and a graph of the results. The question now is:

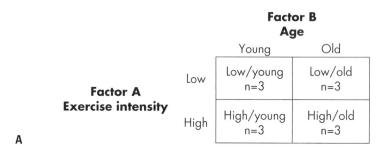

A

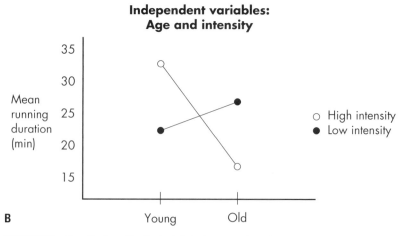

B

FIGURE 7.5 Results from the factorial design experiment.

How do you answer when your professor asks you about the effects of exercise on the aging process?

INTERPRETING FACTORIAL DESIGNS

Factorial designs yield two types of information. The first concerns the individual contributions of the independent variables to the results of the experiment and these are called **main effects.** Main effects are defined as the differences among the treatment conditions of a factorial design that are attributed to a single factor. In our hypothetical experiment, there are results for two main effects: (1) exercise intensity, and (2) age. The second type of information is the **interaction** between the independent variables. Interaction is defined as the *combined* effect of two or more independent variables on the dependent variable. Thus our 2×2 factorial design will yield three results: (1) the main effect for exercise intensity, (2) the main effect for age, and (3) the intensity by age interaction.

An important advantage of factorial designs over a series of separate experiments is the ability to obtain interaction between variables information. Information on interactions is not available from separate simple experiments. Interactions are very important because most behaviors are usually influenced by more than one factor. In this particular experiment, the interaction test answers the question: are the effects of intensity of training constant across age groups?

Although the concept of interaction can be confusing at first, we are affected by interactions on a daily basis. Suppose, for example, that you are at school. It's just about noon, and you are thinking about whether or not to have lunch. A wide range of factors enter into the final decision: how hungry are you, how much money you have, how much time you have before your next class, do you need to spend some time at the library, is there anyone else to have lunch with, and so on. If you are hungry (*yes*—no), you have some money (*yes*—no), and you have some time (*yes*—no), you will probably choose to eat lunch (dependent variable). If you are hungry (*yes*—no), but have no money (yes—*no*), and no time (yes—*no*), you would probably choose not to eat lunch. Hunger, money, and time are each factors, and the combined effect of all of the three contributes to your lunch decision.

Interaction is defined as the combined effect of two or more factors on the dependent variable. When an interaction effect is present, the effect that one independent variable has on the dependent variable depends on the level of the second independent variable. Interaction essentially tests whether the effect of one independent variable is constant across the levels of another independent variable.

Based on the results in Figure 7.5, what do we know about the effects of exercise intensity and age on exercise duration? The answer is, "It depends," because in this experiment we found an interaction to be present. The young rats were able to run for a longer duration when trained under high intensity conditions, but the old rats ran longer with low intensity training. To answer the question, you must first ask a question, "How old are the subjects?" If they are young, high intensity works best and if they are old, low intensity works best.

Outcomes of 2 × 2 Factorial Designs When Interactions Are Not Present

A 2 × 2 factorial design has two independent variables, each with two levels. There are several possible results with this design: (1) there may or may not be an interaction (intensity by age), (2) there may or may not be a main effect for the first independent variable (intensity), and (3) there may or may not be a main effect for the second independent variable (age). The actual decision as to whether or not any of these effects really exist and are not just the result of chance differences between groups is made through the use of a statistical technique known as the Analysis of Variance (ANOVA). If ANOVA determines the results are not due to chance, the effects are said to be statistically significant. These statistical procedures will be described in Chapter 11.

Graphs are a good way to evaluate the results from factorial designs. The four graphs in Figure 7.6 illustrate some possible outcomes of our 2 × 2 factorial design when *no* interaction is present. The dependent variable, exercise duration, is scaled on the vertical axis (y-axis). In Graph A there is no main effect for either intensity or age on exercise duration.

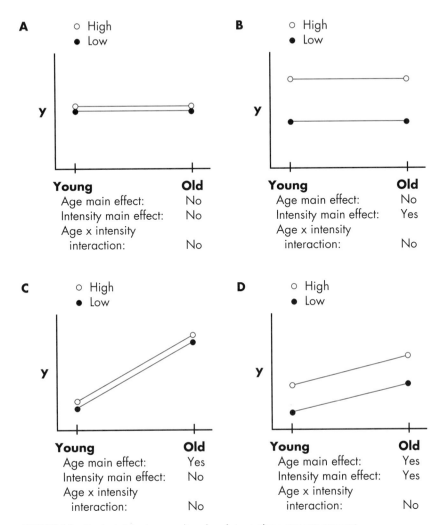

FIGURE 7.6 Factorial design results when interactions are not present.

Compare Graph A with Graph D where there was a main effect for both intensity and age.

Notice that in these four graphs, the lines are *parallel,* indicating *no interaction.* When no interaction is present, the independent variables act independently of one another. That is, exercise intensity affects exercise duration, and age affects exercise duration, but these two factors do not influence each other (opposite from the conclusion in our hypothetical experiment).

Outcomes of 2 × 2 Factorial Designs When Interactions Are Present

Compare the graphs in Figure 7.6 with those in Figure 7.7. The most obvious difference is that the lines in Figure 7.7 are *not parallel* indicating that an *interaction is present.* In each case, the effect of intensity on exercise duration depends on the age of the subjects (and vice versa).

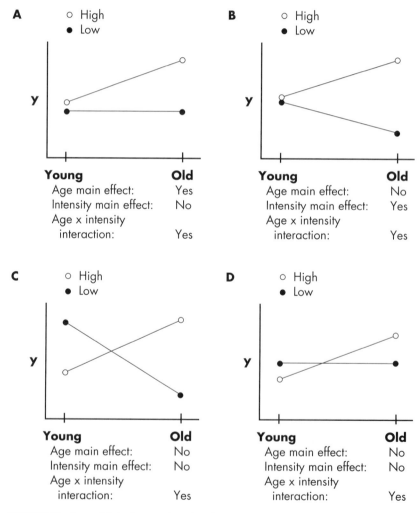

Young		**Old**
Age main effect:		Yes
Intensity main effect:		No
Age x intensity interaction:		Yes

Young		**Old**
Age main effect:		No
Intensity main effect:		Yes
Age x intensity interaction:		Yes

Young		**Old**
Age main effect:		No
Intensity main effect:		No
Age x intensity interaction:		Yes

Young		**Old**
Age main effect:		No
Intensity main effect:		No
Age x intensity interaction:		Yes

FIGURE 7.7 Factorial design results when interactions are present.

EVALUATING THE RESULTS OF FACTORIAL DESIGNS

In a 2×2 factorial design, results for three effects are evaluated: the two main effects, and the interaction. Researchers make decisions on these three effects following a logical sequence. The first result evaluated from a factorial design is the interaction. The interaction result receives priority because the next step of the evaluation depends on this result. If an interaction is present, the researcher analyzes and interprets the results with respect to the *combined effects* of the two independent variables. If no interaction is found, the results of the two independent variables are evaluated as if two separate single factor experiments were conducted. Evaluation of the interaction result is crucial because it reveals if the two variables are connected to one another or if they are independent of one another with respect to their impact on the dependent variable.

FURTHER FACTORIAL DESIGNS

A 2×2 is the simplest factorial design; it has two independent variables each with two levels resulting in four treatment conditions. By adding one more level to one of the independent variables, the design becomes a 2×3 and thus results in six separate conditions. Again, let's return to our hypothetical experiment with the rats. Recall that when appropriate, additional information can be gained by setting the independent variables at more than two levels. Rather than a 2×2 design, a 3×3 design as in Figure 7.8 may be used without increasing the complexity of the experiment beyond a manageable scope. As you can see, this design has nine conditions or cells that represent each combination of the two independent variables.

    The only other difference between this design and the original 2×2 is the greater number of subjects needed. With three subjects in each condition, the 2×2 design needs 12 subjects. A 3×3 needs 27 subjects. The total number of effects tested remains the same at three: (1) the exercise intensity by age interaction, (2) the main effect of exercise intensity, and (3) the main effect of age.

		Factor B Age	
	Young	Middle-aged	Old
Low	Low/Young	Low/middle-aged	Low/old
Moderate	Moderate/young	Moderate/middle-aged	Moderate/old
High	High/young	High/middle-aged	High/old

Factor A Exercise intensity — rows: Low, Moderate, High

FIGURE 7.8 A 3 × 3 design.

An experimental design becomes more complex when adding independent variables. For example, in the exercise duration experiment we could add a third independent variable such as gender (male vs. female), or diet (high fat vs. low fat), or both. Complex designs with three or more independent variables allow researchers to examine the effects of many variables which can lead to the understanding of the complex interplay of the many variables that influence behavior. The disadvantages of complex designs are primarily twofold: first, as independent variables are added to the experiment, the complexity of managing the experiment increases rapidly, and second, interpreting the results of complex designs (particularly significant interactions) can be very difficult.

For example, the simplest factorial design with three independent variables is a 2 × 2 × 2 design with one dependent variable and three independent variables, each with two levels. Theoretically, there is no limit to the number of independent variables in a factorial design, and also there is no limit on the number of levels for each independent variable. In practice, the more complex the design, the more difficult it is to conduct the experiment and the more difficult it is to interpret the results. As we saw in the exercise duration experiment, if we add levels or independent variables to a design, it usually increases the number of subjects and the amount of testing and measuring of subjects. Conducting complex experiments requires more time and cost than one or two factor experiments. A three-factor design with two levels for each factor has nine conditions, a four-factor design also with two levels for each factor has 16 separate conditions.

In addition to larger numbers of treatment conditions with complex designs, as the number of independent variables increases, the number of effects also increases rapidly. If the three independent variables in a $2 \times 2 \times 2$ design are labeled A, B, and C, then the results of this design will include one three-way interaction (A × B × C), three two-way interactions (A × B, A × C, and B × C), and three main effects (A, B, and C) for a total of seven separate effects. A four factor experiment will have 15 effects including one four-way interaction, four three-way interactions, six two-way interactions, and four main effects! Adding to the complexity, subjects can be exposed to treatments in a wide variety of ways ranging from independent groups (each treatment combination is administered to a unique group of subjects), repeated measures (the same subjects are exposed to various levels of one independent variable and/or to various levels of different independent variables), and mixed groups designs (some independent groups and some repeated measures groups). We will discuss this further later in this chapter. In spite of the complexities of designs with three, four, or even more independent variables, you will find many examples of sport and exercise sciences research utilizing complex designs.

Recall the Shank and Haywood (1989) study on baseball players presented in Chapter 5. In that experiment skill level, pitch delivery and pitch type were independent variables. Skill level was an independent groups factor because different individuals appeared in the levels of this variable, but pitch delivery and pitch type were repeated measures because the same subjects were assessed for each level of these two variables.

MULTIPLE DEPENDENT VARIABLES—
THE NEXT COMPLEXITY

So far we have presented information regarding increasing the complexity of a design by changing the number of levels for the independent variable(s) or the number of independent variables, or both. One might also consider increasing the number of dependent variables to be analyzed. As alluded to earlier, the use of a single variable is not really very representative of the real world. Independent variables are likely to have effects on more than a single outcome or dependent variable. Therefore, the researcher might be interested in using more than than one dependent variable in an experiment. The proper statistical procedure when one has multiple dependent variables is to conduct a Multivariate Analysis of Variance (MANOVA). All the previous discussions regarding factorial designs hold true with MANOVA analysis. The main difference is that there are multiple outcomes that must be considered. In a MANOVA each subject will have a score for each dependent variable (MANOVA is described in Chapter 11).

An important consideration in MANOVA is to measure different variables that are related in some way. The MANOVA is then used to determine whether or not significant differences exist between groups or this cluster of related dependent variables.

SUBJECT ASSIGNMENT AND FACTORIAL DESIGNS
Independent Groups Design

In an independent groups factorial design, separate groups of subjects are assigned to each condition of the experiment. Design A in Figure 7.9 illustrates an independent groups factorial design. The subjects in each cell are different from the subjects in every other cell. If a researcher determines that 10 subjects are necessary for each condition, then a total of 40 subjects is needed (4 cells × 10 subjects = 40 subjects).

Repeated Measures Design

In a repeated measures design, the same subjects participate in more than one of the treatment conditions. Design B in Figure 7.9 shows a 2 × 2 factorial design with repeated measures in all four cells. Recall that a repeated measures design needs fewer subjects than an independent groups design. Based on 10 subjects per cell, the independent groups design needs 40 subjects, while the repeated measures design only needs 10 subjects. Also remember, counterbalancing is used with

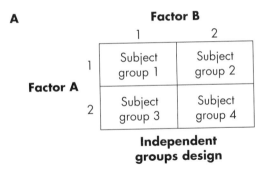

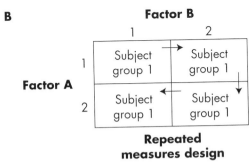

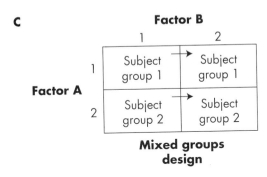

FIGURE 7.9 **A,** Independent groups design. **B,** Repeated measures design. **C,** Mixed groups design.

repeated measures design to control order effects. The arrows (design B) are only meant to illustrate that the same subjects experience all four treatment conditions; in reality, the order of receiving the treatments would be counterbalanced among subjects.

Mixed Design

Design C in Figure 7.9 depicts a mixed design factorial experiment. This design is a hybrid of the independent groups and repeated measures designs. The subjects in condition A_1 would experience both B_1 and B_2. A separate group of subjects would be assigned to condition A_2 and would experience both B_1 and B_2. The two separate groups in the A_1 and A_2 conditions are the independent groups element of the design. For example, Factor A might be gender. The design also has a repeated measures element because each A group experiences both levels of the B factor. As with the repeated measures design, counterbalancing is necessary for the repeated measures treatments. Using the 10 subjects in each treatment condition criteria, this mixed design would require 20 subjects.

The decision to use independent groups or repeated measures (or some combination) is usually dependent on what the levels of the independent variables are. For example, if the independent variable is gender and the two levels are male and female, this factor will obviously require independent groups. Also, if the independent variable is methods of teaching skiing and the two levels are short ski and long ski, independent groups would be required because after learning to ski using one method, a subject would no longer be a novice in being exposed to the second method.

On the other hand, suppose a number of subjects have been trained to perform a level positioning task for a motor behavior experiment. It might be possible to assess the effect of different sets of instructions, or different amounts of feedback or different environmental conditions (all independent variables) with the same subjects exposed to all the possible levels of these factors.

In general, if subjects are not compromised in any way by being exposed to more than one level of an independent variable, repeated measures designs offer increased power (the ability to detect statistically significant differences if they exist). Repeated measures designs also require fewer numbers of subjects than an equivalent independent groups design.

FACTORIAL DESIGNS WITH MANIPULATED AND CATEGORICAL VARIABLES

Experiments involving a factorial design often combine the use of manipulated and categorical independent variables. **Categorical variables** include factors such as gender, age, class standing, or any other distinctive subject characteristic.

Suppose, for example, we wanted to compare the benefits of strength training programs using isokinetic versus isotonic equipment in men and women. The first independent variable, training method (isokinetic and isotonic) is a manipulated variable because we select the levels to be used, and the second independent variable, gender (men and women), is a categorical variable (and not manipulated in the standard sense). Figure 7.10 shows an independent groups design (a unique set of subjects in each cell) for this study. The mode of strength training can be manipulated, but the gender of the subjects cannot. The categorical independent variable, gender, is formed by selecting two groups based on their gender, then these subjects are randomly assigned to one of the two strength training groups. Experiments employing this type of design are very common in sport and exercise sciences. Subject variables such as gender, age, athletes versus nonathletes, experts versus novices, and others serve as the basis for many studies in exercise physiology, motor learning, and/or sport psychology.

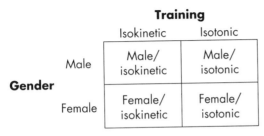

FIGURE 7.10   A factorial design with manipulated and categorical independent variables.

UNDERSTANDING EXPERIMENTS

As a student new to the world of research reports, decipher-
ing the details of an experiment can be difficult. One method
of developing the knowledge necessary to interpret experiments is to read some research reports systematically and
write out the details of the design. Use the following box as a
guide. The items listed in the box below will usually be
explained in the Methods section of a research report.

Identifying the independent variables and the dependent variables is usually not too difficult. You will probably
have to examine the procedures section carefully to identify
all of the control variables. Investigators do not always explicitly list the control variables. They assume that you should be
able to determine what the control variables are, based on
their descriptions of the study. Look for factors that could be

---

Checklist to Help Identify the Experimental Design

Identify the independent variables

1 Name the independent variables that were *manipulated.*
2 Determine the number of levels of each independent variable.
3 Name the independent variables that were manipulated and the
   independent variables that were categorical.
4 Find the total number of treatment conditions.
5 Write the operational definition for each independent variable.

Identify the dependent variables

1 Name the variables that were *measured.*
2 Find out how each dependent variable was measured.
3 Write the operational definition for each dependent variable.

Identify the control variables

1 Name the variables that were held *constant.*

Identify the design of the experiment

1 Learn how the subjects were selected and assigned to groups.
2 Specify the design: independent groups, repeated measures, or
   combined model.

a manipulated variable, but were held constant. In some cases, the investigators state very clearly whether the design was an independent groups, repeated measures, or combined design, while in other cases they do not. If they do not, you will have to examine the procedures section carefully, looking for statements about whether measurements were taken on all the subjects only once, or if measurements were taken on the subjects two or more times each.

Identifying this kind of information in research is a skill; the more experience you gain, the easier it will become. It is not unusual for students to find the distinctions between the different types of variables and designs confusing at first. By continuing to work at it, you will garner the necessary skills and knowledge to understand research reports.

SUMMARY

Experiments can range from simple to complex. In this chapter we discussed some of the general ways that experiments become additionally complex. Two common changes are increasing the number of levels of an independent variable, and/or increasing the number of independent variables. The benefit of increasing the complexity of an experiment is the potential of gaining comprehensive findings. The cost of increasing complexity is the potential difficulty of managing a complex experiment and interpreting complicated findings.

One of the most important reasons for conducting experiments with two or more independent variables is to determine if variables interact with each other. The presence of an interaction shows that an important relationship exists between variables. The existence of complex relationships, if they exist, cannot be shown in experiments with one independent variable.

You will find that many studies in sport and exercise sciences use moderately complex experimental designs with two or three independent variables. Moderately complex experiments provide a nice compromise between simple and very complex experiments. They are efficient—they can show relationships between variables but are also manageable.

EXERCISES

1 If an experiment has two independent variables (IVs) and IV1 has 2 levels and IV2 has 3 levels:
   a How many treatment conditions are there?
   b Assume that 15 subjects are required in each treatment condition.
      1 How many subjects total are needed if an independent groups design is used?
      2 How many subjects total are needed if IV1 is treated as independent groups and IV2 is treated as repeated measures?
      3 How many subjects total are needed if both IV1 and IV2 are treated as repeated measures?
2 A study was conducted on the rate of violent acts (fighting, pushing, hitting) by elementary school children while playing sports. The researcher used three IVs: grade (second, fourth, sixth), gender (male, female), and sport (basketball, volleyball).
   a For each IV, decide whether it appears to be an independent groups IV or a repeated measures IV.
   b How many students total are needed if 10 subjects are required in each treatment condition?
   c Which of the independent variables are categorical IVs and which is a manipulated IV?
   d How many conditions are there in the study?
3 Suppose you want to investigate if caffeine is an effective ergogenic aid for endurance exercise. You decide to test two levels of caffeine and a placebo (placebo, 1-dose, 2-doses) and measure running time to exhaustion. You consider using a repeated measures design and realize that it is important to control for possible treatment order effects by counterbalancing.
   a How many possible treatment orders are there?
   b Write out all possible treatment orders for the conditions P, 1-D, and 2-D.
   c What would be the main disadvantage of a repeated measures design for this type of study?

ANSWERS

1 a $2 \times 3 = 6$ conditions

  b 1 6 conditions $\times$ 15 subjects = 60 subjects

    2 2 levels of IV1 $\times$ 15 subjects = 30 subjects (15 for IV1, level 1 and 15 for IV1, level 2. Both groups experience each of the three levels of IV2).

    3 15 (all 15 experience each of the 6 treatment conditions).

2 a Independent groups—Grade and Gender Repeated measures—Sport (all grades and genders play both sports)

  b 3 grades $\times$ 2 genders = 6 conditions $\times$ 10 subjects = 60 subjects

  c Catergorical IVs—Grade and Gender
Maipulated IV—Sport

  d 3 (grade) $\times$ 2 (gender) $\times$ 2 (sport) = 12 conditions

3 a 6 orders (3! $3 \times 2 \times 1 = 6$).

  b P, 1-D, 2-D; P, 2-D, 1-D;
1-D, P, 2-D; 1-D, 2-D, P;
2-D, 1-D, P; 2-D, P, 1-D;

  c If the same subjects are tested repeatedly, the training effect of the exercise could affect their running times in addition to any possible caffeine effects.

Qualitative Research

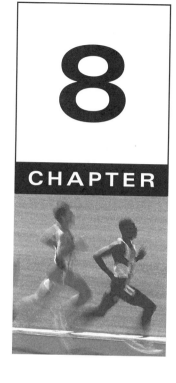

8

CHAPTER

LEARNING GOALS

After reading this chapter you will be able to:

1 Explain the differences between qualitative and quantitative research techniques.

2 Distinguish between observation and ethnography.

3 Define the term *feminist methodology.*

4 Give examples of how the human experience can be described through a "personal voice."

5 Distinguish between descriptive and analytic history.

6 Identify which subdisciplines in exercise and sport use qualitative techniques.

7 Give an example of a research question a qualitative study might address.

TERMS

Ethnography
Descriptive history
Analytical history
Feminist methodology
Personal voice
Autobiography

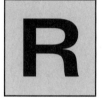esearch that closely follows the steps of the scientific method is not always the most effective way to understand topics in our academic discipline. Well-controlled laboratory settings, statistical procedures, and numerical representations often fail to capture the emotions, values, and other cultural dimensions typically associated with sport and exercise. For example, traditional quantitative or "number crunching" techniques may help us to determine answers to questions such as how many and what types of individuals are participating in physical activity or whether participation rates have increased or decreased over the years. But these numerical techniques cannot capture the role of the "human experience" and thereby overlook questions such as *why* some people are passionately involved in physical activity and of course, conversely, *why* others cling strongly to a "sedentary lifestyle."

Also, traditional "scientific" approaches are often unable to address the complexities of our rapidly changing social and political world. Such topics as gender bias in sport, exploitation of college athletes, and the commercialization of the fitness industry are among the new political and social issues that are of increasing interest to the disciplinary study of sport and exercise. While quantitative approaches can document the extent or degree of social or political inequities potentially present in our sport and exercise world, qualitative approaches allow us to add depth and meaning to such realities.

Qualitative approaches, for the most part, are found in subdiscipline areas related to the social sciences (such as sociology of sport, anthropological study of play) and humanities (such as history of sport, philosophy of sport, sport literature). The qualitative approach to sport and exercise, although a rather new trend, is one of the fastest growing areas of study within our field. A summary of the differences between quantitative and qualitative approaches is presented in Table 8.1.

As suggested in Chapter 2, qualitative research relies heavily on observation in natural settings. On the surface these methods are often viewed as having little or nothing in common with the research techniques associated with quantitative

TABLE 8.1 **Characteristics of Qualitative Contrasted with Quantitative Studies**

Qualitative	Quantitative
The investigator has chosen a topic or issue to study. Task is to discover, hypotheses emerge	Investigator goes much further, delimiting the study, selecting variables, making predictions, etc. His/her task is to verify or refute. Hypotheses are stated in advance
The sites/individuals chosen for the study governed by topic . . . sites/individuals/cases relatively few in number	Sample size is governed ideally by considerations of statistical "power." "N" is preferably large
The investigator is the principal "instrument" for data collection	The investigator should remain anonymous and neutral vis-à-vis the research site/subjects. He/she gathers data via intermediary instruments like questionnaires, tests, structured observation schemes, etc.
The research process is designed to intrude as little as possible in the natural, ongoing lives of those under study	Intrusion may be extreme in that *subjects* may be *paid* to participate in a *laboratory simulation.* At a minimum those being studied will be aware that they are part of an "experiment"
Investigator aware of his/her own biases and strives to capture the subjective reality of participants	Investigator assumes an unbiased stance; safeguards are employed to maintain objectivity
Investigator uses "wide-angle lens" to record context surrounding phenomena under study. Focus may shift as analytical categories and theory "emerge" from the data	Context is seen as potentially contaminating the integrity of study. Procedures employed to reduce extraneous factors
Typical study lasts some months, perhaps years	Typical study lasts some hours, perhaps some days
Report utilizes narrative format, there is a story with episodes	Report is expository in nature, consisting of a series of interlocking arguments

From Lancy DF: Qualitative research in education: an introduction to the major traditions, New York, 1993, Longman Publishers.

studies. This extreme thinking, of course, is an overstatement since all research share a common goal—of increasing our understanding of a body of knowledge. But qualitative research does follow a different set of procedures than do our more scientifically-controlled studies. While quantitative procedures often include carefully designed laboratory experiments, validated and measured protocols, standardized written tests, numerical representations, and statistical analysis, qualitative approaches focus on the inclusion of open-ended interviews, detailed analysis, and subjective interpretation in scoring systems. Even though qualitative scientists approach tasks differently than quantitative scientists, the fundamental difference between the two does not rest in the methods and procedures but in the different ways in which the research questions are asked. In the next section we will elaborate on the qualitative method by discussing a number of recent research examples. Let us look at some qualitative research examples found in sport and exercise literature. For the sake of classification we will consider examples of qualitative studies from four areas: sociological inquiry, historical inquiry, gender analysis, and literary analysis.

SOCIOLOGICAL INQUIRY

Research that incorporates both a systematic observation strategy and a depthness of insight and understanding into what is being observed is known as **ethnography**. Ethnographic techniques, originally developed from the field of cultural anthropology, are popularly used within the subdiscipline of sociology of sport. Alan Klein (1986), for example, conducted a 4-year study of body builders in Southern California (see the first box on p. 193). Using the tools and insights of ethnography he found that the image the body-building subculture projects is different from what actually goes on.

In a second example, Eastman and Riggs (1994) examined the idiosyncratic sport rituals engaged in by viewers of televised sports (see the second box on p. 193). Using a combination of actual observation of sport viewers and the results of interviews with adult sport viewers they found that

Pumping Irony: Crisis and Contradiction in Bodybuilding

Alan M. Klein

While the projection of ideal images is very important in American culture, it is in the subculture and sport of bodybuilding that it gets carried to the extreme. A 4-year study of bodybuilding's mecca—Southern California— revealed a fundamental set of discrepancies between what the subculture projects as ideal and what actually goes on. These discrepancies are examined to determine which ones result from changes that have taken place in bodybuilding and which are structural to it. It is shown that as the sport/subculture altered its image to achieve cultural respectability, it inadvertently created new problems. The shifts are examined within the context of studies of deviance and point to the need for long-term ethnography in sport sociology.

From Klein AM: Sociology of Sport Journal 3(2):112, 1986.

Televised Sports and Ritual: Fan Experiences

Susan Tyler Eastman and Karen E. Riggs

Examination of idiosyncratic sports rituals engaged in by viewers of televised sports revealed complex patterns of negotiation and participation in the televised events. In addition to being well-recognized tools for defining group membership, personal rituals revealed the creation of multistranded connections between fans and teams or players, despite separation by an electronic wall. Personal rituals revealed a balancing of the need for suspense with a need for reassurance, and extended to superstitions and part-play/part-serious efforts to influence game outcome. Exploration of private sports-viewer rituals illuminates the ways individuals alter their experiences of televised sports in order to gain social and cultural empowerment.

From Eastman ST and Riggs KE: Sociology of Sport Journal 11(3):249, 1994.

sport fans' behaviors formed an important social bond with their respective teams and by so doing gained social empowerment (feelings of being in control).

In both cases the researcher combines skills of keen observation with a knowledgeable background in the subject and develops what is known as "thick description." The mere recording or chronicling of events (what happened, where, and when) only gives us an accumulation of facts. The addition of a level of "expertise" in the subject on the part of the researcher adds credibility to their "subjective interpretation" of the events. The reader of ethnographic studies should be mindful of the scholarly background of the researcher(s) (for example, previous publications, etc.), as well as the clarity and comprehensiveness of their written presentation.

HISTORICAL INQUIRY

The current body of information concerning sport and exercise is often best understood after addressing questions such as: Have forms of physical activity always been done this way? Did past societies perceive sport and exercise differently than we do today? Are there patterns in sport and exercise that change over time? For answers to these questions we can look to the work and methods of the historian. Although some sport historians may examine the medieval period, others may examine a very recent context (such as the Persian Gulf War). Understanding the "historian's craft" gives us great insight into describing and explaining events. Historical studies can be broken down into two categories: **descriptive history** and **analytical history**. By descriptive we mean work that through great attention to detail focuses on the identification of persons, places, and events with the goal to recreate the accuracy of the experiences in the past—experiences that because of time and other factors seem to have been lost. For example, McElroy and Cartwright (1986) examined the little-known professional sporting enterprise that existed in sixteenth-century London several centuries before what many historians have identified as the birth of modern sports. Using both surviving legal documents and play scripts, including the works of William Shakespeare, they described a world of professional sport. Although it included violent animal contests, it can be described as a sporting enterprise very similar to today's world of large arenas, large paying crowds, and significant financial backing.

Analytical history, on the other hand, takes the description one step further and asks questions (such as: Are there patterns to these events? Why did these events happen?). One outstanding example of analytic history is Roberta J. Park's (1991) study of nineteenth-century attitudes toward exercise, where she goes beyond the mere description of the lives of two fitness leaders, Lilian Welsh and Dudley Allen Sargent. Through a combination of detailed description and insightful interpretation, Park demonstrates how each leader represented a "tightly gendered world" in a time when societal attitudes toward and thereby opportunities for women were very different than those for men. For readers of historical research in exercise and sport, topics that have been "hidden from history" are becoming the mainstream line of inquiry.

Examining and interpreting past events, past cultures, and old ways of doing things presents real challenges to the historian. The actual participants may no longer be living, written records may have disappeared, and perhaps more problematic, the written records that have survived may be a misrepresentation of the role of sport and exercise in that society. For example, studies of sporting forms in early America often focus on the battle between puritan or "blue" laws and recreation on Sundays. Such studies often report surviving documents of criticism, court and criminal records, angry letters, and so forth. Not unlike in today's world, good news goes unreported while bad news finds its way into the printed record. The reader of history must proceed cautiously, and as suggested in the proceeding chapter, be mindful of the authenticity (external evidence) and the interpretation (internal evidence) of the data. The process of credibility is not complete until we consider the completeness of the evidence. In order to do this we must understand the historical context.

Recreating past histories presents a real challenge to the historian who has not lived within that time period. In reading history one must always ask if it is the true "historical context" or "truth," the historian's own historical context. Such challenges require the historian to work very closely with primary sources (evidence belonging to the time period), and be very cautious piecing together what little primary evidence may be available. For example, Wiggins (1980) examined the play of slave children on southern plantations during the nineteenth century. Most slaves could not read or write and therefore likely would not have left a written record. Wiggins cleverly used slave narratives collected through oral interviews in the 1930s to reconstruct the life on the plantation. Wiggins cautions us that a number of the slaves were well into their later years in life when they were interviewed and may have been subject to memory losses. Although the results of this study need to be taken cautiously, this work has been praised for using the single best source available.

Messner and Solomon (1993) did not have the problem of "lost history." In their analysis of boxing champion Sugar Ray Leonard's alleged wife beating in 1991, their interest focuses on whether the newspapers created history rather than whether the abusive behavior actually occurred (see the box below).

Outside the Frame: Newspaper Coverage of the Sugar Ray Leonard Wife Abuse Story

Michael A. Messner and William S. Solomon

This article analyzes the print media's ideological framing of the 1991 story of boxer Sugar Ray Leonard's admission of having physically abused his wife and abused cocaine and alcohol. We examined all news stories and editorials on the Leonard story in two major daily newspapers and one national sports daily. We found that all three papers framed the story as a "drug story," while ignoring or marginalizing the "wife abuse" story. We argue that sports writers utilized an existing ideological "jocks-on-drugs" media package that framed this story as a moral drama of individual sin and public redemption. Finally, we describe and analyze the mechanisms through which the wife abuse story was ignored or marginalized.

From Messner MA and Solomon WS: Sociology of Sport Journal 10(2):119, 1993.

GENDER ANALYSIS

During the last two decades, our field has focused more attention on women in sport and exercise settings. This interest in women's topics is consistent with a growing qualitative research tradition known as **feminist methodology** or gender analysis. Although the word *feminist* evokes different meanings to different people, feminist methodology focuses on the study of women, taking into consideration their needs, interests, and experiences. As pointed out by feminist researcher Renate Duelli Klein (1983), feminist methodology does not simply compare women to men but embraces the concept that women's experiences, ideas, and needs are valid in their own right.

Feminist methodologies also explore how women are influenced by the world in which they live with a recognition that often the sporting world is not particularly "gender friendly." As indicated in the box below, Kane and Disch (1993) developed a detailed case study concerning a highly publicized locker room incident between a female sports reporter and professional football players.

Sexual Violence and the Reproduction of Male Power in the Locker Room: The "Lisa Olson Incident"

Mary Jo Kane and Lisa J. Disch

Numerous media commentators have deemed the sexual harassment locker room incident between Lisa Olson and the New England Patriots to be an embarrassing case of mismanagement. Our analysis challenges this popular assumption; we argue that the event represents an overt manifestation of male power by means of sexual violence against women. The response to Olson suggests that in an era where women's entry into sport has challenged men's exclusive hold on that domain, the locker room, like the playing field, must be understood as contested terrain. For men to maintain control over the terrain of the locker room, the female sportswriter must be displaced from her role as authoritative critic of male performance and reassigned to her "appropriate" role of sexual object. In light of the importance of sport, and the status of the locker room as an inner sanctum of male privilege, the incident between Olson and the Patriots was not mismanaged at all but, in fact, handled effectively.

From Kane MJ and Disch LJ: Sociology of Sport Journal 10(4):331, 1993.

Feminist methodology often relies on **personal voice—** women telling their own stories. The story may be filled with inaccuracies, exaggerations, fears, and misguided intentions, but it is precisely these "human frailties" spoken from someone who has experienced the events that give this work meaning far beyond what mere numbers can give. Although the emergence of the female sports **autobiography** lags behind examples in other fields, examples of women's personal voice can be found in studies such as the one in the box below. Weiller and Higgs (1994) used an open-ended questionnaire format which allowed the subjects, 52 former participants in the recently highly publicized professional baseball league, to recount their own stories.

The All American Girls Professional Baseball League, 1943-1954: Gender Conflict in Sport?

Karen H. Weiller and Catriona T. Higgs

The increase of women workers in industry during World War II coincided with an increase in sport participation and competition. From 1943 to 1954, the All American Girls Professional Baseball League (AAGPBL) allowed talented women athletes a chance to play professional baseball. The purpose of this study was to examine the nature of women's professional baseball and its connection with the social, cultural, and economic roles for women in society. An open-ended questionnaire allowed former players to respond to the social and cultural forces that impacted on women in society and sport during this era. The players of the AAGPBL were respected and admired professional women athletes in a male-dominated sport.

Appendix

Questionnaire Items

1. How old were you when you first participated in softball/baseball?
2. Were your parents/family supportive of your involvement in softball/baseball?
3. Were your friends/peer group supportive of your involvement in softball/baseball?
4. When you played in the AAGPBL, how did you feel women were treated (a) in society? (b) in sport?
5. How old were you when you started playing in the AAGPBL?
6. What were your reasons for becoming involved in the AAGPBL?

From Weiller KH and Higgs CT: Sociology of Sport Journal 11(3):289, 297, 1994.

The All American Girls Professional Baseball League, 1943-1954: Gender Conflict in Sport?—cont'd

7 What were some of the restrictions imposed upon you as a professional woman athlete?

8 How did you feel about these restrictions?

9 How much money did you earn as a professional woman athlete? Did you have any supplemental income? If so, from where?

10 How long did you play in the AAGPBL?

11 What was your reason for leaving the sport?

12 Did you continue to play after the league disbanded? If so, for how long?

13 At the present time, how do you feel women are treated (a) in society? (b) in sport?

14 How do you feel society would receive a professional woman's baseball league today?

15 In your opinion, is it easier to be a professional woman athlete today? Why or why not?

Note: Demographic information was also requested:

1 age, place of birth

2 place of residence (current and when AAGPBL member)

3 present occupation

It would be incorrect to assume that feminist methodologies are only used by female researchers. The Sugar Ray Leonard example and the participant observation study outlined below are two good examples of male researchers interested in exploring women's issues in sport. The box on p. 200 does not include women as observed subjects, but the analysis of male bonding has strong repercussions for women.

LITERARY ANALYSIS

Our final area of qualitative research tradition focuses on a popular written cultural form—fictional accounts of fantasy and story known as sport literature. Among the products of sport literature are short stories, play scripts, and poems but certainly the most popular is that of the sport novel. Some traditional authors consider sport fiction as "pulp" and clearly

Fraternal Bonding in the Locker Room: A Profeminist Analysis of Talk About Competition and Women

Timothy Jon Curry

A profeminist perspective was employed to study male bonding in the locker rooms of two "big time" college sport teams. Locker room talk fragments were collected over the course of several months by a participant observer, a senior varsity athlete, and by a nonparticipant observer, a sport sociologist. Additional data were collected by means of field observations, intensive interviews, and life histories and were combined to interpret locker room interaction. The analysis indicated that fraternal bonding was strongly affected by competition. While competition provided an activity bond to other men that was rewarding and status enhancing, it also generated anxiety and other strong emotions that the athletes sought to control or channel. Moreover, peer group dynamics encouraged antisocial talk and behavior, much of which was directed at the athletes themselves. To avoid being targeted for jibes and put-downs, the men engaged in conversations that affirmed a traditional masculinity. As a result their locker room talk generally treated women as objects, encouraged sexist attitudes toward women and, in its extreme, promoted rape culture.

Procedures

Fragment 6

Athlete 1 to 2: I've got to talk to you about [whispers name]. They go over to an empty corner of the locker room and whisper. They continue to whisper until the coaches arrive. The athletes at the other end of the locker room make comments:

Athlete 3: Yeah, tells us what she's got.

Athlete 4: Boy, you're in trouble now.

Assistant coach: You'll have to leave our part of the room. This is where the real men are.

Fragment 11

Assistant Coach 1: [announcement] Shame to miss the big [football] game, but you have to travel this week to keep you out of trouble. Here are the itineraries for the trip. They include a picture of Frank's girlfriend. [Picture is of an obese woman surrounded by children. Frank is one of the best athletes on the team.]

Assistant Coach 2: Yeah, when she sits around the house, she really sits around the house.

Assistant Coach 3: She's so ugly that her mother took her everywhere so she wouldn't have to kiss her good-bye. [group laughter]

From Curry TJ: Sociology of Sport Journal 8(2):119, 128, 130-132, 1991.

inferior to the great works of literature. A well-known writer, Mark Harris, considers his well-received series of four sport novels as "an apprenticeship for his more serious fiction." The fact remains that literary giants such as F. Scott Fitzgerald, Ernest Hemingway, and William Shakespeare freely turned to sport to set in motion their fictional tales. During the last decade sport novels have begun to receive attention and respect from the literary world. English professor Michael Oriard (1983), in speaking of what defines a sport novel, clearly resounds why this literary genre is now gaining popularity.

> "A definition of the sports novel, then, as one in which no substitutes for sport would be possible without radically changing the book, also embodies the most basic criterion for judging its quality. . . . The good sports novelist understands and demonstrates that baseball itself is "about" more than "baseball," football about more than the game on the field. The point is not for the novelist to recognize that baseball and football players are people, too, but that as baseball and football players they are particular kinds of people whose necessary concerns and activities touch their culture in important ways."(14)

The interest in sport fiction is a twentieth century phenomenon and the potential for its appeal is outlined in the study of a popular sports novel though perhaps overshadowed by its Hollywood version, still remains one of the classics in the literary world (see the box on p. 202).

Fictional accounts of our sporting world include the emotional dimensions associated with winning and losing. One such study of the importance of game outcome can be found in Everett T. Smith's (1984) study of versions of defeat in baseball autobiographies. Smith in framing his study noted how first-hand descriptions of baseball experiences often include words such as "fail," "defeated," "downfall," and "disaster." Using a literary framework he then details the persistent theme of failure in five baseball autobiographies, among them two of the most successful athletes of the twentieth century—Ted Williams and Ty Cobb. Although sport autobiographies do not always "stick to the facts," the dimension of "literary license," whether by sport novelist or sport autobiographer, makes these "personal stories" a valuable source.

Sport Literature, Literary Criticism, and Historical Inquiry

Mary McElroy and Kent Cartwright

The twentieth century novelist has discovered America's love of sport. Juvenile literature abounds in sport topics; popular fiction features athletes past and present, and some novels focused wholly on sport have now achieved the distinction of contemporary classics. Sport provides the novelist with a metaphor powerful enough both to explore the ambiguities of present life and to reveal the enduring structure of the American experience. In so doing, the novelist can also illuminate for us the appeal of sport itself. No sport is so broadly appealing or so typically American as baseball. Baseball seems to embrace the American spirit, captures the shared dreams of a culture and has even produced a novel that for three decades has been accepted as a contemporary classic. Bernard Malamud's *The Natural,* is explored in some detail as an example of how the study of fiction can benefit the sport historian. At first glance *The Natural* offers tantalizing but unlikely material for the sport historian. *The Natural* tantalizes because its incidents are drawn from specific legends and facts of baseball. Yet while many "real events" are alluded to none are explored in depth; while the Golden Age of baseball is a source of fictional detail the material remains unsorted in time and place, an alphabet soup of different decades, characters, teams and circumstances. What possible benefit can imaginary literature have, then, for the sport historian? While a novel should not be held to historical accountability it still stands in recognizable relation to life. We cannot fully understand and appreciate the ambience of a time period and the coherent shape of its events with historical facts alone: for such a sensibility we need the kind of information the novelist may provide. Malamud for example, is the first writer about baseball to have explored in depth the historical and cultural allusions imbedded in the pastoral rituals of the game; a basic myth that is not only American but is embodied and refashioned incessantly throughout the history of Western culture. Baseball as elaborated by Malamud captures a truth, a shape to experience, that is perhaps more central to our heritage than sport historians have ever expected. *The Natural* also considers the relationship between sport and the social and moral context in which it exists. Roy Hobbs, the novel's protagonist fails as a result of his inability to live up to the myths of natural harmony, integrity, and innocence that baseball embodied. In the final section of this paper we explore the response from the reader and how that response may be reflective of American attitudes toward baseball. Malamud in creating an encounter between the worlds of social reality and baseball myth provides a commentary on the pervading attitudes of America towards heroes and toward their customary modern vehicle, athletics.

From McElroy M and Cartwright K: Sport literature, literary criticism, and historical inquiry, Manhattan, Kan., 1982, North American Society for Sport History Proceedings.

SUMMARY

The tools and "research questions" of qualitative methodology have allowed various subdisciplines in our field to address and appreciate physical activity in ways unavailable through traditional quantitative strategies. Qualitative studies allow us to examine the impact of the complexities of social conditions in our society on the sport and exercise scene, and help us more fully appreciate the place of sport and exercise within the richness of culture and values. Such approaches give center stage to the role of human experiences and perceptions in understanding sport and exercise.

EXERCISES

1 Observe the process by which teams are selected in an urban school yard pick-up game mindful of gender or racial biases.
2 Record and interpret images of war and violence in the speech patterns of football coaches.
3 Check your university library for documents related to physical education and sports programs at your university. Determine any gender differences.
4 Interview first-time participants in a local road race and determine why they chose to participate.

Other Types of Research

9

CHAPTER

LEARNING GOALS

After reading this chapter you will be able to:

1 Explain the difference between a survey and a census.

2 Describe the differences between nonsampling errors and sampling errors.

3 Discuss the relationship between survey bias and survey precision.

4 Explain why it is important to report the margin of error statistic from a survey.

5 Describe the main factors that affect survey reliability and survey validity.

6 Discuss the advantages and disadvantages of using questionnaires, personal interviews, or telephone interviews when conducting a survey.

7 Explain the difference between a closed question format and an open question format.

8 Describe the goals and methods of case study research.

9 Explain the meaning of the terms *external evidence* and *internal evidence* and how these forms of evidence are used in historical research.

10 Give an example of a primary data source and a secondary data source.

11 Describe how the relationship between two variables is described by a correlation coefficient.

12 Explain why the coefficient of determination is reported along with a correlation coefficient.

13 Describe the methods used by researchers who conduct case study research.

14 Define the term *epidemiological research.*

TERMS

Survey
Census
Margin of error
Likert scale
Epidemiology
Primary data
Secondary data
External evidence
Internal evidence
Meta-analysis

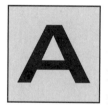s mentioned previously, the categorization of research into types is somewhat arbitrary. Although it would be possible to set up categories of research from a variety of perspectives (for example, types of hypotheses involved, types of statistical analyses used, etc.), it is most common to use data-collecting methods as the basis for the categories.

SURVEY RESEARCH

Surveys and public opinion polls are examples of descriptive research designed to gather information on habits, opinions, or attitudes. Surveys can take the form of a complete **census** (entire defined population) or a sample (a subset of a population). A complete census, particularly when working with a large population, is rare. One exception is the United States Population Census taken at 10-year intervals. The government makes every effort to contact all members of the population, even though they acknowledge it is not actually possible. Most surveys are administered to a sample selected from a population. The information derived from the sample is then used to estimate true population characteristics.

Surveys are not necessarily limited just to people—wildlife biologists, for example, survey animal populations. One goal of these surveys is to gauge the health of the population by estimating the total number of animals.

Conducting survey research appears comparatively simple: questions are written, a group of people is sampled, the data are tallied, and the findings are described. In fact, designing a survey instrument and developing the accompanying procedures to yield dependable information are quite challenging. Gathering meaningful information is difficult because survey research is particularly susceptible to two types of errors: *nonsampling errors* and *sampling errors.*

Nonsampling Errors

We must recognize that the information obtained from a survey depends on the questions that are asked, on how the respondents react to the questions, and on what respondents choose to reveal about themselves. Researchers are somewhat limited in their ability to assess the quality of the findings because there usually is no way of checking the accuracy or truthfulness of the responses. Nonsampling errors have several sources including any differences in the way the researcher and the respondents interpret questions, the inability or unwillingness of the respondents to provide correct or honest information, mistakes made when recording or coding the responses, and missing responses.

Nonsampling errors can be classified into four general categories: *processing errors, response errors, missing data errors,* and *data collection methods errors* (Moore, 1991). Processing errors arise from mistakes in handling the data such as coding responses or entering scores into a computer. These errors are mainly procedural in nature and sources can range from simple mistakes to intentional alterations. Response errors happen when subjects provide incorrect information. Subjects may intentionally give false or misleading answers, may make honest mistakes, or may not understand a question. Missing data errors happen when a subject refuses to participate, cannot be located, or fails to answer all the questions. If we end up with a 75% return rate on a survey, the 25% who did not respond represent a source of potential error. It is difficult to know precisely why some individuals do not respond. Data collection errors are those errors that stem from the methods and procedures used by the researcher in conducting the survey. This includes several potential sources such as the wording of the questions, the timing of the survey, the survey technique used (oral versus written), and others. Of these, the researchers can adopt procedures to minimize procedure and data collection errors. Controlling response and missing data errors is more difficult because they depend on the behavior of the respondents.

Sampling Errors

Sampling errors are those errors resulting from any differences between the data obtained from the sample, and the data that would have been obtained from a complete census. In other words, any errors when inferring a population characteristic based on a sample is called sampling error. An example of this type of error was presented in Chapter 5 involving the 1936 presidential election prediction by the *Literary Digest.*

Another type of sampling error deals not with the sample of individuals selected as respondents but rather with the sample of questions selected to be asked of the respondents. The issue is whether or not the sample of questions selected adequately represents the domain of interest.

The findings from survey research are sometimes criticized because of either the wording of the questions, the questions asked (or not asked), or both. Survey researchers try to word questions so they are not ambiguous, misleading, or biased. Nevertheless, respondents are sometimes confused by the wording of a question. A question on a survey commissioned by the American Jewish Committee and conducted by the Roper Organization in 1992 provides an example of this. The wording question was criticized because it contained a confusing double negative. The original question and results follow below:

> As you know, the term Holocaust usually refers to the killing of millions of Jews in Nazi death camps during World War Two. Does it seem possible or does it seem impossible to you that the Nazi extermination never happened?
>
> | | |
> |---|---|
> | Possible | 22% |
> | Unsure, don't know | 12% |
> | Impossible | 66% |

Because of the controversy that grew out of this finding, the Roper Organization revised the wording of the question and conducted a new poll in April, 1994. The reworded question and new findings are below:

> Does it seem possible to you that the Nazi extermination of the Jews never happened, or do you feel certain that it happened?
>
> | | |
> |---|---|
> | Possible it never happened | 1% |
> | Unsure, don't know | 8% |
> | Certain it happened | 91% |

As you can see, the two findings are very different. The findings from the first survey suggested that most people believed the Holocaust never happened. The finding from the second survey suggested that about 90 percent of the population is certain that the Holocaust happened. The goal of both questions was the same, yet, because of the wording, each resulted in very different findings.

SURVEY PRECISION AND BIAS

Two factors that are important in survey research are *precision* and *bias.* The findings from a survey are said to be biased if one opinion is emphasized to the exclusion of other opinions. Survey precision is a measure of consistency of the findings. If similar findings are achieved on repeated surveys, the precision of the survey is said to be high. If findings are inconsistent, then precision is low.

The target in Figure 9.1 illustrates the concepts of bias and precision (adapted from Moore, 1991). Assume that the center of the target represents the true population characteristic. As the survey researcher, your goal is to hit the center of the target with the findings from the survey. As the findings move away from the center, they less accurately represent true population characteristics. A survey that is imprecise tends to hit the target in different places. A survey that is biased tends to consistently miss the center of the target.

Precision and bias operate simultaneously. A survey can be biased or unbiased, and it can be imprecise or precise, or any combination of the two. Target A shows high precision because all responses are clustered together, and low bias because the responses are close to the center of the target. Target B is just the opposite—precision is low because the measurements are scattered, and bias is relatively high because all measurements are off to one side of the target. The goal of any sampling strategy is to achieve low bias and high precision.

Although precision and bias are important, they are difficult to measure. The most common method is to administer the survey to several separate samples and compare the results. However, this usually is not a viable alternative for most surveys as a result of time and resource constraints. Instead, bias is assumed to be low and precision high if the survey questions are worded carefully and if appropriate sampling methods are used.

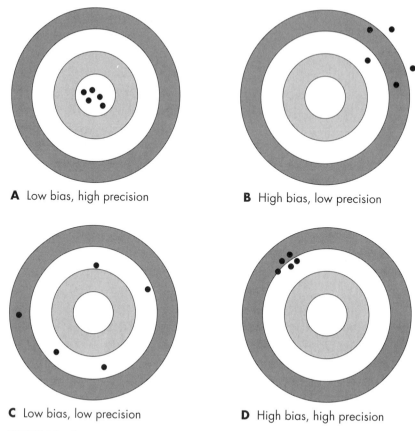

A Low bias, high precision

B High bias, low precision

C Low bias, low precision

D High bias, high precision

FIGURE 9.1 Survey bias and precision. Adapted from Moore DS: Statistics: concepts and controversies, ed 3, New York, 1991, W.H. Freeman and Company.

MARGIN OF ERROR

The next time you see the results of a survey in the news, pay special attention to the **margin of error** or sampling error information. The margin of error statistic indicates a range of values within which the true population values should lie. For example, *Time* magazine reported the results of a telephone survey of 800 Americans on health-care reform (Goodgame 1994). The results are shown in Table 9.1.

Included with the findings, a ±3.5% margin of error statistic was reported. How do we interpret these findings, especially with regard to the margin of error? The results

TABLE 9.1 Health Care Reform Survey		
Do you think the country's health care system needs a great deal of reform?		
	April 1993	**Aug.-Sept. 1994**
Great deal	63%	51%
Only some	34%	38%
No reform at all	3%	9% ("not sure" omitted)

Margin of error ±3.5%.
Data compiled from *Time,* Sept. 14, 1994, pp. 40-42.

August and September show that 51% of those surveyed felt that the health care system needs a great deal of reform. Since this result is based on a sample, we know the population value should be something close to 51%, but is probably not exactly 51%. Instead, we can say that in 19 cases out of 20, poll responses should differ by no more than 3.5 percentage points in either direction from what would be observed if the entire population of interest were questioned. In other words, we can be 95% confident that the true population value lies within a range from 47.5% to 54.5% (51% ± 3.5%). The same margin of error can be applied to each of the results; for example, we can infer that 5.5% to 12.5% of the population feel that no reform is necessary. Keep in mind that these results represent a snapshot of public opinion during the time when the survey was conducted. The April 1993 results indicate that public opinion on these question was very different at that time.

SURVEY RELIABILITY

Two additional considerations are important when evaluating the results of a survey: the reliability and the validity of the results. Survey reliability is related to sample size. In general, the larger the sample size, the greater the reliability (assuming the use of appropriate sampling methods). Suppose, for example, that you conducted a survey on exercise habits and sampled 1% of the students enrolled at your school. All other factors being equal, these findings would be less reliable than a survey where 10% of the students were sampled.

SURVEY VALIDITY

Survey validity, on the other hand, is concerned with how representative the sample is of the parent population. While sample size is important, the sample representativeness is ultimately most important when one considers the accuracy of the survey. Recall the *Literary Digest* survey discussed earlier. Although the sample was very large, it was not representative of the entire voting population.

CONDUCTING A SURVEY

Done well, survey research requires a lot of planning and thought. One of the first decisions made by the researcher is choosing a method for distributing the questions. The three most common methods are mailed questionnaires, personal interviews, or telephone interviews. In this section we will discuss some of the advantages and disadvantages of each method.

Questionnaires

Mailed questionnaires have traditionally been the most commonly used distribution method for survey research. Advantages of questionnaires include low relative cost; they can be distributed over a wide geographic area; a large number of surveys can be distributed at the same time; and a wide range of question formats can be used. The main disadvantage of mailed questionnaires is that many subjects, for whatever reason, fail to return the survey. These "missing data" present problems, particularly if the results are biased as a result of some unknown factor. In addition, conducting a large survey with mailed questionnaires can be time consuming because of the time it takes for the respondents to receive and then return the questionnaires.

Personal Interviews

An alternative to mail questionnaires is interviews, either in person or over the telephone. The main advantage of interviews is that the respondents can give detailed answers and ask for clarification if a question is unclear. In addition, response rates are generally high for personal interviews.

Personal interviews also have some disadvantages: they are usually limited to a narrow geographic range; they are time consuming to conduct; and they typically are limited to smaller samples than mailed questionnaires. In addition, there is the problem of consistency and neutrality on the part of the interviewers. This concern applies to both how the interviewer interacts with the subjects, and how the interviewer interprets and records the answers. Finally, subjects may be hesitant to reveal information in person that they might reveal anonymously in writing.

Telephone Interviews

Telephone interviews are similar to personal interviews with the main advantage that phone interviews are not limited to the immediate locale and they are relatively inexpensive to conduct. Similar to personal interviews, a wide range of question formats can be employed and the respondents can ask questions, although open-scale questions should be kept to a minimum. The main disadvantage is that telephone surveys should be relatively short. In addition, the questions should be easy to read and understand since the respondent has to rely on someone reading the questions to them. If the telephone interview involves questions requiring interpretation and evaluation by the interviewer and if multiple interviewers are used problems in consistency can arise. Training sessions for the interviewers can help control this problem. Because of the wide geographic access and the speed of information gathering, telephone interviews are the most common method for public opinion polls. For example, surveys taken during election years are usually conducted via telephone interviews. Table 9.2 summarizes some of the main features of the three methods.

With the advent and increasing availability of computer networks, we predict that a future survey method might involve the use of E-mail surveys. This will require investigation of the feasibility, reliability, validity and accuracy of such procedures. However, E-mail surveys could have several advantages: distribution costs would be very low, the time required to send and receive the questionnaires could be reduced, and the data could be directly imported into data

TABLE 9.2 Common Methods of Conducting Survey Research	Mailed questionnaire	Personal interview	Telephone interview
Data collection costs	Moderate	High	Moderate
Amount of assistance needed to conduct	Low	High	High
Opportunity to clarify questions	Low	High	High
Response rates	Moderate	High	Moderate
Perceived anonymity	High	Low	Moderate
Opportunity to clarify answers	Low	High	High
Chance of interviewer bias	None	Moderate/ High	Moderate
Length of survey	Moderate/ Long	Long	Short/ Moderate
Time needed to complete the study	Long	Short	Long
Large samples	Best	Worst	Best

analysis software. The main disadvantage at the present time is the relatively limited pool of potential respondents because not everyone has an E-mail address.

SURVEY QUESTION FORMATS

Survey questions are written in any one of several formats depending on the type of interview, the goals of the survey, and the characteristics of the target population. Question formats can be categorized into two general groups: closed question format and open question format.

Closed Question Format

The closed question format provides a predefined range of responses from which the respondent must select an answer. The closed question format ranges from categorical answers that provide only two options, to many-choice scaled answers that provide a range of answers. The **Likert scale** question format is popular and you have no doubt seen questions written in this style. A Likert scale provides the respondent with several choices on a scale so they can grade their responses. Examples of closed-scale questions are shown in the box below.

Closed scale questions are probably the most commonly used survey question format because they are the easiest to analyze statistically. Responses can be coded, entered into a computer, and analyzed. The main disadvantage of closed scale questions is that the respondent is limited to a defined set of responses. The respondents may not be able to fully express their opinions when confined to a limited range of questions

---

Examples of the Closed Question Format

Categorical Responses

College athletes deserve full financial scholarships:

     Agree_____   No Opinion_____   Disagree_____

College athletes should be paid in addition to their scholarships:

     Yes_____   No_____

Likert scale

College athletes should be paid in addition to their scholarships:

Strongly Agree   Agree   Uncertain   Disagree   Strongly Disagree
    ( )   ( )   ( )   ( )   ( )

Athletes should meet all university entrance requirements:
(10 = very important : 1 = not important)

      10   9   8   7   6   5   4   3   2   1

Ranked list

Rank order the most important reasons for supporting college athletics:
(1 = most important, 4 = least important)

To win competitions   _____

To support future professional athletes   _____

For university prestige   _____

For university pride   _____

and answers. The researcher never knows if "the right question" or the "right responses" were presented to elicit the information sought. In addition, responses to closed scale questions are "shallow." This means that the respondents cannot elaborate on their answers. Our opinions are often more complex than those responses listed in a closed scale question.

Open Question Format

The open question format consists of questions requesting short answers or essays. The respondents give answers in their own words. Once the survey is complete, the researcher categorizes the responses according to a certain set of criteria. Some examples of the open scale questions are shown in the box below.

The main advantage of open questions is the opportunity for the respondent to give a personalized answer. The main disadvantage is the difficulty the researcher has in interpreting and categorizing the responses in a consistent and reliable manner. In addition, it can be very time consuming to read and categorize a large number of open scale questions. Finally, it is difficult to apply statistical analysis methods directly to open scale questions.

Examples of the Open Question Format

Open Question Format

Discuss the most important reasons for supporting college athletics.

What is your opinion of paying college athletes a salary?

How do you think college athletics are affected by the financial demands placed on the institutions?

Writing Survey Questions

Probably the most difficult aspect of conducting a survey is writing the questions. The primary goal when writing questions is to word the questions so they have the same meaning for all subjects. You have probably taken multiple-choice exams where a few of the questions were unclear to you. In other words, you were not sure exactly what the question was asking. The same confusion can exist in a survey.

Researchers attempt to write clear questions by recruiting "experts" to provide feedback, by answering a draft version of the survey. Their feedback can be used to clarify and improve the questions. Researchers do not expect their first draft to be perfect and realize it may require several drafts before a satisfactory survey is written. Usually they attempt to keep each question as short as possible and center it on only one idea or issue. They try to word the questions clearly to minimize ambiguity, and use questions that convey neutrality on their part to avoid biasing answers. The box on p. 218 outlines the steps that should be followed when preparing a survey. Appendix B contains a sample cover letter and survey. The sample survey shows how different question formats can be combined to make the survey interesting for the respondents.

STEPS IN CONDUCTING SURVEY RESEARCH

Survey research, like any other form of research, is best conducted following a systematic plan. The box on p. 219 provides an outline for completing a survey.

If the response rate in a survey research is low, it is important to contact some of the nonrespondents to determine why they did not respond. The reasons may or may not be related to the purpose of the study. The conclusions to be drawn may be affected by knowing why individuals failed to respond to the survey instrument.

NATIONAL AIR AND SPACE MUSEUM SURVEY

The Smithsonian National Air and Space Museum in Washington D.C. surveys the visitors of an exhibit titled "Where Next Columbus?" about the history of space exploration. Two

---

Preparing a Survey

1 Choose a question format.
  - Open scale
  - Closed scale
      Categorical
      Likert-scale
      Ranked list
  - A combination of formats
2 Write the instructions and the first draft of the questions.
3 Evaluate the questions. Correct any of the following types of questions:
  - Double-barrel questions
      "Do you believe that there are equal opportunities for minorities and women in college athletics?"
  - Loaded questions
      "All scholarship athletes should be required to participate in team prayer before games."
  - Biased questions
      "I agree that college athletes should be paid a salary."
  - Double negatives
      "I do not support the argument that a salary should not be paid to college athletes."
4 Pretest the survey.
5 Revise and pretest again if necessary.
6 Write a final draft of the instructions and questions.

---

touch-screen computers are located at the exit of the exhibit and conduct the survey. The survey consists of several closed scale questions on issues related to space exploration. The survey is voluntary and self-administered. Table 9.3 shows the questions and the response percentages from more than 105,500 respondents who had participated as of July, 1994.

More than 105,500 respondents certainly constitutes a very large sample; however one might question whether or not this sample is truly representative of the opinions of the citizens of the United States. For example, should this information be used by the federal government when planning further space exploration? Is this sample representative of the American voting public and does it express the voting population's true wishes for future space exploration?

Conducting Survey Research

1 Define the objectives of the survey.
 • Gathering information on a single group of people
  Opinions or attitudes
  Behaviors or activities
 • Making comparisons among groups of people
2 Define the population of interest.
3 Develop the sampling strategy.
 • Sample size
  Determine the number of subjects needed
  Determine the target response rate
 • Choose a sampling method
  Simple random sample
  Stratified random sample
  Cluster sample
  Quota sample
4 Select an interview method.
 • Mail
 • Telephone
 • Interview
5 Plan a timetable for the information gathering phase.
 • Set first contact date to mail the surveys or begin interviews
 • Set follow-up contact date for unreturned surveys
 • Set the last day for accepting surveys
6 Administer the survey.
7 Reduce the data.
 • Determine the coding plan for the responses
 • Enter data into the computer
 • Account for missing responses
8 Analyze the data.
 • Identify the specific statistical analysis methods to be used
  Calculate the selected descriptive statistics
  Calculate the selected inferential statistics
 • Write a summary of the analysis
9 Complete the written report of the survey.

To answer these questions, we should consider aspects about the respondents to the survey. The National Air and Space Museum is the most popular tourist attraction in the Washington, D.C. area, and Washington, D.C. is one of the most popular tourist destinations in the country. Based on this, it might be

TABLE 9.3 **Survey Results from "Where Next Columbus"**

1 Do you think we should explore space?

1) Yes	85%
2) No	10%
3) Undecided	5%

2 What do you think is the *best* reason for exploring space?

1) Increase knowledge and search for life	60%
2) Establish settlements or space colonies	11%
3) Gain economic benefits	8%
4) Maintain national prestige and leadership	6%
5) Encourage international cooperation	7%
6) Other	8%

3 What concerns you *most* about space exploration?

1) Risks and danger	22%
2) Cost	22%
3) Urgent needs and problems on Earth	26%
4) Competition among exploring nations	8%
5) Environmental impact on other worlds	12%
6) Other	10%

4 Where do you think we should explore?

1) Moon	9%
2) Mars	13%
3) Other planets in the solar system	12%
4) Stars	9%
5) All of the above	48%
6) None of the above	9%

5 How do you think we should explore space?

1) Observe from earth	8%
2) Send robots	17%
3) Send people	15%
4) All of the above	53%
5) None of the above	7%

6 Do you think there is life on other worlds?

1) Yes	50%
2) Probably	30%
3) Probably not	10%
4) No	10%

Data from the Smithsonian National Air and Space Museum, Washington, D.C.

TABLE 9.3 Survey Results from "Where Next Columbus"—cont'd	
7 Do you think we should settle on Mars?	
1) Yes	41%
2) No	32%
3) Undecided	27%
8 What percentage of a nation's budget do you think should be spent on space exploration (the U.S. spends about 1%)?	
1) None	10%
2) < 1%	21%
3) 1 to 5%	48%
4) > 5%	21%

safe to assume that the museum attracts a representative cross-section of the population. However, the museum is also an extremely popular attraction for visitors from other countries. Thus the survey includes opinions from tax-paying citizens and noncitizens as well. The Air and Space Museum also tends to attract people who are particularly interested in aviation and space exploration. In addition, after touring the exhibits, the visitors might be "inspired" by space exploration and may be inclined to respond more favorably. Therefore, the respondents to the survey might be biased towards those individuals who support these efforts and the associated costs. Members of the population who are not interested in space exploration may not be inclined to visit this museum to the same extent as those who favor exploration. As a consequence, those who do not favor space exploration may not have their views represented to the same degree as those who do favor exploration.

CASE STUDY

A form of qualitative research, the *case study,* has as its purpose an extremely detailed examination of a particular individual, group, phenomenon, or event. This is usually accomplished through in-depth interviews, extensive observation, exhaustive records review, or combinations of all of the above techniques.

While the goal of case study research is virtually to know all there is to know about the particular person, group, or topic being investigated, it is also used to uncover previously unknown information. This "new" information can then either be added to the corpus of knowledge, or as is common with many types of research, it is used as a beginning point for further investigation. This additional investigation may take the form of another case study, an experimental research project, or any other type of appropriate inquiry (see the box on p. 223).

A difficulty with case study research, of course, is the concern of representativeness. It is not always possible to conclude on the basis of a case study that the findings generalize to the population from which the individual, group, phenomenon, or event was chosen. A solution to this problem is to conduct multiple case studies, but this is rare since the object of a case study is usually selected for its uniqueness, not its representativeness of some population.

Methods Associated with Case Studies

Bogdan and Biklen (1982) liken the design of a case study to a funnel. It starts wide and finishes narrow. The researchers begin by identifying all possible people or locations where relevant data might be located. By continuing to modify the topic as information is located, a focus develops and this eventually dictates the manner for collecting data.

The major data gathering techniques of interviewing, observing, and examining records are used to varying degrees depending on the topic being studied. For example, to trace the history of a particular organization over time, a researcher would rely extensively on interviews and examination of records but probably not on observation. In contrast the study of a particularly successful curriculum or individual might rely on all three techniques, particularly observation.

EPIDEMIOLOGICAL RESEARCH

Epidemiology is a branch of medical science that deals with the study of the incidence and distribution of disease in a

Example of a Case Study in Sport and Exercise Science

Acute Exertional Anterior Compartment Syndrome in an Adolescent Female

Allan Fehlandt, Jr. and Lyle Micheli

Abstract

Acute compartment syndromes usually occur as a complication of major trauma. While the chronic exertional anterior tibial compartment syndrome is well described in the sports medicine literature, reports of acute tibial compartment syndromes due to physical exertion, or repetitive microtrauma, are rare. The case of an adolescent female who developed an acute anterior compartment syndrome from running in a soccer game is described in this report. Failure to recognize the onset of an acute exertional compartment syndrome may lead to treatment delay and serious complications. Whereas the chronic exertional anterior compartment syndrome is characterized by pain that diminishes with the cessation of exercise, the onset of the acute exertional anterior compartment syndrome is heralded by pain that continues, or increases, after exercise has stopped. Compartment pressure measurement confirms the clinical diagnosis and helps guide treatment. True compartment syndromes require urgent fasciotomy.

From Fehlandt A and Micheli L: Medicine and Science in Sports and Exercise 27(1):3-7, 1995.

population. Examples of concerns for epidemiologists are noting increases and decreases of a disease over time, seeking possible connections between characteristics of humans and the presence or absence of a disease, and determining the geographical boundaries of a disease. The types of variables a sport and exercise sciences epidemiologist considers are varied. They include demographic variables such as age, gender, and ethnic group; social characteristics such as level of education or socioeconomic status; physiological traits such as those revealed by blood analysis and fitness levels; genetic information such as muscle fiber type and even personal traits such as nutritional information, drug use, and physical exercise patterns.

Although some epidemiological research is descriptive in nature (in other words, what changes have occurred in the percentage of deaths that are caused by coronary heart disease in women in the United States over the past 20 years?), the most interesting studies are those seeking to determine possible causal relationships between disease states and other variables. Epidemiological studies were responsible for uncovering the relationship between increased exposure to asbestos and increasing incidence of cancer, and for demonstrating that the increased presences of fluoride in the water is related to a decreased incidence of cavities in the teeth.

Epidemiological research is nonexperimental and therefore the drawing of cause-and-effect relationships is sometimes dangerous. In other words, because this type of research relies on data that already exist in nature which cannot be manipulated (such as the use of control variables in an experiment), there is always the possibility of discovering associations that are not cause-and-effect related. For example, it has been determined that bald men have a slightly elevated risk of coronary heart disease (CHD). It is unlikely that the lack of hair on the scalp is responsible for an increased chance of a heart attack. It may be that both CHD and baldness are genetically connected in some way but presently we do not know why this relationship exists—only that it does.

By its nature epidemiological research is more concerned with groups than it is with individuals. Although the final conclusions from epidemiological research may be applicable to individuals (for example, it is relatively well confirmed that regular physical activity provides positive health benefits), it is usually the use of large data sets that leads to these conclusions.

Methods of Epidemiological Research

Most epidemiological research falls into one of two types. The first is focused on the identification of relationships between a disease and a population characteristic. Although relatively sophistical statistical procedures are often employed in determining the existence and strength of such associations, this type of research is principally conducted by using rather mechanical procedures. The second type of epidemiological research is much more creative and interpretive in nature. It involves the inferential process of collecting data to confirm or negate hypotheses related to the possible relationship between a population characteristic and a disease.

An interesting feature of epidemiological research is that it can be done over a relatively short period of time, such as a study to determine the specific cause of an outbreak of food poisoning, or it can take place over an extended period of time. Two often cited longitudinal epidemiological studies in the area of sport and exercise science are the Framingham study and the Harvard Alumni study. The Framingham study (see the box below) originated in 1948 with 5209 subjects between the ages of 28 and 62 (Dawber, Kannel, and Lyell 1963). The Harvard Alumni study began in 1962 with almost 17,000 alumni originally involved (Paffenbarger, Hyde, Wing, and Hsieh 1986).

Example of Epidemiological Research

Impact of Left Ventricular Structure on the Incidence of Hypertension

The Framingham Heart Study

Wendy S. Post, Martin G. Larson, and Daniel Levy

Background: Left ventricular hypertrophy is often found very early in the course of hypertension. It is not known whether increased left ventricular mass contributes to the pathogenesis of hypertension. The purpose of this study was to examine the impact of left ventricular mass and other echocardiographically assessed cardiac structural features on the incidence of hypertension.

Methods and Results: Subjects for this investigation included participants in the Framingham Heart Study and the Framingham Offspring Study who were normotensive at the baseline examination (systolic blood pressure, <140 mm Hg; diastolic blood pressure, <90 mm Hg; not receiving antihypertensive medications) and free of coronary heart disease, congestive heart failure, valvular heart disease, hypertrophic cardiomyopathy, diabetes mellitus, and renal insufficiency. The study sample included 1121 men (mean age, 44.4 years) and 1559 women (mean age, 45.6 years). Four years after the baseline examination, 202 men (18.0%) and 257 women (16.5%) were hypertensive (systolic blood pressure, ≥140 mm Hg; diastolic blood pressure, ≥90 mm Hg; or use of antihypertensive medication.

From Post WS, Larson MG, and Levy D: Circulation 90(1):179-184, 1994.

Probably the most common topic for epidemiological research in sport and exercise science is the search for relationships between physical activity on fitness and health. According to Blair (1993) more than 100 large population-based studies of this kind have appeared in peer-reviewed literature in the past 30 years. We recommend this article for an excellent summary of current knowledge in this area.

HISTORICAL RESEARCH

Understanding the present relies on knowledge of the past. Historical research provides us with this knowledge. This type of research is done through an examination of data like any other type of research. The data in this case take the form of recorded observations, photographs, memorabilia, written records, letters, artifacts, portraits, diaries, and film. Audio and videotape may be data in studies of recent history. Recall from Chapter 8 that historical research is normally qualitative in nature and is based on descriptions rather than numerically based data (see the box on p. 227).

Methods

The two main concerns in conducting historical research are collecting the data and interpreting them. In the collection of the data it is important whenever possible to obtain **primary data.** These are data closest to the event. Examples would be information recorded by those who actually participated in the event or the expressions of eye witnesses. **Secondary data** include those sources that are at least once removed from the actual event. Each successive telling of a story usually alters the details to some degree. Although secondary sources are used in historical research, they should be avoided if it is possible to track down a primary source.

Let us assume that you have been given the assignment of investigating the history of the development of health related fitness tests used in public schools in the United States. Information about this phenomenon can be found in many measurement textbooks but most of these would be considered secondary sources because the authors did not participate in the development of these tests, but rather are writing

Example of Historical Research in Sport and Exercise Science

From Pitch to Putt: Sport and Class in Anglo-American Sport

Steven A. Reiss

Class has always been one of the paramount issues in sport historiography. During the period 1983-1992, historians have continued to debate the role of class in sport history, particularly its relationship to modernization, industrialization, and urbanization. Scholars have focused on such concerns as agency and hegemony, cultural diffusion, socialization, crowd composition and behavior, and social mobility. This essay examines how scholars have dealt with class as an independent and dependent variable in the United States, Great Britain, and Canada, whose sport historiography is in each case firmly based on their national scholarly traditions. Thus grand theory, particularly Marxism, and its sophisticated variants, remains a major feature of British literature, moderately so in Canada, and is largely avoided, if not rejected, in the United States. Class remains *the* central issue in British sport historiography, while Canadians are nearly equally concerned with other factors like colonialism, ethnicity and nationalism, and Americans consider class not much more prominent than race and ethnicity as a major feature of industrial capitalism and urbanization.

From Riess SA: Journal of Sport History 21(2):138, 1994.

what they have learned or read about this occurrence. Primary sources would include minutes of the meetings of organizations at which these tests were developed or articles authored by the individuals involved in these projects.

The second task of interpreting the data consists of two parts. The first part is usually titled **external evidence.** This has to do with authenticity of the data. The researcher must be confident that the document (painting, artifact, or other primary data) is genuine. External evidence, sometimes referred to as external criticism, is crucial to the credibility of historical research. Carbon dating, handwriting analysis, and even statistical analysis of the lengths of sentences have all been used to authenticate historical data.

As you might have guessed, the second part of interpretation is titled **internal evidence** (or internal criticism). This has to do with determining the meaning embedded in the data. Precisely what did the author of a particular document mean by the words spoken or written? When you read historical research you must be continually alert and question how the researcher reached conclusions from the evidence available. The ability to glean the true meaning from historical sources is not easily attained. It relies on a knowledge of the events occurring simultaneously and in near proximity with the habits and idiosyncrasies of the author of the source. Development of these traits takes time, practice, an open mind, and persistence.

CORRELATIONAL RESEARCH

All research designs could be considered correlational in one sense. We are always seeking to identify how variables are related to each other. However, the term *correlational research* is generally applied to studies employing specific correlational statistics to examine possible relationships among variables. Two primary uses of this type of research are *exploration* and *prediction.*

In exploratory research the goal is often simply to determine which variables in a data set might be related to each other. Although the researcher may have some ideas and hypotheses in mind, the goal is usually not involved with demonstrating why variables are related to each other as much as to determining if they even are correlated in any way. In predictive research the purpose is usually to determine how well a variable or a set of variables can be used to predict another variable.

The correlation coefficient is the statistic that reflects both the direction and the strength of the relationship between two variables. The value of the coefficient ranges from +1.0 (a perfect positive) to −1.0 (a perfect negative) correlation. A value of 0.0 signifies no correlation between two variables. The closer the coefficient is to the value of 1.0, the stronger the association between the two variables. The sign (+ or −) reflects the direction of the relationship. If the sign is positive it means that the high scores on one variable are associated with the high scores on the other variable. If negative, it indicates that the high scores on one variable are connected to the low scores on the second variable. Care must be taken in interpreting the direction because not all high scores represent the best achievement (for example, golf scores or the time to run 50 yards are instances where lower scores reflect better performance).

The correlation coefficient not only indicates mathematically the strength and direction of a relationship between two variables but is also used in prediction studies. If two variables were perfectly correlated, it would result in a correlation coefficient of 1.0 (either + or −). In this situation perfect prediction is possible. All subjects having a particular score on the first variable would have equal scores on the second variable (not equal to their first variable scores but equal to each other on the second variable). Pretend for a moment that a perfect correlation exists between height and weight. This would mean that anyone 6 feet tall would weigh exactly the same as any other person of this same height. Of course there is not a perfect correlation between height and weight because people of the same height vary in weight. However, because tall people "tend" to weigh more than short people, one would expect a positive correlation between these two variables but only modest in "strength."

One method of attaching meaning to the value of a correlation coefficient is to square it, thus producing a statistic called the coefficient of determination. The coefficient of determination tells us the amount of variability that exists in one variable because of the variability in the second variable to which it is correlated. For example, if the correlation coefficient between height and weight for a given sample of individuals was .70, the coefficient of determination would be .49 (.70^2). This can be interpreted to mean that 49% of the variability in weight scores is due to the fact that the individuals vary in height (or vice versa). This also means that 51% of the variability in weight scores is due to factors other than height. Notice that even with a correlation coefficient as high as .90 between two variables, nearly 20% of the variability exhibited in the scores on one variable are not accounted for by the variability in the related variable.

There are many types of correlation coefficients and which one is appropriate in a given situation depends on the level (nominal, ordinal, internal, or ratio) of measurement (these terms will be explained in the next chapter), whether or not the variables are related in a linear fashion, and the number of variables involved. If *two* variables are being correlated, a bivariate correlation coefficient is appropriate but if *several* variables are being correlated to determine how well they correlate as a package with another variable (or another set of variable), multivariate correlational statistics are appropriate. Another decision in determining the appropriate statistical test to use involves determining the shape of the possible relationship. Researchers usually draw a picture (called a scatterplot) to examine whether or not a straight line (linear) or a curved line (curvilinear) best fits the data and thus which types of coefficient should be calculated.

Methods for a Correlation Study

Whether exploratory or predictive in nature, the first step in a correlational study is to identify the variables that are thought to be connected to the behavior or characteristics of interest. This is usually done through literature review or observation. Next comes the selection of the subjects to be studied. The importance of this step revolves around the knowledge that correlation coefficients are situation-specific. That is, the same correlation between variables would not be expected under varying conditions or types of subjects involved. For example the correlation between height and weight would not necessarily be the same for elementary aged females and high school aged males. Thus the choice of subjects used in a correlation study dictates the specific group to which generalizations may be made (see the box on p. 231).

Regular sampling procedures, described elsewhere in this text, are required if generalizations are to be made beyond the set of subjects actually used (as in prediction, for example).

Measurement of the subjects on the variables selected is the next step. As with any research study, care and precision in taking these measurements help increase data reliability and validity.

Analyzing the data comes next, and as mentioned, the particular statistical technique employed will depend on the measurement level of the scores obtained, the purpose of the study (for example, exploration or prediction), and other factors. The various correlational statistics and when they are used will be presented in Chapter 10.

Example of Correlation in Sport and Exercise Science

Fanship and the Television Sports Viewing Experience

Walter Gantz and Lawrence A. Wenner

Employing a uses and gratification paradigm, we expected that audience experience with televised sports would vary on the basis of fanship, with fans having a qualitatively different, deeper, and more textured set of expectations and responses than nonfans. Fans were expected to respond in similar ways, regardless of gender. Telephone interviews were completed with 707 adults residing in Los Angeles and Indianapolis. Fanship was operationalized using cognitive, affective, and behavioral bases. In this study, fanship made a difference, with fans clearly more invested in the viewing experience. Male and female sports fans reacted and responded in almost identical ways, although men generally were an insignificant shade more involved than women. However, since more males are fans, the televised sports viewing experience in many households may not be shared, even when husbands and wives watch the same TV sports program.

Relationship between Fanship and Exposure Motivations

| | Pearson Correlation Coefficients | | | Mean Responses | | | | |
	Males	Females	Total sample	Males Nonfan	Fan	Females Nonfan	Fan	Total sample
It's something to do with friends or family	.07	.02	-.02	3.2	3.5	4.1	4.1	3.8
It gives me something to talk about	.24	.29	.27	2.6	4.4	1.4	3.7	3.2
It gets me psyched up	.29	.37	.34	2.9	5.2	1.2	4.5	3.5
It's a good way to let off steam	.27	.31	.31	2.3	4.3	0.9	3.5	3.0
It lets me relax and unwind	.30	.37	.38	4.5	6.8	2.7	6.0	5.1
I like the drama and tension involved	.33	.40	.40	5.1	7.3	3.0	6.9	5.7
It's something to do when there's nothing else going on	.09	.06	.06	4.0	4.6	3.7	4.1	4.2
It's something to watch when there's nothing else on TV	.05	.01	.01	3.8	4.4	3.8	3.8	4.0

From Gantz W and Wenner LA: Sociology of Sport Journal 12(1):56, 66-67, 1995.

CORRELATION AND CAUSATION

The existence of a correlation between two variables cannot be taken alone as proof that one is causing the other to occur. For example, if we determine the existence of a correlation between years of being in physical education classes and being healthy, it would be tempting to advocate that exposure to physical education makes you healthy. While this may be true, just the existence of this correlation does not prove it. For example, it may be that some individuals have more exposure to physical education classes because they stayed in school longer, thus becoming better educated, resulting in higher paying jobs and thus greater access to health care. In other words, behind the seemingly straightforward correlation between any two variables may be connections to a third variable or even a fourth, fifth, and so on. Statistical methods exist to explore these types of possibilities but it is important for researchers to remember that the discovery of a correlation does not prove the existence of a cause-and-effect relationship, it only provides for the possibility. It usually requires experimental research designs to eventually confirm or deny the causal relationship.

META-ANALYSIS

Empirical research is pouring in from all directions. This is true in many fields of inquiry including sport and exercise science. How does one make sense of it all? It seems impossible to organize it and combine it in any lucid and meaningful way.

One approach is to integrate studies narratively. Occasionally a reviewer will undertake the task of accumulating a large number of studies focusing on a single topic but concluded from a variety of directions and attempt to draw integrative conclusions. These reviews are often helpful and insightful. Their worth, of course, is heavily dependent on the ability of the reviewer.

Meta-analysis is a quantitative approach for analyzing the conclusions drawn from a large number of empirical studies. As with any statistical analysis its purpose is the reduction of information and generalization. Meta-analysis, however, uses other studies as data points rather than individual measurements of subjects.

Method

Studies relating to the question of interest are located throughout an exhaustive literature search. For each study located, relevant information dealing with the types of treatments administered, pertinent information about the subjects used, nature of the experimental design, and the effect size is gathered. The effect size is the treatment mean minus the control mean divided by the standard deviation of the control group. The effect size numerically represents the effect of the study. These measurements are then treated statistically to determine overall conclusions.

The above paragraph is somewhat misleading in that the work involved, the decisions to be made, and the issues to be resolved are much more complex than just listing the steps conveys. For example, the material in Chapter 4 of this book should give you some sense of the enormity of the task of reviewing the literature. For an excellent treatment of this research method we recommend "Meta-Analysis in Social Research" by Glass, McGraw, and Smith (1981).

SUMMARY

The methods employed by researchers are usually dictated by what questions they seek to answer, the availability and form of the data they require, as well as many practical considerations such as availability of subjects, costs, and skills of the investigator. Many research questions could be examined from a variety of directions equally effectively while others may have just one or two effective methods. For example, it would be ethically objectional to propose an experimental study to determine if smoking causes cancer by assigning some human subjects to a smoking group and others to a control group. A correlational or epidemiological method would be appropriate in this case. No matter what methods are employed, assuming moral appropriateness, the keys for you to evaluate are the completeness and precision with which the research was conducted.

EXERCISES

1 Look for surveys in some popular news magazines, such as *Time* and *Newsweek.* Read through the article and determine how well issues such as survey bias, precision, reliability, and validity are addressed. Look to see if margin of error statistics are reported. If so, do the findings show clear differences in opinions?

2 Try searching SPORT Discus for historical epidemiological or case study research in sport and exercise science. Pick one or two studies that appear interesting and then read in further detail.

3 Ask your professors if they employ any of the research methods discussed in this chapter. If so, ask them to recommend some reports for you to read using these methods.

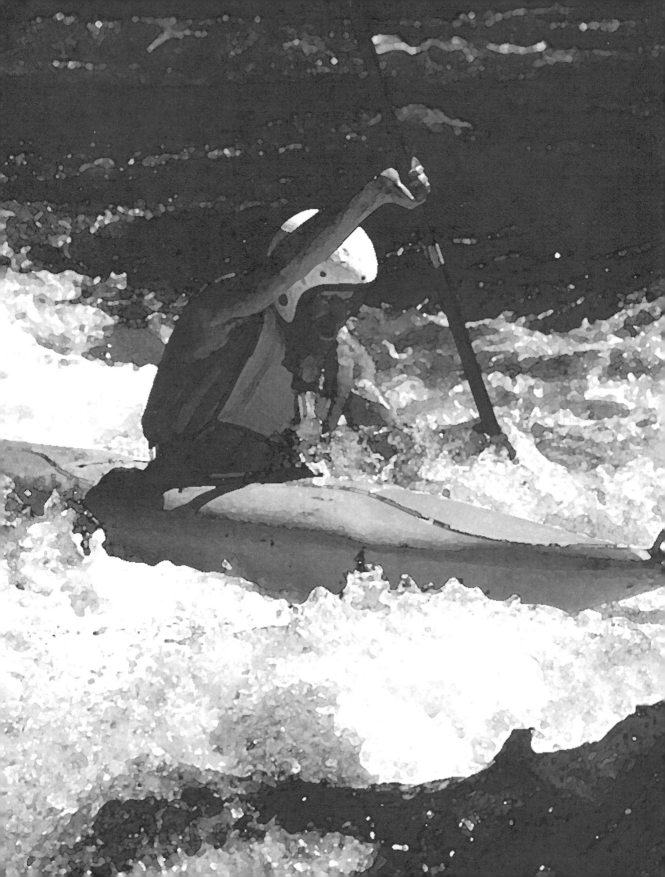

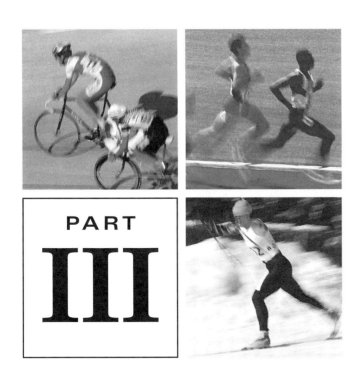

Results

Measurement, Data Analysis, and Reporting

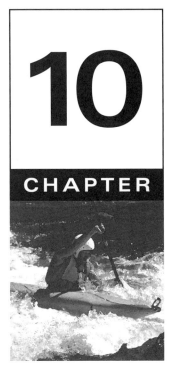

10

CHAPTER

LEARNING GOALS

After reading this chapter you will be able to:

1 Describe nominal, ordinal, interval, and ratio measurement scales.

2 Define the term *reliability*.

3 Discuss the common methods for assessing reliability.

4 Define the term *objectivity*.

5 Define the term *validity*.

6 Explain the difference between content validity, concurrent validity, predictive validity, and construct validity.

7 In general terms, distinguish between descriptive statistics and inferential statistics.

8 Explain the differences between the mean, median, and mode.

9 Describe how the range, semi-interquartial range, and the standard deviation are used in data analysis.

10 Explain how a correlation statistic describes the relationship between two variables.

11 Discuss how the results section of a quantitative research report would differ from the results section of a qualitative report.

TERMS

Measurement scales
Mean
Standard deviation
Correlation
Reliability
Objectivity
Validity

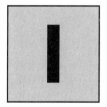n the Results section of a research report the investigator presents the findings from the statistical analysis of the data (in quantitative research). Likewise, the "data" (such as text, words, quotes, etc.) in qualitative research are also presented in the Results section. We will present information about the Results sections for various types of research paradigms in this chapter. Many students find the statistical information in a quantitative Results section initially the most difficult to understand. Our approach is to describe some of the most commonly used statistical methods in sport and exercise research to help you understand the Results section of a quantitative research report and to describe the results in a qualitative manuscript or presentation.

QUANTITATIVE MANUSCRIPT RESULTS

Typically one of the first things reported in the Results section is information about the nature and character of the outcome variables that were studied. This includes summary information that describes the sample characteristics (often presented in tabular format). Next, information about the reliability and validity of the measures is typically included. This is done to convince the reader of the quality of the instrumentation, judges, observers, tests, and so forth. This is followed by summary information that describes the sample characteristics (often presented in tabular format). The investigator is attempting to describe the subjects and the nature of the work as fully as possible. The following outlines the general presentation of a quantitative research Results section:

Scaling properties
Descriptive statistics
   Central tendency
   Variability
   Correlation
Measurement and instrumentation
   Reliability
   Validity

We will review the quantitative Results section in the order suggested on p. 240.

MEASUREMENT ISSUES
Scaling Properties

Quantitative researchers use numbers to summarize and report their results. Measurement varies from simple to complex depending on certain rules or principles. **Measurement scales** refer to the level of information obtained through the measurement process. It is important to realize that not all numbers are identical in nature or purpose. Depending upon the nature of the particular number that is reported as a result of the research process, certain numerical calculations may or may not be legitimate. Determining the scale of measurements helps to better understand the numbers reported by researchers.

Nominal scale—The simplest level of measurement is called *nominal* measurement. The nominal level of measurement permits only the making of statements of sameness or difference. For example, level of class standing (freshman, sophomore, junior, or senior), gender (male or female), or health risk factor (smoker or non-smoker) are all nominal measures. Referring to the nominal scale as a measurement scale is, in a sense, a little misleading. The nominal scale might be better thought of as a classification scale. Note that it is inappropriate to think about averaging or summing such numbers. For example, it makes no sense to think of the "average gender" simply because males are coded "0" and females are coded "1." It is, however, appropriate to speak about the frequency with which a particular number occurs (such as, there are 10 males and 12 females).

Ordinal scale—The *ordinal* scale adds a second level of information not present with the nominal scale—an indication of rank-order among scores. Thus the ordinal scale of measurement permits the ordering of subjects (or scores) in addition to statements of sameness or difference. When you look at the baseball standings in the newspaper and see that the Giants are in first place, the Rockies are in second place, and the Dodgers are in third place, you are looking at an ordinal measurement scale. The advantage of the ordinal scale is that we can make judgments about one thing compared to another. For example, we can usually tell if the temperature outdoors today is warmer or colder than yesterday, Yet, we have a difficult time judging if the difference is 3° or 5°. We recognize that the temperatures are different (classification) and we sense that today is warmer (ordering) than yesterday. The disadvantage of the ordinal scale is it does not provide any information on exactly how far apart each unit being measured is from another. Just looking at the baseball standing by rank order does not tell us if the Giants are one game, three games, or 10 games ahead of the second-place team.

Interval scale—The *interval* scale contains even more information than the ordinal scale. The interval scale contains information on interval width and order, but a score of 0 does not indicate a complete absence of the quality being measured. Many tests of motor ability or motor skill are interval scale measures. For example, if one student scored 20 on a tennis skills test, and another student scored 40 on the same test, we could conclude that the second student is more skillful (order) and that the second student scored 20 points higher on the test than the first (distance between scores), but we cannot say the second student is twice as skilled as the first because a score of 0 does not mean that there is complete absence of any tennis skill. Another example of an interval scale is temperature in Fahrenheit. We know the difference between 10° and 20° is the same difference as the difference between 40° and 50° (equal units) but since 0° F does not mean a complete absence of heat we can not say the 40° is twice as warm as 20°.

Ratio scale—The *ratio* scale contains the most information of all the measurement scales. Physical measures such as weight, volume, distance, or time are ratio scale measures. Because the ratio scale does have a "true" zero point, it is possible to state that a 10 pound weight is twice as heavy as a 5-pound weight or a ball thrown 50 yards went five times farther than a ball thrown 10 yards. The ratio scale of measurement permits statements about ratios, such as one variable is twice another, in addition to statements of sameness or difference, greater or less than, and equality of intervals. Referring back to the baseball standings example, the column that shows how many games behind the first place team the other teams are is a ratio scale measure. Baseball standings, as well as those for other team sports, provide information about each team with ordinal, internal, and ratio scale measures. The boxes below and on p. 244 illustrate the detail that authors use to describe the measures obtained in their studies. Note that each author presents the score values and interpretation. The "total" score used in each of these studies was interval in scale.

An Examination of Personal/Situational Variables, Stress Appraisal, and Burnout in Collegiate Teacher-Coaches

Betty C. Kelley and Diane L. Gill

Following Smith's (1986) cognitive-affective model of stress and burnout in athletics, this investigation examined (a) the relationship of personal/ situational variables (social support, gender, and years of experience) to stress appraisal and (b) the relationship of stress appraisal (perceived stress, coaching issues, and role conflict) to burnout. Male (n = 99) and female (n = 115) teacher-head basketball coaches from NCAA Division III and NAIA colleges completed established measures of burnout, perceived stress, teacher-coach role conflict, and social support and a measure of coaching issues developed for this study. Multivariate analyses supported the hypothesized relationships. Specifically, greater satisfaction with social support, less experience, and gender (females higher) were related to stress appraisal, and all stress appraisal variables were positively related to burnout. Contrary to previous studies, these teacher-coaches reported moderate to high levels of burnout.

Measures

Coaching Issues Survey: The Coaching Issues Survey (CIS) is a 32-item instrument developed for this investigation to assess the stress associated with various coaching issues. The CIS is based on the 60-item Degree of Stress instrument developed by Hunt (1984). Respondents rate the degree of stress attributed to each coaching issue on a 6-point Likert-type scale ranging from "no stress" (0) to "extreme stress" (5). Initial content validity was assessed with 14 dual-role teacher-coaches from colleges in the upper Midwest who completed the 60-item survey and participated in an in-depth interview to develop the revised 32-item measure.

Continued.

From Kelley BC and Gill DL: Research Quarterly for Exercise and Sport 64(1):92-102, 1993.

An Examination of Personal/Situational Variables, Stress Appraisal, and Burnout in Collegiate Teacher-Coaches—cont'd

Respondents' survey and interview responses were similar on the issue of "what causes stress for themselves within the sport-specific environment of coaching." Respondents also identified issues that they thought "did not belong or were out of place." Items were discarded if less than half of the respondents did not perceive stress on this item, and items were added based on open-ended responses and interview data. The revised 32-item CIS was then pilot tested for this study with 52 NCAA Division III coaches. Coaches consistently expressed the opinion that the items included in the final survey were relevant to the general coaching situation and were, for the most part, highly characteristic of their own situations. Four sample items from the CIS are "understanding my athletes' emotional responses and motivations"; "budget limitations hampering recruiting"; "not successfully fulfilling my responsibilities outside my coaching duties (teaching)"; and "placing pressure on myself to win." Internal consistency was demonstrated with an alpha coefficient of .89.

Psychological Consequences of Athletic Injury among High-Level Competitors

Matthew H. Leddy, Michael J. Lambert, and Benjamin M. Ogles

Injury prohibiting continued athletic participation has been hypothesized to have a predictable emotional impact on athletes (Rotella and Heyman, 1986). However, the psychological impact of injury has not been well documented. This study examined the psychological reactions to injury among 343 male collegiate athletes participating in 10 sports. All athletes were assessed using measures of depression, anxiety, and self-esteem during preseason physical examinations. Injured athletes along with matched controls were later assessed within one week of experiencing an athletic injury and 2 months later. A 4 × 3 (Injury Status × Time of Testing) repeated measures multivariate analysis of variance (DM MANOVA) revealed that injured athletes exhibited greater depression and anxiety and lower self-esteem than controls immediately following physical injury and at follow-up 2 months later. These findings supported the general observation that physically injured athletes experience a period of emotional distress that in some cases may be severe enough to warrant clinical intervention.

Continued.

From Leddy MH, Lambert MJ, and Ogles BM: Research Quarterly for Exercise and Sport 65(4):347-354, 1994.

Psychological Consequences of Athletic Injury among High-Level Competitors—cont'd

Instrumentation

In order to assess the psychological impact of injury, three widely used clinical instruments were administered to all subjects: the Beck Depression Inventory, the State-Trait Anxiety Inventory–Form Y, and the Tennessee Self-Concept Scale. Clinical instruments were selected, as opposed to sport-specific measures, in order to investigate the clinical impact of injury on athletes. Trait measures of anxiety and self-esteem were included to assess the potential impact of injury on more dispositional psychological characteristics of athletes. Since sport participation may be an important part of an athlete's identity, injury may have an impact on more stable psychological characteristics. In addition, a demographic and training questionnaire was administered to all subjects.

Beck Depression Inventory (BDI): The Beck Depression Inventory (Beck, Ward, Mendelson, Mock, and Erbaugh, 1961) is a 21-item self-report inventory that measures the intensity of common depressive symptoms and attitudes. Each symptom is rated for intensity from 0 to 3. A total score is then calculated by summing the ratings for each of the 21 items. Total scores range from 0 to 63. Higher scores reflect the presence of more intense depressive symptoms.

The types of scales differ in the amount of information they provide and this leads to potential restrictions in the use of mathematical operations and the interpretations of the actual numbers obtained. The ratio scale provides the most information, followed in descending order by the interval, ordinal, and nominal scales. In addition, the measurement scale partially determines the choice of possible statistical analysis. Table 10.1 shows the four measurement scales and the descriptive statistics normally used with measures made on these scales.

DESCRIPTIVE STATISTICS AND DATA ANALYSIS

Data consist of scores or values taken on objects or subjects. Statisticians have developed methods used to summarize and describe data. They have also developed methods that allow them to draw conclusions and make statements about causal

TABLE 10.1	Four Measurement Scales and Descriptive Statistics			
Level of measurement	**Purpose of the measure**			
	Central tendency	**Variability**	**Individual position**	**Association**
Nominal	Mode	Number of cases	Uniqueness	Chi-square
Ordinal	Median	Range	Percentile rank	Rank-order correlation
Interval and ratio	Mean	Standard deviation	Standard scores	Pearson's Correlation

relationships. These two activities are accomplished using descriptive statistics and inferential statistics.

What Are Descriptive Statistics?

Descriptive statistics are the methods used to report a data set in summarized form. When you read the sports section of the newspaper, descriptive statistics are used to convey information about such things as batting averages, average points per game, and many others. In health, sport, and exercise research, statistics are used extensively to describe the behavior of the subjects in experiments or in other forms of research. Our discussion of the most common descriptive methods begins in the next section on measures of central tendency.

The term *statistics* has several meanings. The academic discipline of statistics is a branch of mathematics providing researchers with methods used to analyze data. These methods include actions such as organizing, summarizing, or manipulating data so we can describe the characteristics of the data and draw conclusions. Statistics also provide us with facts about a sample of subjects that served in an investigation such average age, height, and so on. Statistics are also information. Take a look in the sports section of the newspaper and you'll find a wealth of statistical information. Or, look at the Results section of a journal article and you will also find tables, figures, and other numerical information. Both the statistics in the sports section and the statistics in the Results section serve the same purpose—they provide the reader with information.

Inferential Statistics

Descriptive statistics are easy to understand and are used commonly in everything from advertisements to newspapers to research reports. As common as descriptive statistics are, the appearance of inferential statistics in lay literature is as equally rare. The term *inferential* is the adjective form of the word infer, which means to conclude from facts. Inferential statistics are used to support statements of fact based on information gathered from research. Essentially, the researcher gathers data on a sample and infers to the population from which the sample data were obtained. Our discussion on inferential statistics continues in Chapter 11.

MEASURES OF CENTRAL TENDENCY

One of the most important and useful characteristics of a data set is the location of its center point. Because the definition of the center point varies, several measures of central tendency exist. The computational procedures for obtaining three of them—the median, the mean, and the mode—and the advantages and disadvantages of each are presented below.

The Median

The *median* of a distribution is the point on the score scale below and above which 50% of the scores fall. The median, usually represented by the symbol Mdn, is the 50th percentile (P_{50}) of a distribution. A percentile represents the percentage of observations that fall at or below a given point. If you score at the eighty-fifth percentile on an examination, that means that 85% of the individuals scored the same value as you or below. The median is determined by locating the middle point of a distribution. With data arranged in chronological order, this is merely a counting procedure. The formula, (N + 1)/2, where N is the total number of scores, can be used to determine the location of the median. Notice that when the number of scores (N) in a distribution is odd, the middle point, as determined by this formula, will be a whole number. For example, if a distribution contains 15 scores, the middle point is the eighth score [(15 + 1)/2 = 8]. Thus, if the 15 scores are arranged in chronological order, the eighth score from the bottom (or top) is the median. However, when the number of scores in a distribution is even, the middle point is not a whole number. If, for example, a distribution contains 16 scores, the middle point is the 8.5th score [(16 + 1)/2 = 8.5]. Since, in reality, there is no 8.5th score, the median is taken to be midway between the eighth and ninth scores.

The median, by its definition, is related to the *position of the scores* rather than the *actual values* of the scores. This fact is illustrated by noticing that the median for each of the two following distributions is the same:

Distribution A	1, 2, 6, 12, 14	Mdn = 6
Distribution B	1, 2, 6, 12, 114	Mdn = 6

From this example it can also be seen that the value of an extreme score (114 in distribution B) does not alter the value of the median. Because the median is not affected by extreme score values it is often referred to as the "most typical" score in a distribution. You will discover that in most sport and exercise studies, the median is usually not reported unless the data deviate greatly from a normal distribution (for example, the data are skewed).

The Mean

The **mean** of a set of scores is simply the arithmetic average of the scores, or in other words, the point on the score scale that corresponds to the sum of the set of scores divided by the number of scores in the set. The mean is what you probably think of as the average. Unlike the median, it is not necessary that the scores be listed in chronological order to facilitate computation of the mean. It is only necessary to determine the algebraic sum of all the scores in the distribution and the number of scores contributing to that sum. The symbolic representation of the definition of the mean is:

$$\bar{X} = \frac{\Sigma X}{N}$$

where

$\bar{X}$ (read, X bar) = symbol for the mean
Σ = the sum of
X = each individual score in the distribution
N = the total number of scores in the distribution

The most important characteristic of the mean is the fact that *every score* in the distribution affects the value of the mean. A change in any score will change the value of the mean. Previously two distributions were presented to show that the value of an extreme score has no effect on the value of the median. Notice, however, the effect of this same extreme score on the mean:

		Median	Mean
Distribution A	1, 2, 6, 12, 14	6	7.0
Distribution B	1, 2, 6, 12, 114	6	27.0

Of course, if the score that changes is not an extreme score but rather one close to the mean, the value of the mean will not change dramatically, but it will nevertheless change. Consider the following two distributions and means:

		Mean
Distribution A	1, 2, 6, 12, 14	7.0
Distribution C	1, 2, 8, 12, 14	7.4

The property of being affected by every score in a distribution results in the mean being the most sensitive of the three measures of central tendency. It is this characteristic that makes it the most valuable in a mathematical sense. You will see that the mean is by far the most commonly reported measure of central tendency in sport and exercise research. Scores must be measured at the interval or ratio level to use the mean as a measure of central tendency.

The Mode

The *mode* of a set of scores is simply the value of the most frequently occurring score. An inspection of the data (more easily accomplished if the data are arranged in numerical order) is all that is needed to determine the mode.

In a distribution where each score only occurs once (as in 1, 2, 6, 12, 14) or every score occurs more than once but with the same frequency (as in 1, 1, 2, 2, 6, 6, 12, 12, 14, 14), a mode cannot be determined. In a situation where two adjacent or nearly adjacent scores occur with equal frequency higher than the frequency of other scores, the mode is usually considered to be the mean of the two equally occurring scores. (The mode for a set of scores containing the values 1, 1, 2, 2, 6, 6, 6, 7, 7, 7, 12, 12, 14, 14 would be considered to be 6.5.) However, when two scores that are not close together both occur with the same frequency (higher than for other scores), the distribution is described as *bimodal.* In other words, both scores would be considered modes. In a practical sense, the mode is of limited value because it is subject to judgment and does not lend itself to algebraic manipulation. Because the mode is a relatively crude measure of central tendency, it has little meaning unless the number of scores in the distribution is quite large. As such, it is uncommon to report the mode in a research article.

Comparison of the Median, Mean, and Mode

The word *average* is a common term used to indicate a measure of central tendency. Although to most the word *average* is synonymous with the mean, the median and mode are also classified as averages. When reporting data it is important to specify which average has been computed. It is equally important to determine which average is being referred to by others reporting results. The example below demonstrates this importance.

A realtor was interested in influencing potential customers into buying a particular house. Attempting to indicate the desirable features of the area in which the house was located, the realtor informed potential customers that the average yearly income of the seven families on the block where the house was located was over $50,000. In fact, the yearly incomes of the seven families were $20,000, $24,000, $26,000, $28,000, $28,000, $30,000, and $200,000. It is true that the mean yearly income of the seven families was over $50,000, but it is also true that only one of the seven families had an income over $50,000. In this case, as a result of the presence of an extreme score, the median income ($28,000) represents a less misleading average.

Selection of an Average

In almost all cases in sport and exercise research, the mean is preferred and is reported most often. It is easily calculated, exactly defined, and amenable to algebraic manipulation. When extreme scores such as the $200,000 yearly income in the example above are present in a set of data, the median becomes the proper average. The mode, the least useful average, is seldom reported in research, but does have uses. For example, a clothing company needs to know which size of a given garment is sold most often and can tune their orders based on this information. However, where a mean or median can be usefully calculated, the mode is seldom used.

In summary, the value of the median is not influenced by the particular values of the data but by their order and frequency. The value of the mean is not affected by the order of the data but by their values and frequency. Finally, the value of the mode is not influenced by the particular value or order of the data but only by their frequency.

MEASURES OF VARIABILITY

Thus far the characteristics of central tendency have been examined. Central tendency yields some valuable information but it is not sufficient in itself to completely describe a data set. The average only paints part of the picture that we need to fully appreciate the characteristics of a data set. Consider the following two sets of scores:

| Distribution D | 2, 28, 50, 50, 72, 98 |
| Distribution E | 41, 47, 50, 50, 50, 53, 59 |

The mean, median, and mode for both distributions are all equal to 50, but the two sets of scores have obvious differences. It becomes apparent that other characteristics must be examined to describe a set of scores adequately.

The most evident difference between distributions D and E is the disparity in the distance between extreme scores. This characteristic is referred to variously as dispersion, deviation, spread, scatter, and variability. As with central tendency, there are several statistics used to describe this characteristic.

The Range

The *range* is the measure of variability represented by the highest number in the data set minus the lowest number in the set. As such, calculation is simply a matter of determining the highest score and the lowest score and finding the difference between the two scores: high score – low score (the range is also sometimes found by high score – low score + 1). This is actually a more precise mathematical definition of the range but as the distance between the highest and lowest score increases the +1 becomes less significant. Regardless of which is used, the range is dependent on only two scores in a distribution—the highest and the lowest.

Although the range is the simplest measure of central tendency to obtain, it is also the least adequate. Its weakness lies in the fact that it does not account for the variability among any scores in a distribution except the two extreme scores. Because of this, two sets of data could vary greatly in respect to the compactness of their scores and yet have the same range. Further, the range is a misleading indicator of variability when an unusually low or high score occurs in the data.

The Semi-Interquartile Range

To overcome some of the weaknesses of the range as a measure of central tendency, the distance between two specified points within a distribution is sometimes used to describe the characteristic dispersion of the scores. The most common measure of this type is known at the *semi-interquartile range.*

The semi-interquartile range is half the distance between the 75th and the 25th percentile scores. The initial step in calculating its value is to determine what score points in the distribution correspond to the 75th and 25th percentiles. Calculation is similar to that for the median (the 50th percentile), except the points we are determining are such that 25% and 75% of the scores fall below them:

$$\text{Semi-Interquartile Range} = \frac{\text{75th Percentile} - \text{25th Percentile}}{2}$$

The semi-interquartile range functions more adequately than the range as a measure of variability because it is more stable; that is, it is less likely to be influenced by extreme scores. However, the semi-interquartile range has two serious shortcomings that limit its usefulness as a statistic to describe variability. It does not take into account the value of each individual score within the data, and it would be possible for two distributions to have very similar semi-interquartile range values and yet end scores that vary widely. Therefore, except when a crude but fairly stable measure of variability is all that is required, it is seldom worth the extra effort to calculate the semi-interquartile range even though it is in some ways an improvement over the range. Because of this, the semi-interquartile range is not reported very often in research. It is most often seen when the median is reported as the measure of central tendency (for example, with skewed data).

The Standard Deviation

Ideally a measure of variability should reflect the distance between each score in the distribution and the center of the distribution. One possible way to obtain such a value would be to determine the amount by which each score deviates from the mean. These deviation values could then be summed to obtain an indication of the variability of the distribution since, if the scores were widely scattered, the resulting sum would be greater than if the scores were all fairly close to the center of the distribution. However, if this procedure is followed in a strict algebraic sense, the resulting sum will *always equal zero.*

For example, consider the following distribution:

Scores	Mean	Deviation
14	7	7
12	7	5
6	7	−1
2	7	−5
1	7	−6
		$\Sigma = 0$

To remove this problem, the squared values of the deviations could be used. The squares are summed and then divided by the number of scores in the distribution. (The denominator is actually N − 1 but this won't make much difference with large samples.) To return to the units of the original scores, the square root of the resulting quotient is obtained. The measure is named the **standard deviation** and is symbolically defined as follows:

$$SD = \sqrt{\frac{\Sigma x^2}{N-1}} \qquad x = (X - \bar{X})$$

where

SD = standard deviation
Σ = the sum of
x^2 = each deviation score, squared
N − 1 = the total number of scores in the distribution minus one
X = the mean

The following example, using the distribution above, is provided to clarify the computational procedures in determining the standard deviation from the definitional formula:

Scores	Mean	Deviation	Deviation squared
14	7	7	49
12	7	5	25
6	7	−1	1
2	7	−5	25
1	7	−6	36
$\Sigma = 35$		$\Sigma = 0$	$\Sigma = 136$

$$SD = \sqrt{\frac{\Sigma x^2}{N-1}}$$

$$= \sqrt{\frac{136}{5-1}}$$

$$= \sqrt{34}$$

$$= 5.83$$

Direct calculation of the standard deviation using the definitional formula presented above can become a tedious task. Fortunately, through algebraic manipulation of the definitional formula, it is possible to arrive at a computational formula that yields the sum of squares of the deviations without actually determining each deviation value:

$$SD = \sqrt{\frac{\Sigma X^2 - N \bar{X}^2}{N-1}}$$

where

SD = standard deviation
Σ = the sum of
X^2 = each score squared
$N - 1$ = the total number of scores minus one
$\bar{X}^2$ = the mean, squared

The example below shows that the computational formula and the definitional formula produce the same results:

Scores	Scores squared
14	196
12	144
6	36
2	4
1	1
$\Sigma X = 35$	$\Sigma X^2 = 381$
$\bar{X} = 7$	

$$SD = \sqrt{\frac{381 - 5(7^2)}{5-1}}$$

$$= \sqrt{\frac{381 - 245}{5-1}}$$

$$= \sqrt{\frac{136}{4}}$$

$$= \sqrt{34}$$

$$= 5.83$$

The definitional and computational formulas presented here are used to describe the variability of a data set from data taken from a sample from the population. Inferential statistics, which will be discussed in more detail later, is concerned with estimating population values based on values obtained from samples of the population. As explained in Chapter 5, in most research it is impossible to measure every member of a population (nor is it necessary), so a sample is obtained and estimates about the population are made from the sample data. When working with population values the denominator (N − 1) is changed to N. This difference is pointed out because most hand calculators provide separate keys for calculating the population standard deviation (denominator is N) or the sample standard deviation (denominator is N − 1). The notation used on the calculator varies from brand to brand, so you should consult your operating manual. For most research oriented class assignments or projects you will use the sample standard deviation formula (N − 1).

It is important to note that if the standard deviation is added to and subtracted from the mean, approximately 68% of the scores will be included. The following is approximately true for a normal distribution:

$$X \pm 1SD = 68\%$$
$$X \pm 2SD = 95\%$$
$$X \pm 3SD = 99.7\%$$

Obviously, most scores will lie within ± 3SD of the mean.

Considerations of Measures of Variability

Interpretation of measures of variability is more difficult than that of measures of central tendency. The standard deviation, with all its mathematical niceties, is far more easily defined in terms of symbols than in terms of words. Measures of variability reflect the average amount of *deviation* from a center point among the scores in a distribution, whereas measures of central tendency reflect an average *position* in the distribution. Put another way, a measure of central tendency represents a particular point; a measure of variability represents a particular distance.

In research it is essential to report both a measure of central tendency and a measure of variability. For many reasons, in most research studies the two values reported are the mean and the standard deviation.

CORRELATION

The techniques previously explained for arranging, describing, and interpreting data primarily involve one set of scores. Sometimes researchers are interested in comparing two or more sets of scores. For example, the health, sport, or exercise researcher may be interested in determining the relationship between strength gains and the diameter of muscle fibers during a weight training program. Or, the researcher might investigate whether free-weights are more or less effective than weight machines for efficient strength gains. Various measures of association are used to test whether or not these relationships are significant. Our purpose here is to present correlational statistics which are descriptive in nature. We will return to the correlation as an inferential statistic in Chapter 11.

Correlation Techniques

When measures of two traits are obtained for a group of subjects it may be noticed that the scores for each subject tend to be related in some way. For example, they may have approximately the same relative position in each distribution.

The **correlation** coefficient can be used as a method of quantifying these relationships. The correlation coefficient includes all the values from +1.00 to −1.00. The sign indicates the direction of the relationship (positive or negative). The absolute value of the coefficient indicates the strength of the relationship (the typical evaluation is strong 1.0 − .80; moderate .79 − .50; weak .49 − .20; or poor .19 − 0.0). A perfect correlation is indicated by a coefficient of 1.00 (either positive or negative). A correlation coefficient of 0.00 indicates that no correlation exists (the two variables are unrelated to each other).

For example, what do you think the correlation is between grade point average and the number of hours studying? Is more time studying associated with higher or lower grades? Will long hours of studying always result in high scores? Will no studying always result in low grades? Or, is time studying unrelated to grades? The scatter plots in Figure 10.1 show some of the possible relationships between study time and grades. Which of these do you think is the most

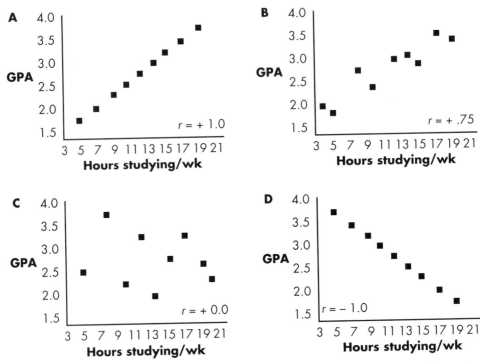

FIGURE 10.1 Scatter plots showing some possible relationships between time studying and GPA.

accurate? The axes in a scatter plot list the values for the two variables being studied. An intepretation is then based on the relationship identified. Each of the scatter plots in Figure 10.1 results in a different interpretation. The box on p. 259 illustrates the author's reporting of correlations (*r*).

Calculation of Correlation Coefficients

Karl Pearson, an English statistician, introduced a measure of relationship called the Pearson Product Moment Correlation Coefficient, *r*. Various formulas are available for calculating *r*—the formula given below represents a commonly used variation:

$$r = \frac{S_{xy}}{S_x S_y}$$

Perceived Exertion and Affect at Varying Intensities of Running

Edmund O. Acevedo, Karl F. Rinehardt, and Robert R. Kraemer

Results

Descriptive characteristics

Descriptive characteristics revealed that all subjects demonstrated a high level of fitness. This is represented by VO_{2max} values (males = 76.77 ± 4.40 ml · kg⁻¹ · min⁻¹ and females = 59.55 ± 6.40 ml · kg⁻¹ · min⁻¹), body compositions assessed by underwater weighing techniques (males = 10.04 ± 3.28% fat and females = 20.24 ± 5.36% fat), and training distances per week (males = 123.80 ± 49.30 km and females = 106.90 ± 46.00 km). In addition, running speeds (RS) demonstrated the running ability of these subjects. For males, RS ranged from 5.97 ± .07 min/mile to 4.51 ± .08 min/mile. For females, RS ranged from 7.19 ± .19 min/mile to 5.57 ± .13 min/mile.

Correlational analyses

Ratings of perceived exertion and the FS were strongly and negatively correlated after RS1 ($r = -.80$) and moderately after RS2 ($r = -.58$) and after RS5 ($r = -.59$). Thus, those runners who rated RPE higher tended to rate affect more negative after running at low and high intensities. However, this was not the case following runs that were at moderate speeds ($r = -.23$ for RS3 and $r = -.16$ for RS4). Across all workloads, RPE and the FS were highly correlated to HR ($r = .75$ and $r = -.63$, respectively) and moderately with La ($r = .55$ and $r = -.42$, respectively).

From Acevedo EO, Rinehardt KF, and Kraemer RR: Research Quarterly for Exercise and Sport 65(4):372-376, 1994.

where

S_{xy} = covariance of the X and Y variable
S_x = standard deviation of the X variable
S_y = standard deviation of the Y variable

where

$$S_{xy} = \frac{\Sigma XY - N\overline{X}\,\overline{Y}}{N-1}$$

where

ΣXY = sum of each X score times its corresponding Y score
N = number of pairs of scores
$\overline{X}\,\overline{Y}$ = mean of the X variable times the mean of the Y variable

Since we usually calculate the mean and standard deviation of a data set, this formula allows us to find r with only a few more calculations. The following data are height and weight measurements taken on 10 elementary school children.

Height and weight data for 10 subjects

Subject	Height (X)	Weight (Y)	XY
1	50	49	2450
2	52	62	3224
3	55	69	3795
4	53	65	3445
5	54	72	3888
6	56	78	4368
7	57	70	3990
8	57	73	4161
9	58	75	4350
10	56	83	4648
	Mean = 54.80	Mean = 69.60	Sum = 38319
	SD = 2.53	SD = 9.43	

The values necessary to determine r for the 10 pairs of measurements are as follows:

$$S_{xy} = \frac{38319 - [10\,(54.8 \times 69.6)]}{10 - 1}$$

$$= \frac{38319 - 38140.8}{10 - 1}$$

$$= \frac{178.2}{9}$$

$$= 19.80$$

$$r = \frac{19.80}{2.53 \times 9.43}$$

$$= .83$$

The resulting correlation between height and weight for the 10 students is +.83. The fact that the sign of the correlation is positive is not surprising if an examination is made of the data and of the graph below. As children grow taller, they tend to weigh more. The strength of the relationship

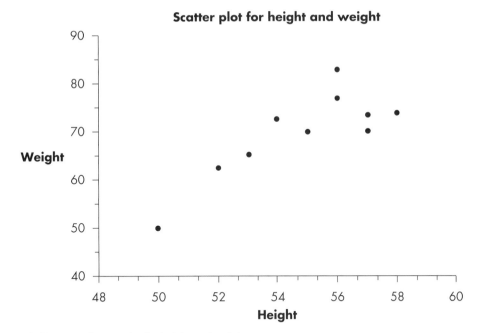

FIGURE 10.2   Scatter plot for height and weight.

between the two traits is given by the absolute value of the correlation coefficient, namely .83, which in most situations would be considered a strong correlation. In other words, there is a predictable, but not a perfect relationship between height and weight.

Figure 10.2 is called a scatter plot and provides a visual image of the relationship between two sets of scores. Each point on the scatter plot represents a pair of scores for one subject. Subject 1 is 50 inches tall, weighs 50 pounds and is represented by the lower left point on the graph. From the scatter plot, it is easy to see that as height increases, generally so does body weight.

INTERPRETATION OF CORRELATION COEFFICIENTS

Two parts of the correlation coefficient, the sign and the actual value, require interpretation. As mentioned previously the sign of a correlation coefficient indicates the direction of the relationship, and the value of a correlation coefficient denotes the degree to which the sets of scores are related.

Sign

A positive sign preceding a correlation coefficient signifies a relationship in which the high scores in one distribution are associated with the high scores of the second distribution. A negative sign in front of a correlation coefficient signifies that the high scores in one distribution are associated with the low scores in another. The sign of a correlation coefficient indicates nothing about the strength of the relationship that exists between the sets of scores. A negative correlation can have a positive meaning if a low score indicates a good performance in one set of the scores (for example, golf scores).

Absolute Value

The absolute value of the correlation coefficient denotes the strength of the relationship that exists between sets of scores. Once the correlation is obtained it is necessary to interpret this value.

If only general descriptions of the degree of relationship are required, visual inspection of a scatter plot will probably be sufficient. But being more precise, even with the correlation coefficient, is difficult. With the exception of $r = .00$ and $r = \pm1.00$, various word descriptions are used to describe an association between sets of scores. Often researchers will present the square of the correlation coefficient which is known as the *coefficient of determination*. The coefficient of determination represents the percent variation in one of the variables that can be accounted for by the other variable. For example, if the correlation between hydrostatically determined body density and skinfold is .80, the coefficient of determination (.64) is interpreted as "64% of the variation in hydrostatically determined body density can be accounted for by differences in skinfolds" (and 36% of the variation is accounted for by other factors).

Purpose of Obtaining Correlation Coefficients

If two separate correlations are calculated and identical values of .80 result, for example, the same degree of relationship is present between each of the two sets of scores. However, depending on the purpose for which the two correlation coefficients are calculated, one might be considered high while the other, even though equal in value, might be regarded as only fair. For example, when correlation coefficients are used to report reliability, objectivity, or validity, higher values are usually expected for reliability and objectivity than for validity. This is because reliability coefficients result mainly from correlations of a test with itself whereas validity coefficients usually result from a correlation between a test and another measure of the same characteristic.

Methods of Obtaining Correlation Coefficients

Whether the value of the correlation coefficient is calculated through the use of the Pearson Product Moment Correlation Coefficient or some other calculating method, the differences in the actual value obtained generally will be only slight. However, any formula requires two sets of scores for which the correlation coefficient is calculated. The procedures for obtaining the two sets of scores can vary and the interpretation of the meaning of a particular value of the correlation coefficient is influenced by how these scores are obtained. Because some results are ordinal in nature, it is sometimes necessary to calculate a "rank order correlation" which is an estimate of the correlation coefficient based on the fact that the data are not interval or ratio in nature. Generally, rank order correlations can be interpreted and thought of in the same way as the typical Pearson Product Moment Correlation Coefficient.

Variability of Scores Affects the Correlation

Another factor influencing the interpretation of a correlation coefficient is the variability of the scores involved. Generally, if the variability of the scores is small the correlation coefficient will be less than if the variability of the scores is large. Consequently higher correlation coefficients can be expected to occur when measures are obtained from a heterogeneous group of subjects rather than from a homogeneous group. For example, consider an experiment with two groups of subjects, one skilled and one novice, both containing 10 people. The task is a 50 centimeter arm movement with a 100 millisecond

TABLE 10.2   Arm Movement Data for 10
Subjects—Goal = 100 Milliseconds

| Subject | Skilled subjects | | Novice subjects | |
	First trial	Second trial	First trial	Second trial
1	97	98	80	84
2	102	99	82	83
3	100	99	85	80
4	102	100	89	87
5	97	99	93	95
6	101	97	95	94
7	99	97	101	102
8	103	100	106	100
9	97	99	110	112
10	99	102	110	101

movement time goal. Assume that the skilled group contains subjects who can complete the movement very accurately and consistently, and the novice group contains subjects who vary from poor to excellent in their movement skill. Table 10.2 shows hypothetical data for the two groups.

The value of the correlation coefficient between the two trials in the skilled group is .17, which is considerably less than the value of .93 obtained with the novice subjects. Therefore, to interpret the meaning of a correlation coefficient it is important to be aware of some characteristics of the group from which the measurements or scores were obtained.

Exactness of Scores

Some measurements in health, sports, and exercise research can be made very accurately but others cannot. This factor too must be considered when interpreting correlation coefficients. For example, response times are relatively consistent among individuals and can be measured quite accurately with electronic equipment. Because of their nature, however, some traits such as competitiveness, anxiety, sportsmanship, and others cannot be assessed with great accuracy. As a result of its lack of precision, a test to measure competitiveness may classify a subject high one time and average another, whereas a subject who shows a fast response time on one trial will likely show a fast response time on the second trial. It is thus more difficult to achieve high correlations when inexact measures are used than when relatively precise scores can be obtained.

CONSIDERATIONS OF CORRELATION COEFFICIENTS

Three important considerations about correlation coefficients should be understood. First, a correlation is specific to the group, time, and conditions under which it is obtained. A correlation coefficient calculated on a set of scores obtained from a different group of subjects, or from the same group of subjects but at a different time, or under different conditions will probably differ somewhat from the original correlation coefficient. Therefore when considering the information conveyed by a correlation coefficient, the specific situation from which it was derived must also be considered.

A second and perhaps more important consideration regarding correlation coefficients is that, although it indicates the existence of a relationship between two sets of scores, the correlation coefficient does not necessarily imply that a cause-and-effect relationship is present. For example, a strong correlation exists between the heights of elementary school children (25 inches, 30 inches, and so on) and grade level (first grade, second grade, and so on). Logically, of course, height is not "caused" by grade level, nor is grade level "caused" by height.

A high correlation coefficient suggesting a cause-and-effect relationship may be due to the fact that both traits involved in the correlation are related to another trait (or to several other traits). For example, if a correlation coefficient between a measure of softball throwing ability and a measure of reading ability of elementary school children was calculated, the value obtained would likely be fairly high. Obviously, the ability to throw a softball well does not cause students to read well or vice versa. Instead, both of these abilities increase with age, reading as a result of training in school, and softball throwing to growth and experience.

This influence of an unobserved or unrecognized factor is termed the *third variable problem.* Any number of other "third" variables may be responsible for an observed relationship. Researchers working with correlation statistics are careful to consider alternative explanations to explain relationships between variables and to search for hidden variables.

Lastly, it is important to realize that the correlation coefficient only estimates the *linear relationship* between the variables. If the variables are curvilinearly related, the correlation coefficient might still be close to zero. A simple way to check for possible curvilinearity is to develop a scatter plot.

MEASUREMENT AND INSTRUMENTATION

Once descriptive statistics are presented, the researcher attempts to convince the reader of the quality of the data collected for analyses. Quantitative research is based on empirical observations and data collection. Observations are generally recorded by making measurements. Measurement in health, sport, and exercise research takes many forms; we can measure muscular strength, cardiorespiratory function, the center of mass of object, response time, opinions, comprehension of information, direct observation, and many others. We can even measure how well a measurement instrument works. In some health, sport, and exercise studies, measurement is a matter of finding the appropriate method or laboratory instruments to measure the variables in which we are interested: oxygen and carbon dioxide gas analyzers, force plates, or computers can provide researchers with physical measurements in exercise physiology, biomechanics, and motor learning. In areas such as sport psychology or sport sociology, the researcher may need to devise an instrument to measure the variables of interest. Health and recreation researchers may obtain measurements in the cognitive and affective domains. These measures, too, have to be as free from error as possible. *Measurement,* the act of assessing, is defined as the process of assigning numerical or symbolic values to members of a group for the purpose of distinguishing among the members on the basis of the degree to which they possess the characteristic being assessed. Measurement allows us to describe objects or variables somewhat precisely and to make comparisons with other variables or treatment conditions accurately and objectively. Unfortunately, the measurement process is not perfect.

Researchers may introduce measurement error due to inconsistent methods or procedures. For example, consistent body fat measurements using skinfold calipers require a certain level of skill on the researcher's part. If the measurements are taken in an inconsistent manner, reliability will be reduced. Research equipment can affect the reliability of the measurements. For example, the oxygen and carbon dioxide gas analyzers found in the exercise physiology lab are commonly left on 24 hours a day so that the operating temperature remains constant. This is done to maintain a constant operating environment and thus improve reliability and validity. Objectivity is particularly important when different raters or observers are used and in qualitative research studies.

There are three primary concerns when obtaining measurements: the reliability, the objectivity, and the validity of the measurements. Each of these will be considered below.

RELIABILITY

Reliability concerns the consistency or dependability of measurement. If the same score is obtained when a measurement is repeated, the measurement is said to possess high reliability.

Reliability is related to precision and the reduction of measurement error. Some traits can be measured more precisely and thus more reliably than others. For example, the distance of a long jump can be measured quite precisely whereas it is difficult to estimate one's motivation to participate in sports. Anytime a measurement is made some error is introduced, so it is recognized that any obtained score is composed of two elements, the true score component and an error component:

$$X_o = X_t + X_e$$

where X_o is the observed score, X_t is the true score, and X_e is measurement error. An important goal in measurement is to reduce measurement error as much as possible by employing careful and accurate methods. For example, when you take a multiple choice exam, your final score (X_o) is comprised of your knowledge of the topic (X_t) plus correct guesses, incorrect guesses, your mistakes, and mistakes by the grader (X_e).

Various methods have been devised for obtaining reliability estimates to accommodate the fact that various sources of errors in measurement are possible. For example, the complexities of most physical movements do not allow them to be performed the same way physiologically and anatomically every time. In addition, individual motivation states and interest levels may cause different performances. The inconsistencies in repeated measurements caused by these differences are not caused by measurement error but nevertheless must be noted when determining the appropriate reliability coefficient.

Inconsistent application of instructions and scoring procedures, differences in environmental conditions, and changes in equipment used between test administrations are examples of measurement errors that can reduce reliability. The degree to which any of these occur and thus alter scores from one administration to the next will affect the reliability of a test.

Reliability coefficients are of two general types—*interclass* and *intraclass.* Interclass reliabilities are based on the correlation between trials and intraclass reliabilities are based on variation across trials. There are important differences in reliability coefficients. Foremost among these differences is the interpretation of the reported reliability.

CALCULATING RELIABILITY COEFFICIENTS

To examine the consistency of a measuring procedure it is necessary to obtain at least two sets of scores (that is, two or more trials). The conditions under which the scores are obtained and the time between their collection introduce differing error components and thus necessitate various methods of estimating reliability. The value of the reliability coefficient will be between 0.0 and 1.00, with 0.0 indicating no reliability and 1.00 reflecting perfect reliability. Generally, researchers desire reliabilities in excess of .80. The exact reliability desired depends upon the type of instrumentation used and the relative importance of the decision to be made with the data. More important decisions reflect the need for greater reliability.

Test-Retest Method

If a test is administered twice to the same group of subjects, a correlation coefficient computed between the resulting two sets of scores will serve as an indicator of the test's reliability. A high correlation would be possible only if the subjects' scores remained consistent from one administration to the next. Since this correlation reflects stability over time, it is often referred to as *stability reliability.*

In evaluating a reliability coefficient obtained by the test-retest method, it is important to know the time interval between testing. If the test is re-administered immediately, it would be logical to assume that such factors as environmental conditions and test administration procedures would not affect the reliability coefficient although such factors as fatigue or motivation might. If a substantial amount of time occurs between testings, the fatigue factor might be eliminated but other factors, such as increases in skill because of practice, changes in strength, or differences in the environmental conditions, might affect the reliability coefficient.

If the time between testing does not exceed two or three days, the test-retest method is one of the best ways to assess the reliability of a physical performance test. If the time between testing exceeds 3 or 4 days, changes in subjects' abilities might begin to affect the reliability coefficient, and these changes should not be considered a measurement error. The test-retest method is time consuming because the entire test must be re-administered to obtain the second score to use in calculating the reliability coefficient.

Split-Halves Method

To estimate the reliability of a measuring instrument by the split-halves method, the test is split into two parts. Each part is scored and the resulting two sets of scores are correlated. A written test provides a good example. Suppose you administer a knowledge test consisting of 50 items and you want to estimate the test's reliability. You could administer the entire test a second time but this is not very feasible. The split-halves method provides an alternative method of determining reliability. Note, however, that this is not stability reliability because you are not testing the instrument's consistency across time since both half-scores would be obtained at the same time. With the split-halves method, the sum of the scores for the odd-numbered trials (items) and the scores for the even-numbered trials (items) are used as the two sets of scores. The even-odd split is usually adopted so that the effects of learning from being tested and fatigue are equally represented in both sums of the score for each individual. Thus two scores (an odd total and even total) are available for each subject and instrument reliability can be estimated.

Splitting the test in two parts raises an important issue about the obtained reliability. Test reliability is related to test length. Longer tests are generally more reliable than shorter tests. Since the reliability coefficient obtained using the split-halves method is based on half the length of the test, the coefficient should be "stepped up" to reflect the actual length of the test. To accomplish this it is necessary to apply the Spearman-Brown Prophecy formula. The split-halves method and application of the Spearman-Brown Prophecy formula are best explained through an example.

Suppose a simple response time test consists of 12 trials. To determine the reliability of this test the sum of each subject's score on the odd-numbered trials (1, 3, 5, 7, 9, 11) can be correlated with the sum of the scores on the even-numbered trials (2, 4, 6, 8, 10, 12). Assume for illustrative purposes that the correlation coefficient obtained is .74. Each of the two scores for each student consists of the sum of six trials; however, since the test actually consists of 12 trials, the value of .74 is substituted into the Spearman-Brown Prophecy formula to obtain an estimate of what the reliability coefficient would be if a 12-trial test were administered twice and the test-retest method used.

The formula is:

$$r_{(est)} = \frac{2 \times r_{(obt)}}{1 + r_{(obt)}}$$

where

$r_{(est)}$ = estimated reliability of the full test
$r_{(obt)}$ = correlation obtained using the split-halves procedure

For the above example we obtain:

$$r_{(est)} = \frac{2 \times .74}{1 + .74}$$

$$r_{(est)} = \frac{1.48}{1.74}$$

$$r_{(est)} = .85$$

One-Mile Walk Test: Reliability, Validity, Norms, and Criterion-Referenced Standards for Young Adults

Allen Jackson and Jeffrey Solomon

The reliability estimates are provided in the table below and demonstrate excellent reliability estimates for a three-trial test. Using the last two trials, which would eliminate any significant effects between trials for the total sample, males, and females, the reliability estimates were also excellent. The practical application of this test might be one practice trial and only one performance trial. Using the Spearman Brown prophecy formula, the reliability estimates would still be acceptable, as shown in this table.

Reliability Estimates and Confidence Intervals

Number of trials	Total N = 41 r_{xx}	Total N = 41 0.95 CI	Males N = 21 r_{xx}	Males N = 21 0.95 CI	Females N = 20 r_{xx}	Females N = 20 0.95 CI
3	0.96	0.92–0.98	0.95	0.87–0.98	0.95	0.87–0.98
2	0.95	0.91–0.97	0.95	0.87–0.98	0.93	0.84–0.97
1	0.90	0.83–0.94	0.90	0.77–0.96	0.87	0.71–0.93

From Jackson A and Solomon J: Medicine, Exercise, Nutrition and Health 3:317-322, 1994.

Note that the reliability for the 12 trials is greater than that for the 6 trials.

The advantage of the split-halves method is that it eliminates retesting simply for the purposes of obtaining a reliability coefficient. However, the split-halves methods does not allow for day-to-day changes since all the scores are obtained on the same day. Thus it tends to overestimate the reliability obtained using the test-retest method. The box above illustrates the use of the Spearman-Brown Prophecy formula to estimate the reliability of two and one trials of the one-mile walk test.

Internal Consistency Reliability

A method of determining the internal consistency of subject responses to items is termed *internal consistency reliability*

A Study of the Nutrition Knowledge of Allied Health Students

Saroj M. Bahl, Stephanie Hamilton, and Patricia Ormesher

A seven-page questionnaire was used as the survey instrument. The survey had two components: a demographic data component and a nutrition-knowledge test. The demographic information included questions, such as age, sex, program, year of educational program, previous and current nutrition education. This portion also included a question regarding the subject's degree of satisfaction with nutrition education in the professional curricula and, if dissatisfied, a question on preferred modalities for gaining such knowledge. The nutrition test consisted of 50 multiple-choice questions related to basic nutrition principles, sources of nutrients, and function of nutrients. The questions measured four cognitive levels of Bloom's taxonomy: recall, comprehension, application, and analysis. The reliability of the questionnaire was 0.86, by the Kuder-Richardson-20 (KR_{20}) formula. This questionnaire has been validated and used as a tool for determining the understanding of nutrition subject matter of potential nutrition educators. Details of the validation design have been discussed in a study that included nutritionists, home economists, nurses, health and physical educators, college graduates, and elementary educators.

From Bahl SM, Hamilton S, and Ormesher P: Health Values 17(5):3-8, 1993.

(also called alpha reliability). This is an intraclass reliability and does not determine the "stability" reliability. Rather, the alpha is high (for example, approaching 1.0) when respondents tend to answer all items near the same end of the scale. For example, if a respondent answers all Likert-type responses near 4 or 5 on the instrument while another answers 1 or 2, the items on the instrument reflect "internal consistency." This does not, however, infer that the instrument is stable over time. Analysis of variance is used to calculate the alpha coefficient. Alpha reliabilities are reported with instruments used in the affective domain. Additional names that are used for the intraclass reliability coefficient are Kuder-Richardson 20 (KR_{20}), Kuder-Richardson 21 (KR_{21}), and Hoyt reliability. The box above illustrates the use of the alpha coefficient (KR_{20}) with a written knowledge test.

Interpreting Reliability Coefficients

Because the various methods of calculating the reliability coefficient reflect different sources of error, an interpretation of the coefficient must consider the method by which it is derived. In general, however, the higher the reliability coefficient, the more consistently does a test measure whatever it does measure. As mentioned above, it is sometimes helpful to think of a measurement or an observed score as being made up of two parts: a true score and an error score. It can be shown that the variance of the observed scores (σ_0^2) is equal to the variance of the true scores (σ_t^2) plus the variance of the error scores (σ_e^2). Within this theoretical model, reliability is defined as the ratio of the variance of the true scores to the variance of the observed score, or

$$\text{Reliability} = \frac{\sigma_t^2}{\sigma_0^2} = \frac{1-\sigma_e^2}{\sigma_0^2}$$

Only when no error is present in the observed score could the value of the reliability coefficient be 1.0 (for example, the variation in observed scores consists only of true score variation). As the amount of error increases, the value of (σ_0^2) increases, and thus reliability decreases. Thus when a test is made up entirely of true score variations, the reliability is 1.0. When there is no true score variability, the reliability is 0.0.

Another method that is useful in interpreting the meaning of a reliability coefficient is to use the reliability coefficient in calculating a statistic called the *standard error of measurement (SEM)*. This statistic is used to determine the amount of confidence that can be placed in a subject's observed score. It is calculated from the following formula:

$$\text{SEM} = \text{SD}_0\sqrt{1-r}$$

where

$$\text{SEM} = \text{standard error of measurement}$$
$$\text{SD}_0 = \text{standard deviation of the observed scores}$$
$$r = \text{reliability coefficient}$$

Using this formula, verify that the SEM for a test having a standard deviation of 10 and a reliability coefficient of .64 is 6.

The SEM is actually the standard deviation. It is the standard deviation of the errors of measurement in the instrument. Since the SEM is actually the standard deviation of the error scores for the group tested, and because error scores are considered to be normally distributed with a mean of zero, the SEM can be used to determine limits within which the individual's true score lies. For example, on a test having a reliability coefficient of .81 and a standard deviation of 9.17, a subject received a score of 54. By calculating the SEM to be 4 and knowing that in a normal curve approximately 68% of the scores are located between one standard deviation above and below the mean, the researcher could assume (with 32% risk of being wrong) that the subject's true score lies between 50 and 58 (54 ± 4). To reduce the risk of being wrong to slightly less than 5%, the values of 2 times SEM could be added to and subtracted from the subject's score (2 × 4 = 8; 54 ± 8 = 46 − 62). Thus, the chance is 95% that the subject's true score lies between 46 and 62.

To be reasonably certain that a subject's true score is "captured," the range of scores becomes increasingly wider. Also, by examining the formula to obtain the SEM, notice that the less reliable the test, the greater the value of the SEM and thus the greater the range of the limits necessary to be certain the true score is contained within it. Researchers generally report the Standard Error of Measurement when reporting the reliability. Morrow and Jackson (1993) provide guidelines that authors should follow when reporting reliability statistics in research reports.

OBJECTIVITY (INTER-RATER RELIABILITY)

Objectivity is actually a form of reliability in which one source of error—that of the differences in test administrators—is examined. Possibly the best way to explain the meaning of the term objectivity is by illustration. Assume that two different researchers each administer separately a muscular endurance test to the same group of subjects. Further assume that all factors that could cause a difference to exist between the two sets of measures are carefully controlled. If these assumptions are correct, the only reason for differences to exist between the measures obtained by the two researchers is the fact that two

---

International Bias Detected in Judging Gymnastic Competition at the 1984 Olympic Games

Charles J. Ansorge and John K. Scheer

The purpose of this study was to determine whether or not a pattern of bias was shown by men's and women's gymnastics judges at the 1984 Olympic Games. To determine whether judges were biased in favor of gymnasts from their own countries and against gymnasts from countries in close competition with their own, the scores of each individual judge were compared to the mean of the other three judges on the panel. Results of six sign test analyses revealed that both male and female judges were biased in their scoring of gymnasts ($p<.001$). Judges scored gymnasts from their countries higher than the remaining members of the panels. Judges also scored gymnasts on teams both immediately ahead and behind their own lower than other judges on their panels.

From Ansorge CJ and Scheer JK: Research Quarterly for Exercise and Sport 59(2):103-107, 1988.

different people administered the test. Thus a measure of the objectivity of this test would be made by comparing the two sets of measures obtained by the two researchers. Objectivity coefficients range between 0.0 and 1.0.

Tests such as measuring height, pulse rate, or strength are reasonably high in objectivity because the procedures for obtaining these measures are fairly standard and the possibility of measurement error is not as great as when administering some other tests. Tests that involve a high degree of subjectivity are the most difficult to maintain high objectivity. In the box above, Ansorge and Scheer (1988) provide an excellent example of the importance of objectivity. They reviewed gymnastic judges' ratings from the 1984 Olympic Games and reported that the judges were biased (that is, not objective) in their evaluations of performances. As a result of this and other supporting research, the International Olympic Committee modified some of the rules and monitoring procedures for judges in an effort to increase scoring objectivity.

VALIDITY

The most common definition of **validity** is the degree to which an assessment process or device measures what it is intended to measure—that is, *the truthfulness of the measurement.* Various types of validity have been defined and methods for their examination and calculation of indexes have been devised. In general, two approaches can be used to examine validity: The qualitative approach involves logic and subjective judgment; the quantitative approach involves statistical evidence. Four types of validity and the approaches used to examine each are discussed below. *Standards for Educational and Psychological Tests* (1985) is an excellent source which describes the nature and characteristics of developing and reporting reliable and valid measurements.

Content Validity

Content validity is assessed by determining the degree to which a measuring instrument or process contains tasks that inherently provide evidence about the traits or capabilities to be measured. The content validity of a measuring instrument is usually examined qualitatively. Content validity is supported from logical evidence. For example, the content validity of a set of survey questions is generally subjectively evaluated by the extent to which the individual items represent a sufficient sample of the objectives of the survey. In other words, by examining a copy of the survey being considered for use, a researcher can estimate the degree of content validity the survey has for a particular study.

Content validity also can be evaluated by logically examining the actions required to complete a physical performance measurement. For example, the content of a maximum oxygen uptake test would seem to be a valid indicator of aerobic capacity, whereas the content validity of a test purporting to measure mental imagery ability may be more difficult to assess. Often, experts in a field are called upon to help evaluate content validity (or expert opinions).

Concurrent Validity

The concurrent validity of a measuring instrument or process is usually assessed quantitatively. To determine the validity of a test it is necessary to compare how well a test measures what it actually measures with what it is supposed to measure. To make such a comparison requires a method of obtaining a *criterion score* that accurately measures what the original test is designed to assess. If this requirement can be met, a correlation coefficient (called a concurrent validity coefficient) between the two resulting sets of scores provides evidence for a type of measurement validity. At this point you may be wondering why, if we have some method for accurately measuring whatever it is we want to measure, we need to check the validity of a new test. This is usually answered by showing that the process for obtaining the criterion measure is too costly or difficult to use. For example, percent body fat can be measured by any one of several methods. The method of underwater weighing is generally considered the criterion (or "gold standard") against which other methods are validated. Unfortunately, underwater weighing takes special equipment. If a high validity correlation is found between underwater weighing and an alternative measurement method, then evidence would exist supporting the concurrent validity of the alternative method. The selection of the criterion measure is critical; unless the criterion scores are accurate measures of the traits desired, the evidence for concurrent validity is not worthwhile.

The *Standard Error of Estimate (SEE)* is used to reflect the degree of error in estimating the criterion. The SEE is a standard deviation. It is the standard deviation of the errors of estimating the criterion score from the other measure. The SEE is:

$$SEE = SD_0\sqrt{1-r^2}$$

where

SEE = standard error of estimate
SD_0 = standard deviation of the observed scores
r = correlation between the criterion and the other measure

If the SEE is 3% and your estimated percent fat is 20%, you can be 68% confident that your actual percent fat is between 17% and 23% (or, 20% ± 3%). You can be 95% confident that your actual percent fat is between 14% and 26% (or, 20% ± 2 × 3%). The box on p. 278 illustrates the concurrent validity of skinfolds to estimate hydrostatically determined percent body fat.

Generalized Equations for Predicting Body Density of Women

Andrew S. Jackson, Michael L. Pollock, and Ann Ward

Abstract

Previous research with women has shown that body composition regression equations derived from anthropometric variables were population specific. This study sought to derive generalized equations for women differing in age and body composition. The hydrostatic method was used to determine body density (BD) and percent fat (%F) on 249 women 18 to 55 years (X = 31.4 ± 10.8 yrs) and 4 to 44 %F (X = 24.1 ± 7.2 %F). Skinfold fat (S), gluteal circumference (C) and age were independent variables. The quadratic form of the sum of three, four and seven S in combination with age and gluteal C produced multiple correlations that ranged from 0.842 to 0.867 with standard errors of 3.6 to 3.8 %F. The equations were cross-validated on a different sample of 82 women with similar age and %F characteristics. The correlations between predicted and hydrostatically determined %F ranged from 0.815 to 0.820 with standard errors of 3.7 to 4.0 %F. This study showed that valid generalized body composition equations could be derived for women varying in age and body composition, but care need to be exercised with women over an age of forty.

From Jackson AS, Pollock ML, and Ward A: Medicine and Science in Sports and Exercise 12(3):175-182, 1980.

Predictive Validity

Another type of validity examined through correlational techniques is predictive validity. If a measuring instrument has high predictive validity, its scores will have a high correlation with some future measure. The typical procedure for assessing predictive validity is to measure several individuals whose future behavior you are interested in predicting. At some later date, you measure the same individual on the trait or quality in question and then see if the scores on the initial measurement correlate highly (or predict) or at all with the second assessment. The assessment made in the future serves as the criterion measure. For example, if there is a high correlation between a battery of tests to predict future success in the National Football League (NFL) and a later measure of how well the tested individuals do in the NFL, the battery would be said to possess predictive validity. The higher the

**Physical Fitness and All-Cause Mortality:
A Prospective Study of Healthy Men and Women**

Steven N. Blair, Harold W. Kohl III, Ralph S. Paffenbarger, Jr., Debra G. Clark, Kenneth H. Cooper, and Larry W. Gibbons

We studied physical fitness and risk of all-cause and cause-specific mortality in 10,224 men and 3,120 women who were given a preventive medical examination. Physical fitness was measured by a maximal treadmill exercise test. Average follow-up was slightly more than 8 years, for a total of 110,482 person-years of observation. There were 240 deaths in men and 43 deaths in women. Age-adjusted all-cause mortality rates declined across physical fitness quintiles from 64.0 per 10,000 person-years in the least-fit men to 18.6 per 10,000 person-years in the most-fit men (slope, −4.5). Corresponding values for women were 39.5 per 10,000 person-years to 8.5 per 10,000 person-years (slope, −5.5). These trends remained after statistical adjustment for age, smoking habit, cholesterol level, systolic blood pressure, fasting blood glucose level, parental history of coronary heart disease, and follow-up interval. Lower mortality rates in higher fitness categories also were seen for cardiovascular disease and cancer of combined sites. Attributable risk estimates for all-cause mortality indicated that low physical fitness was an important risk factor in both men and women. Higher levels of physical fitness appear to delay all-cause mortality primarily due to lowered rates of cardiovascular disease and cancer.

From Blair SN, et al.: Journal of the American Medical Association 262:2395-2401, 1989.

correlation, the more predictive validity the battery possesses. Predictive validity is almost the same as concurrent validity, the only difference being the time interval between the initial measurement and the criterion measurement of scores.

The use of SAT scores to predict success in college is an example of predictive validity. In sport science, predictive validity is demonstrated in the relationship between various lifestyle parameters (for example, dietary intake, hypertension, blood lipids, physical activity, etc.) and the development of heart disease. Note that the criterion (success in college or heart disease development) is measured some time after the measurement of the predictor variable(s). The box above illustrates the use of physical fitness test performance to predict all-cause mortality.

Construct Validity

Such attributes as athletic ability, anxiety, and intelligence are examples of constructs. Although these attributes are intangible, they are believed to exist because they explain observable behavior. For example, some people appear to be very creative; others do not. Thus it seems logical to assume that creativity exists as a construct. Construct validity is the combination of logical and statistical evidence.

The usual approach to evaluating the degree of construct validity of a test is to conduct several experiments in which specific outcomes are hypothesized. For example, Mood (1971) devised a test to measure the construct of physical fitness knowledge and then hypothesized that students enrolled in a large number of classes where they are exposed to information on physical fitness will score higher on the test than students not enrolled in such classes. Confirmation of this hypothesis can be used as one piece of evidence that the test actually measures the construct of physical fitness knowledge but it is certainly far from conclusive proof. The construct validity of a test is generally examined over repeated uses and examination of the results obtained. Construct validation is not only used as an assessment of the test itself but also an appraisal of the existence of the construct. Construct validation procedures are often used to develop evidence for theoretically existing, yet directly unmeasurable constructs (for example, attitude, intelligence, etc.).

Considerations of Validity

Recall the discussions of internal and external validity from Chapter 5 in the Methods section. Internal validity refers to the technical quality of an experiment; external validity is related to application of findings to new situations or populations. Content, concurrent, predictive, and construct validity are concerned with the measurement process, and as such, affect both internal and external validity. When you hear the term validity, it is important to identify in which context the term is used.

Measurement validity is a matter of degree; tests are generally neither completely valid nor completely invalid. The degree to which a test measures what it is intended to measure is a function of many factors. The environmental conditions under which validity is assessed, the attributes (for example, age, gender, and ability level) of the particular group of participants involved, and the criterion measure are among the issues that must be considered when a validity coefficient is presented.

The validity of a test is also related to its reliability. A test that does not result in consistent scores (is unreliable) cannot be a valid measure of a specific trait. The value of the validity coefficient will be between −1.00 and +1.00. Since the validity coefficient is a correlation, you interpret the validity coefficient by considering its absolute value and the coefficient of determination. Thus −1.00 and +1.00 reflect the same degree of validity. −1.00 and +1.00 reflect perfect validity while 0.0 indicates no validity. In practice, validity coefficients normally lie somewhere between the extremes.

Relationship among Validity, Reliability, and Objectivity

The three characteristics of measurement under discussion are related. A test cannot be valid without first being reliable. In other words, if it is possible to demonstrate that a test actually does measure cardiovascular fitness, then the test must necessarily measure cardiovascular fitness consistently or else the demonstration would not be possible. However, a test can be reliable without being valid. For example, the cardiovascular test might give consistent results but upon further inspection the test might be found to be a measure of skeletal muscular endurance of the legs. This test could be considered reliable but not valid for measuring cardiovascular fitness.

A test may be reliable but not reflect objectivity. An example of this situation involves skinfold measurements. One person, with some practice, may become adept at taking these measurements and arriving at consistent results. However, if this person's measurements are compared to those obtained on the same subjects by someone else equally adept, the results might differ considerably. Thus even though both testers are able to take reliable (repeatable) measures, the objectivity of the measurements is low.

Correlation Coefficients in Reliability, Objectivity, and Validity

Definitions of reliability, validity, and objectivity were presented previously. Quantifying these concepts is one of the uses of the correlation coefficient because they all involve determining the degree of relationship between sets of scores. Recall that a concurrent or predictive validity coefficient must be between −1.00 and +1.00. This is identical to the limits for the correlations coefficient. The reliability coefficient can range between 0.00 and 1.00.

QUALITATIVE RESEARCH RESULTS

While the Results section of qualitative research appears quite different from that of a quantitative research report, the contents of the Results section serve the same purpose. The qualitative researcher, like the quantitative counterpart, reports the quality of the data collected (or speaks to issues of reliability and validity) and then reports the results of the "data" collected. The qualitative researcher's data are different from that of the quantitative researcher. The qualitative researcher's purpose is largely to describe the essence, context, text, and being of a particular setting, program, or activity. Thus the Results section "sets the stage" for the reported results.

The quality of the data rests in large part in the researcher's ability to present the data in an unbiased manner. Thus the researcher describes the methods of data collection and provides evidence that the interpretation of the data are consistent when viewed from different perspectives and/or by different researchers. Often, the researcher reports the use of *triangulation* to provide evidence that multiple (typically, three) different means are used to draw essentially the same conclusions when the text, situation, and context are reviewed by independent individuals and/or data sources. Locke (1989) suggests that typical quantitative concerns such as a control group or test-retest reliability have "source checking" and "constant comparison" as qualitative analogies. Analogs to classical test reliability and validity are "credibility, transferability, dependability, and confirmability" in qualitative studies. Since the qualitative researcher is essentially the "instrument," it is necessary to be convinced that similar conclusions would be drawn by other researchers who review the same data. The researcher is developing credibility in the presentation of the results. The development of common themes and conclusions drawn by one researcher should be also identified by another data reviewer.

The actual results for the qualitative Results section are distinctly different from those of the quantitative researcher. The quantitative researcher reports numbers (such as mean and standard deviation) while the qualitative researcher presents actual data (such as text, words, descriptions). Often, direct quotes are used by the qualitative researcher to illustrate representative comments from interviews or text that have been reviewed. These reports provide evidence of the nature of being (or the essence of being) of the particular activity being described. The researcher draws upon common themes to develop theories that are "grounded" in the text. Based upon these descriptions, further studies can be conducted that are either quantitative or qualitative in nature. The boxes below and on pp. 284-285 illustrate the use of qualitative analyses in three distinctly different settings.

Quality of Life of Hospitalized Persons with AIDS

Diane Ragsdale, Joseph A. Kotarba, and James R. Morrow, Jr.

This study explores quality of life from the viewpoint of Persons with AIDS (PWAs) who were interviewed during periods of hospitalization. Quality of life was viewed as the patients' perception of the relative effectiveness of a chosen or ascribed management style in solving the practical problems associated with being ill. Six management styles used by the respondents to improve their quality of life were identified. Results of this study suggest that nurses can improve PWAs' quality of life by supporting their respective management styles.

Description of the study

Setting

A specialized hospital unit for the care of persons with AIDS served as the setting for this study. This unit is located within a 508 bed for-profit community

Continued.

From Ragsdale D, Kotarba JA, and Morrow JR: Image: Journal of Nursing Scholarship 24:259-265, 1992.

Quality of Life of Hospitalized Persons with AIDS—cont'd

hospital located in the southwestern United States. The special diseases unit consists of 60 beds that are located on two floors. Each floor has three wings or "pods" which contain 12 patient beds. One of the pods is used for offices and treatment protocols. All the rooms are private (one patient to a room) and face the nurses' station that is centrally located. Visiting hours were unlimited and accommodations can be made for significant others, family members or friends to stay in the patient's room overnight if they desire.

Findings

Participants

The participants were 13 males and one female, all caucasian except for one Hispanic. Their ages ranged from 26 to 61 years. Areas of employment varied; seven were blue collar workers (clerical, computer technicians) and seven were professionals (teachers, managers, artist). Respondents identified the following belief systems: agnostic (1), Jewish (1), Protestant (4), Catholic (4), and no specific religion (4). The respondents were generally well educated. One respondent had a PhD, three had baccalaureates and three had between one and a half and three years of college; six had completed high school and one participant had finished ninth grade.

A Qualitative Study on the Socialization of Beginning Physical Education Teacher Educators

Kay M. Williamson

Few studies have focused on how university faculty learn and understand expectations of their professional role. The purpose of this study was to describe the experiences of five female physical education teacher educators in their first positions as assistant professors in research oriented universities. Data were collected using primarily qualitative methods—weekly journals and in-depth interviews. Quantitative data were gathered to compare organizational factors such as salary, load allocation, equipment, and travel funds. Data yielded five main categories concerning how and what participants learned about their faculty roles. These categories included participants' perceptions of (a) organizational structure and job facilitation, (b) work tasks, (c) support systems, (d) evaluation and feedback, and

From Williamson KM: Research Quarterly for Exercise and Sport 64(2):188-201,1993.

A Qualitative Study on the Socialization of Beginning Physical Education Teacher Educators—cont'd

(e) participants' psychological states. All participants reported experiencing role ambiguity and stress. Clear criteria for job performance, collegial support and mentoring, and regular evaluation and feedback were cited by all participants as important factors for reducing stress and facilitating their roles as faculty.

Response to Work Tasks: The initial months were very traumatic for all participants, which resulted in their questioning their own competence in all facets of the role.

I was insecure about, Do I really know everything I'm supposed to know? I felt a pretender almost. (Anne)

I have found people here think I'm an expert. I don't feel like one, in fact I feel somewhat insecure about the role. It's amazing how I can get in a car and drive [a few hundred miles] and suddenly be regarded as the expert in teacher ed. (Ella)

Using Qualitative Structured Interviews in Leisure Research: Illustrations from One Case Study

Christine Z. Howe

Data analysis

The data were analyzed by triangulating the qualitative data analysis techniques of typological analysis (Goetz and LeCompte, 1984), enumeration (Miles and Huberman, 1984), constant comparison (Glaser and Strauss, 1967), and estimating (Miles and Huberman, 1984). According to Denzin (1978) there are four major kinds of triangulation; methodological triangulation or the use of multiple methods of data collection and/or analysis; theory triangulation or the use of differing perspectives or world views in investigations; data triangulation or the use of a variety of sources of data; and investigator triangulation or the use of several different researchers. The methodological triangulation that occurred here was limited to the four different qualitative data analysis techniques that were appropriate for the interview and observational data collected.

From Howe CZ: Journal of Leisure Research 20(4):305-324, 1988.

CASE STUDY MANUSCRIPT RESULTS

Results from the case study analysis are often combined in a "Results and Discussion" section. This is done because the case study analysis often "tells a story" and it is best to present the details and interpretation of the details in a combined manner. The exact nature and content of the case study results depend upon the nature and extent of the case being reported. A case study could be based upon a single individual (such as the integration of a multiple-disabled student into a traditional classroom setting) or be much more extensive in nature (for example, the accommodations made by an entire university to meet the legislative requirements of the Americans With Disabilities Act). Regardless, the investigator's intent is to describe the context and surroundings of the case being studied. A full description of the "environment" helps the reader best understand the surroundings that impact the case being described. The researcher attempts to combine the environment and the case to fully describe the essence of being the particular case. The boxes below and on p. 287 illustrate case studies.

 Current Treatment of Obesity Exemplified in a Case Study

Diane Wyshogrod

Summary

In a single case study, a 29-year-old man was successfully treated for obesity using a behavior therapy approach. He was taught to monitor his eating, exercise, correct misconceptions and develop appropriate strategies to change these in order to achieve the desired weight loss and develop a healthier lifestyle. As a result of significant changes in eating and exercise habits, significant weight loss occurred during treatment, and continued at 6-month follow up.

Case history

The patient was a 29-year-old employed divorced white male, 5'8" tall and weighing 283 pounds. He wanted to lose about 100 pounds, complaining of weight-related physical problems such as back pain, edema, and the general difficulty moving around. Because he was ashamed of his appearance, he tended to avoid interpersonal situations, making him very lonely. He was anxious and mildly depressed.

From Wyshogrod D: Journal of Behavior Therapy and Experimental Psychiatry 16(2):151-157, 1985.

Psychological Consequences of an Exercise Training Program for a Paraplegic Man: A Case Study

Jonathan F. Katz, Joan C. Adler, Nicholas J. Mazzarella, and Laurence P. Ince

Abstract

Although the psychological benefits of exercise participation have been documented with several clinical and nonclinical populations, one group of individuals that has not been addressed is the physically disabled. The present investigation examines the effects of a 12-week exercise training program on the psychological status (i.e., mood states) of a spinal-cord-injured patient in a rehabilitation hospital. The results of this case study investigation provide tentative support for the hypothesis that vigorous physical exercise can be a useful adjunctive therapeutic strategy in working with the disabled.

Results

It can be seen that R.S. was able to increase all of his physiological parameters within the 12-week exercise training program. His workload increased from 50 watts to 75 watts, a substantial gain; HR, VO_2, and METS also improved with the work performed. In addition, R.S.'s performance tolerance (i.e., maximal exercise capacity) increased in duration by 40% over the course of the training program.

From Katz JF, et al.: Rehabilitation Psychology 30:53-58, 1985.

Inguinal Mass in a College Football Player: A Case Study

Clinical Case Study

Brent S.E. Rich, David O. Hough, Jeffrey S. Monroe, and Sally Nogle

Abstract

A 22-year-old male college football player presented with a 3-week history of a mass in his right inguinal area. Originally thought by the athlete to be a groin strain, evaluation revealed a large indirect inguinal hernia. Surgical evaluation was obtained to confirm the diagnosis of a 4-centimeter opening at the external inguinal ring. The hernia completely and spontaneously reduced in the supine position. The athlete was successfully allowed to participate with the use of a truss and underwent an uneventful surgical repair at the end of the season.

From Rich BSE, et al.: Medicine and Science in Sports and Exercise 25:318-320, 1993.

META-ANALYSIS MANUSCRIPT RESULTS

The term *meta-analysis* refers to a method for statistically evaluating several separate research reports. The initial aspects of a meta-analysis reported are those that describe the obtained Effect Sizes (ESs). The ES is reported in standard deviation units and reflects the effect of the "treatment." The results indicate the total number of manuscripts reviewed, those that met the inclusionary criteria, and the number of ESs calculated. The investigator then presents descriptive information about the ESs categorized by perceived important characteristics (for example, gender, age, type of publication, year of publication, quality of study, etc.). The meta-analyst often uses graphical presentation (referred to as a "box and whiskers") to illustrate the distribution of the ESs. Some researchers then present inferential statistics where mean differences are tested between the various characteristics. For example, is the mean ES for boys significantly different from that of the girls? More will be said about these tests in Chapter 11 where inferential statistics are presented. The following box illustrates a meta-analysis.

Exercise and VO_2max in Children: A Meta-Analysis

V. Gregory Payne and James R. Morrow, Jr.

Despite widespread belief that children are aerobically trainable, studies examining the ability of a child to improve maximal oxygen uptake (VO_{2max}) have yielded inconsistent findings. The present investigation, using meta-analysis, examined the effects of physical activity, gender, experimental design, and sufficiency of exercise on the VO_{2max} of child subjects. Sixty-nine studies examining the effects of training on children were originally located; 28 met criteria for inclusion. From these studies, 70 effect sizes (ESs) were calculated. Some studies employed cross-sectional (XS) designs involving comparisons of intact groups of subjects; the others used a pretest-posttest (PP) design, which followed subjects throughout a specified training program. Average ES indicated a considerable difference between trained

From Payne VG and Morrow JR: Research Quarterly for Exercise and Sport 64(3):305-313, 1993.

Exercise and VO₂max in Children: A Meta-Analysis—cont'd

and untrained subjects though several possible sources of confounding (e.g., subject self-selection) in XS studies were identified. Effect sizes of .94 (±1.00) and .35 (±0.82) were achieved for XS and PP designs, respectively. Further analyses were conducted with the PP design studies. In these studies, subjects improved approximately 2 ml · kg^{-1} · min^{-1}. In the PP studies, effect sizes were not significantly affected by (a) gender, (b) "sufficient" and "insufficient" training protocol, or (c) test mode. Results indicated that reported changes in VO$_{2max}$ in children are small to moderate and are a function of the experimental design used.

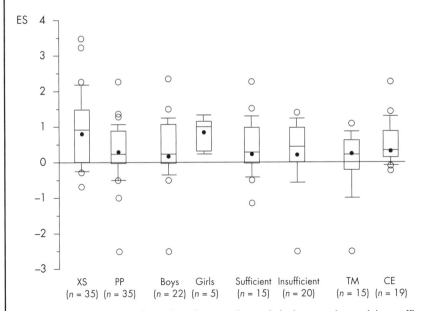

FIGURE 1 Box plots of effect sizes by experimental design, gender, training sufficiency, and test mode.* *Note:* ES = effect size; XS = cross-sectional design; PP = pre- and posttest design; TM = treadmill; CE = cycle ergometer. The box represents the 75th (top), 50th (middle), and 25th (bottom) percentiles. The lines extending from the box represent the 90th (top) and 10th (bottom) percentiles. Effect sizes deviating further than the 90th and 10th percentiles are printed as circles. The mean is represented by the black dot. *Only pre/post designs used for gender, sufficiency, and test mode.

EPIDEMIOLOGIC STUDY MANUSCRIPT RESULTS

Epidemiologists present descriptive statistics that illustrate the number of subjects studied and the length of time over which individuals were studied. Of utmost importance is the definition of the study characteristics in terms of group membership. Important categorical variables might include living-dead, healthy-ill, male-female, no risk-at risk, and so forth. The number of subjects in each of the important divergent groups is presented (typically in tabular form) and then the major statistics reported with epidemiologic research include *odds ratios, relative risk,* and *attributable risk* statistics. These statistics are based upon weighted (by the number of subjects and years of follow-up) ratios that illustrate the risk associated with being in one of the categories over the other. Generally, these statistics are based on the following calculation:

$$\frac{\text{Incidence Rate of Disease in the Exposed Group}}{\text{Incidence Rate of Disease in the Unexposed Group}}$$

For example, if one leads a sedentary versus active lifestyle, what are the risks of dying earlier or developing cardiovascular disease? The rate of disease in the sedentary group is divided by the rate of disease in the active group to determine the odds or risk as a result of being in one group versus the other group. The odds or risks are often then presented in graphic form to illustrate the potential increase in risk from a particular lifestyle behavior. The odds ratios or relative risk descriptive statistics are then followed by inferential statistics, which present the confidence interval, which is an inferential statistic to be presented in Chapter 11. If there is no association (or no increased risk) identified between being in one group or another and the disease state, the odds ratio or relative risk would be 1.0. A higher ratio indicates increased risk by being in one group as contrasted from another. Depending on which group is in the denominator, a ratio below 1.0 could indicate reduced risk. A confidence interval is then used to determine if the actual odds ratio is 1.0, a chance fluctuation from 1.0, or significantly different from 1.0. The box on pp. 291-292 illustrates results from an epidemiologic study.

1993 C.H. McCloy Research Lecture: Physical Activity, Physical Fitness, and Health

Steven N. Blair

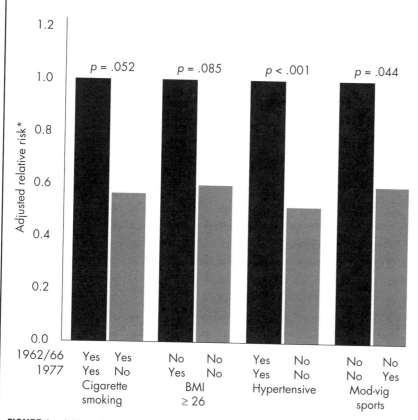

FIGURE 1   Adjusted relative risks (each relative risk is adjusted for age and all other variables in the figure) for coronary heart disease mortality by changes in lifestyle characteristics. (The black bars represent men who had unfavorable characteristics at baseline [in 1962 or 1966] and at follow-up [1977]. The gray bars show the adjusted relative risks for men who made favorable changes on the variable of interest between baseline and follow-up. There were 10,269 men in the cohort, with 130 deaths from coronary heart disease. *Adjusted for age and other factors in the figure. BMI = body mass index; Mod-vig = moderately vigorous. Data taken from Paffenbarger et al., 1993.)

Continued.

From Blair SN: Research Quarterly for Exercise and Sport 64(4):365-376, 1993.

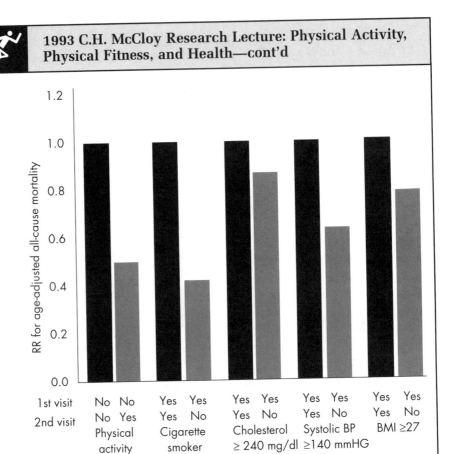

1993 C.H. McCloy Research Lecture: Physical Activity, Physical Fitness, and Health—cont'd

FIGURE 2 Relative risks (RRs) for age-adjusted all-cause mortality are shown for changes in lifestyle characteristics in 10,288 men with two examinations at the Cooper Clinic during 1970 to 1989. (There were 275 deaths during 52,069 man-years of follow-up. The black bars represent men who were at risk on the variable at both examinations, and the gray bars represent men who made favorable changes in risk factors from the first to the second examination. BP = blood pressure; BMI = body mass index.)

HISTORICAL STUDY MANUSCRIPT RESULTS

The historical study results are presented in narrative form and provide the heart of the story being presented. History (the practice of telling a story) research requires the narrator to present extensive descriptions of the background, context, personalities, interactions, environment, and full description of all characters and place them in the context of the historical time. The Results section is the major piece of historical research. Through the use of personal interviews, primary and secondary information sources, videotapes, printed materials, and so forth, the investigator attempts to provide an accurate record of the events for a given period of time. The Results section is often combined with the Discussion section, though the extensive Results section may then be followed with a brief summary of the discussion and implications of the work. The following two boxes illustrate results from historical studies.

The Rise and Demise of Harvard's B.S. Program in Anatomy, Physiology, and Physical Training: A Case of Conflicts of Interest and Scarce Resources

Roberta J. Park

A century ago Harvard University established a comprehensive, scientifically based four-year B.S. degree program in Anatomy, Physiology, and Physical Training. On paper its academic rigor matched—and almost certainly exceeded—the best undergraduate curricula that exist today. Given the recent debates concerning the future of physical education, it is surprising that only Walter Kroll and Ellen Gerber have given any systematic attention to this interesting, albeit transitory, event. The circumstances that surrounded the program's inception and rapid demise merit further examination.

From Park RJ: Research Quarterly for Exercise and Sport 63(3):246-260, 1992.

Prized Performers, but Frequently Overlooked Students: The Involvement of Black Athletes in Intercollegiate Sports on Predominantly White University Campuses, 1890-1972

David K. Wiggins

Connie Hawkins was full of apprehension on entering the University of Iowa in the fall of 1960. He found himself in an alien environment, hundreds of miles away from friends and family for the first time in his life, and far removed from

Continued.

From Wiggins DK: Research Quarterly for Exercise and Sport 62(2):164-177, 1991.

Prized Performers, but Frequently Overlooked Students: The Involvement of Black Athletes in Intercollegiate Sports on Predominantly White University Campuses, 1890-1972—cont'd

the familiar surroundings of Boys High in Brooklyn, where he had established himself as one of the greatest basketball stars in schoolboy history. He was determined, though, to make a go of it at the large, predominantly white midwestern university. Head coach Sharm Scheuerman and his staff painted an idyllic picture of college life that enamored Hawkins and helped offset some of the misgivings he had as an urban black man suddenly living on a white campus in middle America. The coaches, in whom he had placed so much of his trust, assured Hawkins that in exchange for bringing glory to the university by playing basketball, he would be given money, would have access to an active social life, would be treated like royalty by those on campus and in the local community, and would be provided a quality education. Everything would be taken care of for him. All he had to do was remain eligible, play basketball, and life would be wonderful.

PHILOSOPHICAL MANUSCRIPT RESULTS

Philosophic manuscripts typically do not have a traditional Results section. The philosophic research paper does not have typical literature review and methods sections. Rather, the investigator is presenting a case for a particular perspective or developing a concept, theory, or position that is either inductive or deductive in nature. The researcher presents the theoretical groundwork for the presentation, provides differing perspectives, and draws conclusions and attempts to demonstrate that the proposed philosophy or theoretical position is the most strongly supported. The boxes on p. 295 illustrate philosophical works in kinesiology and physical education.

Knowledge and Kinesiology

Steve Estes

Epistemology, or ways of knowing, can be used (a) to show that kinesiology employs different but complementary methods for gaining knowledge and that each method has a role to play in kinesiology, and (b) to show how epistemology can be used to organize an introductory kinesiology course or textbook. The epistemologies used to organize the subdisciplines are rationalism, empiricism, science, and subjectivism. An epistemic approach to a foundations course or textbook allows one to answer questions in the subdisciplines regarding how knowledge is evaluated, how knowledge develops, what method should be used to develop knowledge, and how knowledge can best be taught. The goal is to enable students to understand an increasingly diverse field by literally charting how methods of knowledge creation relate to the subdisciplines that compose kinesiology.

From Estes S: Quest 46(4):392, 1994.

"I Hit a Home Run!" The Lived Meaning of Scoring in Games in Physical Education

Nancy Peoples Wessinger

This paper offers reflections on the lived meaning of "scoring" in the game world of the child. One of the emergent themes in the stories of fourth-grade children was that "feeling good" in the gymnasium results primarily from scoring or helping one's team to win. This was somewhat surprising given that no one was keeping score. What meaning, then, do these experiences of "scoring" have for the child? And how can educators utilize this knowledge? This article explores the lived meaning of scoring for the child using Arnold's (1979) text, Meaning in Movement, Sport and Physical Education, as a stimulus. A brief discussion of implications for teachers follows. An integral part of this paper is the rationale for and description of a method for enabling researchers to gain insights on these topics. A phenomenological analysis that purposefully goes beyond themes to meaning is described.

From Peoples Wessinger N: Quest 46(4):425, 1994.

SUMMARY

In the Results section of a research report, you will find the analysis of the information gathered in the study. In quantitative research, this information is usually expressed numerically with descriptive statistics. In qualitative research, the information is usually presented in a narrative. In this chapter we focused on the most common quantitative methods used to describe numerical information.

The most commonly used descriptive statistics in research are the mean and standard deviation. The mean is the average value of a set of scores: the standard deviation is a measure of variability in a set of scores. In addition to describing each set of scores individually, we can also describe the relationship between two sets of scores with a correlation statistic.

A researcher is not only concerned with presenting the data analysis, but is also concerned with showing that the data are reliable and valid. Reliability is used to assess measurement consistency. Validity is an assessment of the degree to which an assessment process or device measures what it is intended to measure.

The results in a qualitative research report are presented differently than the results in a quantitative report. Qualitative researchers attempt to establish that their findings and conclusions are objective and correct using a variety of techniques including triangulation, source checking, and constant comparison methods.

EXERCISES

1 Identify the scale of measurement for each of the following items:
  a The time needed to take a multiple choice exam.
  b The rank order of football teams at the end of the season.
  c Percent body fat.
  d Scores on a tennis skills test.
  e Political party affiliation.
  f The distance from San Francisco to Honolulu.
  g Gender.
  h Zip code.
  i Score on a history exam.
  j Reaction time.

2 Define the descriptive statistics mean, median, and mode. Describe how each is calculated.

3 Describe a situation under which:
  a the mean would be the appropriate measure of central tendency.
  b the median would be the appropriate measure of central tendency.
  c the mode would be the appropriate measure of central tendency.

4 Define the descriptive statistics range, semi-interquartile range, and standard deviation. Describe how each is calculated.

5 Describe a situation under which:
  a the range would be the appropriate measure of variability.
  b the semi-interquartile range would be the appropriate measure of variability.
  c the standard deviation would be the appropriate measure of variability.

6 Describe how a correlation coefficient shows the strength and direction of a relationship between two variables.

7 Describe the differences between measurement reliability, measurement validity, and measurement objectivity.

ANSWERS

1 a Ratio.
  b Ordinal.
  c Ratio.
  d Interval.
  e Nominal.
  f Ratio.
  g Nominal.
  h Nominal.
  i Interval.
  j Ratio.

Statistics as Evidence

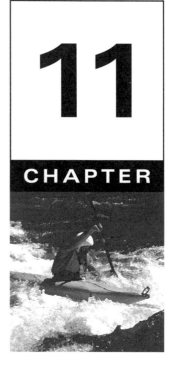

11

CHAPTER

LEARNING GOALS

After reading this chapter you will be able to:

1 Explain the purpose of inferential statistical methods.

2 Outline the five steps of hypothesis testing.

3 Explain the difference between the research hypothesis, the null hypothesis, and the alternate hypothesis.

4 Define the terms *Type I* and *Type II* inference error.

5 Describe how changing a significance level from .05 to .01 affects the chance of committing a Type I error.

6 Describe why it is important to identify the measurement scale of a variable when choosing an inferential statistic.

7 Explain the sources for between groups variability and within groups variability.

8 Describe how the between groups-within groups variability ratio changes as an experimental relationship becomes stronger.

9 Explain the purpose of a p-value in a research report.

10 Explain how to interpret a statistic such as $F(2,30) = 5.50$, $P < .05$.

11 Describe some of the statistical methods used in research to find correlations between variables.

12 Explain the general purpose of a meta-analysis.

TERMS

Inferential statistic
Null hypothesis
Alternative hypothesis
Research hypothesis
Type I error
Significance level
Type II error
Power
ANOVA
Between groups variability
Within groups variability
Multiple comparison tests
ANCOVA
MANOVA
MANCOVA

HYPOTHESIS TESTING

The principal information in the Results Section is the statistical tests conducted by the quantitative researcher. A key to understanding the Results Section of a quantitative research article is understanding the process of hypothesis testing. This chapter will describe the nature and purpose of hypothesis testing and many of the statistical tests researchers use. Researchers use **inferential** statistical tests to be able to infer to a population from a sample that is representative of the population under study. Regardless of the actual test used, it is important to understand that the basic purpose behind all inferential statistical tests is identical. In general, the researcher:

1 Develops a research hypothesis about a relationship between variables.
2 Develops a statistical hypothesis in a null form (in other words, there really is *no* relationship between the variables).
3 Develops an alternative statistical hypothesis if the sample data suggest that the null is not true. This alternative hypothesis typically reflects the actual research hypothesis.
4 Obtains data on the variables of interest from a sample. The researcher actually wishes to infer the results to the original population based on the evidence obtained from the sample.
5 Ascertains the probability of finding the obtained relationship in the sample if, in fact, the null hypothesis is true in the population. If the probability is small of finding such a relationship when the null is actually true, the researcher rejects the null hypothesis (that there is no relationship) and entertains the alternative hypothesis (that there actually is a relationship).

It is important to have an understanding of the concept of hypothesis testing because many of the conclusions drawn by researchers are based on the results of hypothesis tests. In addition, the authors of research articles assume that readers have at least a basic understanding of hypothesis testing and do not take the time to explain the process. As indicated above, hypotheses come in three forms: the research hypothesis, which is a statement about the predicted results of an experiment; the statistical null hypothesis, which is examined through the statistical analysis of the data; and an alternative statistical hypothesis, which is entertained if the results of the data analysis suggest that the null is unlikely to be the actual state of circumstances. Statistical hypotheses are actually concerned with the results of a hypothetical experiment where an infinite number of subjects were tested. Of course this never occurs, but the underlying theory of statistical hypothesis testing is based on this premise. When a statistical hypothesis is stated, it is always done so with reference to the characteristics of a population even though the conclusions are typically based on a sample. Researchers commonly use letters from the Greek alphabet to symbolize population characteristics (usually referred to as parameters). For example, the Greek letter μ (mu) is used to represent a population mean, the letter σ (sigma) represents the population standard deviation, and the letter ρ (rho) is used for the population correlation coefficient. A sample mean is represented by X (X-bar), a sample standard deviation by s, and a sample correlation coefficient by r. As you will see, when a statistical hypothesis is stated, μ is used to represent the mean of a population even though the researcher is working with data that are drawn from a sample.

When stating a statistical hypothesis, the researcher describes two mutually exclusive conditions (the null and its alternative are mutually exclusive). Then based on the data analysis, the researcher will adopt one of the two conditions (either conclude that the null is still believable or reject the null and entertain the alternative hypothesis) as the finding.

It is important to further develop the concept of a relationship between variables before progressing. The purpose behind inferential statistics is to gather information on a sample and then be able to infer from the sample to the population from which the sample was drawn. Obviously, this means that the characteristics of the sample must match those of the population to which the researcher wishes to generalize following the data collection and analysis. The term *relationship* means that having knowledge about one variable tells the researcher something significant about another variable. There are a number of ways that one can find a relationship.

The box below provides some examples. Each of the statistical tests suggested in this box (and many more) will be further illustrated in this chapter.

Notice in this box that there is always an outcome variable and a manipulated variable. Table 11.1 further defines these two variables as independent and dependent variables.

A researcher hypothesizes that there is a relationship between the independent variable and the dependent variable. That is, if the independent variable (X) is changed, the

---

Some Relationships in Exercise Science

1 A researcher believes there is a relationship between instructor gender in a conditioning class and the enrollment patterns of male and female students. Essentially, the researcher thinks that women are more likely to enroll in a class if a woman is teaching and men are more likely to enroll if a man is teaching. Both variables indicate group membership (such as gender of instructor and gender of student). Thus both variables are nominal in scale. The null hypothesis is that there is no difference in the proportion of males and females in each of the instructors' classes. The alternative hypothesis is that the proportion of males and females is not the same for the male and female instructors. This relationship would be examined with a Chi square test.

2 A researcher believes that training a single group of subjects will result in significant change in a physiological parameter (for example, VO_2max). The researcher believes that the mean for the group will increase significantly as a result of the intervention (or training). The grouping variable (pretest and posttest) is nominal in scale and VO_2max is ratio in scale. The null hypothesis is that there is no training effect. The alternative hypothesis is that there is a training effect (or a change in the group's average VO_2max). This relationship is assessed with a dependent (paired) t-test.

3 A researcher believes that there is a significant relationship between one's skinfold measure at the abdomen and one's percent body fat. Both variables are scaled at the interval or ratio level. The null hypothesis is that there is no relationship between these variables. The alternate hypothesis is that there is a relationship between the variables. The existence of a relationship between these two variables could be tested using a Pearson Product Moment Correlation Coefficient.

Some Relationships in Exercise Science—cont'd

4 A researcher believes that a change in resting heart rate is related to the number of times per week that a person trains. The researcher identifies three groups: one that does not train, one that trains three days per week, and one that trains six days per week. The researcher believes that there will be a significant mean difference in resting heart rate among the three groups as a result of the various training regimens. Group is nominal in scale and the outcome measure is interval or ratio in scale. The null hypothesis is that the three groups do not have different resting heart rate mean values following the training period. The alternative hypothesis is that the three groups will differ in resting heart rate following the experiment. This relationship is tested with a one-way Analysis of Variance (ANOVA).

5 Another researcher has a similar belief to that identified in #4 above. However, this researcher believes that the effect of the training regimens (none, or three days per week, or six days per week) will not be the same for both men and women. Thus, this researcher can conduct additional tests of hypotheses. There are actually three different hypotheses this researcher can test (a gender effect; a training effect; and an interaction effect between gender and training frequency). There are two nominal variables (gender [with two levels] and training group [with three levels]) and the outcome variable is interval or ratio in scale. The null hypotheses (there are actually three of them which we will further develop in this chapter) are that gender nor training group have any influence on the subjects' performances. The alternative hypotheses state that there will be differences in the measured variable which is a function of the training frequency group and/or gender. These hypotheses are tested with a two-way ANOVA.

TABLE 11.1   Variable Classification

Independent variable	Dependent variable
X	Y
Presumed cause	Presumed effect
The antecedent	The consequence
Manipulated by researcher	Outcome
Predictor	Criterion

dependent variable (Y) will be affected significantly. The word *significantly* is important here. Statistical significance infers that the observed relationship is not simply due to randomness or chance but is a "true" relationship.

An Example

Let's return to our resting heart rate study for an example. For simplicity, let us assume we have two groups, a no-exercise group (or control) and an exercise (or treatment) group. The research hypothesis is that there is a relationship between training level and resting heart rate. In our resting heart rate experiment, the two conditions proposed by the researcher through hypotheses are: (1) aerobic exercise *will not affect* resting heart rate (the null hypothesis), or (2) aerobic exercise *will affect* resting heart rate (the alternative hypothesis). The first condition is termed the **null hypothesis**. That is, it is hypothesized that there is no (null) relationship between exercise training and resting heart rate. The null hypothesis is written as H_o, where *H* stands for hypothesis and *o* for the null condition. When testing the differences between the means for two groups or conditions, the null hypothesis is written as:

$$H_0: \mu_1 = \mu_2$$

where μ_1 refers to the population mean for group 1, and μ_2 refers to the population mean for group 2. In our heart rate experiment, group 1 would be the control group (no exercise) and group 2 would be the treatment group (aerobic exercise), so we can say:

$$H_0: \mu_c = \mu_t$$

where μ_c represents the control group and μ_t represents the treatment group. Because it is extremely unlikely that the obtained means for the two groups will be numerically identical, the null hypothesis attributes any observed difference to chance variation.

The **alternate hypothesis** is written one of three ways depending on the researcher's educated guess about the outcome of the study:

$$H_a: \mu_c \neq \mu_t$$
$$H_a: \mu_c < \mu_t$$
$$H_a: \mu_c > \mu_t$$

The first hypothesis is called the nondirectional hypothesis (or two-tailed hypothesis), while the second and third hypotheses are directional (or one-tailed hypotheses). In our example, the nondirectional hypothesis predicts that there will be a heart rate difference between the two groups, but does not predict the direction of that difference. The second hypothesis predicts that the control group resting heart rate will be less than the exercise group resting heart rate. The third hypothesis makes the opposite prediction (in practice, only one of the three alternative hypothesis could be stated).

The alternate hypothesis attributes any observed difference among the groups to the effects of the treatment conditions. In other words, the alternate hypothesis suggests that any observed differences between the two groups is due to the effect of the independent variable on the dependent variable and not due to chance factors. The alternate hypothesis actually reflects the researcher's **research hypothesis**. That is, there is a relationship between the variables being studied.

Figure 11.1 shows two hypothetical results. The dots represent the means and the extended lines represent the standard deviations. Experiment A in Figure 11.1 shows a case where we would probably retain the null hypothesis. You can see that although the exercise group's mean resting heart rate is lower than the treatment group, the difference is small and is most likely due to chance variations among the subjects. In Experiment B, the difference in resting heart rate between the two groups is very pronounced. In this case, the null hypothesis would probably be rejected.

In reality, the researcher hypothesizes that there is no statistically significant difference between the mean heart rates. The researcher retains this position until data are gathered which indicate that the differences between the means are probably *not* due to chance. If the data suggest that the differences are probably *not* due to chance alone, the researcher decides to reject the null hypothesis and the alternative hypothesis is presumed to be the true circumstance.

SIGNIFICANCE LEVELS AND ERROR TYPES

In most research the goal, if warranted, is to reject the null hypothesis and demonstrate a relationship among groups

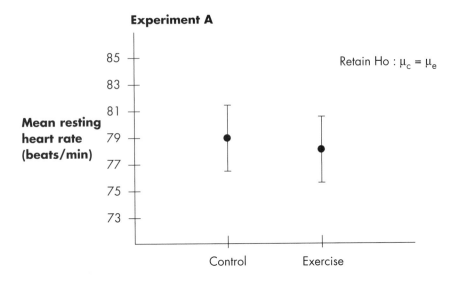

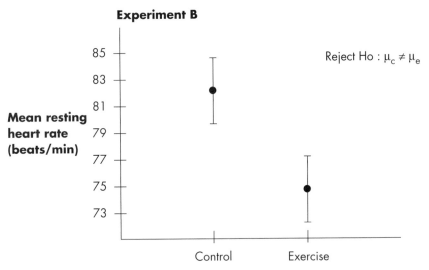

FIGURE 11.1 Hypothetical results from experiments A and B.

beyond what could be expected due to chance variation. However, when conducting hypothesis tests, there is also a possibility that an error may occur. In other words, each time we test a hypothesis, there is a chance that we make the correct decision, and there is also a chance that we make an incorrect decision. There are two types of incorrect decisions and they are referred to as Type I and Type II inference errors.

TYPE I AND TYPE II INFERENCE ERRORS

The decision to reject the null hypothesis is based on statistical evidence. Remember, however, that statistical evidence is never *proof* because statistical evidence is based on probabilities, not absolutes. Hypothesis testing decisions are made without direct knowledge of the *true* relationship in the population. As a result, even though supported by statistical probabilities, the researcher's decision may or may not be correct. Hypothesis testing limits the researcher to two possible conclusions: retain the null hypothesis, or reject the null hypothesis. Table 11.2 shows the decisions that can be made, and the consequences of those decisions. Based on statistical evidence, we reject the null hypothesis or retain the null hypothesis. In the population, one of two states is true; the null hypothesis is correct, or the null hypothesis is not correct. Table 11.2 represents the decisions researchers can make with regard to the null hypothesis. Remember, we never know the exact truth of the null hypothesis.

Correct Decisions

When the researcher rejects the null hypothesis, and the alternate hypothesis is true (cell b), a correct decision is made. In

TABLE 11.2 Hypothesis Testing Decisions: (Correct, Type I, and Type II Errors)		
The decision that was made based on the evidence	The true state in the population	
	Null hypothesis is true (Retain Ho)	Null hypothesis is false (Reject Ho)
Reject the null hypothesis (Reject Ho)	Cell a Type I error (α)	Cell b Correct decision
Retain the null hypothesis (Retain Ho)	Cell c Correct decision	Cell d Type II error (β)

this case, the decision predicts that there is a relationship between the independent and dependent variables. For example, in our resting heart rate experiment, we conclude that the aerobic exercise group has a significantly lower resting heart rate than the control group. When the researcher decides to retain the null hypothesis, and the null hypothesis is true (cell c), a correct decision is also made. In this case, we would say that the resting heart rate for the aerobic exercise group and the control represent two samples from the same population and are not significantly different. That is, there is no relationship between the amount of exercise and resting heart rate.

Type I Errors

A **Type I error** is made when the researcher rejects the null hypothesis when in fact the null hypothesis is true (cell a). In other words, the researcher decides on the basis of the evidence that there is a relationship between the independent and dependent variable when, in fact, the researcher's finding was just a chance deviation from the true circumstances represented by the null hypothesis. In our heart rate experiment, a Type I error would occur if we decided that there was a significant difference in resting heart rate between the control group and the exercise group, when in fact the difference that we observed was due to chance or to some unrecognized factor in our experiment that resulted in the appearance of a difference. A Type I error is also represented by the Greek letter α (alpha). The term **significance level** is commonly used to indicate the acceptable Type I error rate. Researchers normally specify the significance level prior to beginning the study. For example, in our heart rate study, if we set the significance level at .05, we are willing to accept a 5 percent chance of committing a Type I error.

When reading the Results Section of a research report, you will find both p-values (probability values) and treatment index statistics. A p-value is the chance of committing a Type I inference error. When you read, $p < .05$, the researcher believes that there is less than 5 chances in 100 of a Type I error when the null hypothesis is rejected. Actual probability (p) values can range from zero (0.00) to unity (1.00). Neither of these values typically occurs in inferential research. Reported p-values typically range from .05 on the high end, to .001 (or even smaller) on the low end. For example, p =.03 indicates 3 chances in 100 of a Type I error, p <.01 indicates less than 1 chance in 100 of a Type I error. As you can see, the smaller the p-value (.01 versus .05) the lower the chance of a Type I error when the null is rejected.

Type II Errors

A **Type II error** occurs when the researcher retains the null hypothesis, when in fact the correct decision should have been to reject the null hypothesis (cell d). A Type II error is often represented by the Greek letter β (beta). In effect, a Type II error means that the researcher failed to recognize that the independent and dependent variables are significantly related. Researchers rarely give Type II error probabilities in a research report. Determining the actual probability of a Type II error is complex because it depends on various assumptions.

Controlling Type I and Type II Inference Errors

Researchers control the chance of committing Type I and Type II errors in several ways. As mentioned earlier, the way to reduce the chance of a Type I error is to reduce the significance level. If the significance level is .05, then there are 5 chances in 100 of a Type I error. If the significance level is lowered to .01, then the chance of a Type I error is reduced to 1 in 100. The tradeoff to reducing the chance of a Type I error is increasing the chance of committing a Type II error and decreasing **power**. Power is a statistical term and is defined as the chance of rejecting the null hypothesis when the null hypothesis is false. In other words, power is the opposite of a Type II error. The greater the power of a test, the greater the chance of correctly rejecting the null hypothesis (power is equal to 1-β). It is helpful to think of the power of a study as a type of microscope. The greater the power of the microscope, the greater one's ability to see true relationships between variables. Researchers should design a study with sufficient power so that they are able to identify relationships between independent and dependent variables if there truly is a relationship.

The probability of a Type II error can be affected through the combination of several methods. The simplest approach to reduce Type II errors would be to increase the significance level (for example, from .05 to .10). However, this is not normally a viable option since significance levels are stated at the inception of a study and should not be changed to fit the results of the data analysis. Other methods of decreasing the chance of a Type II error (and increasing power) include increasing the number of subjects, increasing the treatment effect, decreasing measurement error, and using more sensitive experimental designs. As mentioned previously, these are all options that cannot usually be adjusted as the experiment is being conducted, and clearly cannot be changed after the data collection has been completed. Therefore, these factors need to be considered before beginning the data acquisition.

THE EXPERIMENT

The first step in designing and conducting an experiment is to propose a research hypothesis, then develop the independent variable(s), identify the dependent variable(s), set the control variables, recruit subjects, and then collect the data. After gathering all the data, the researcher calculates descriptive statistics which include the means and standard deviations for each group and perhaps constructs some graphs. The exact nature of the analysis depends on the research and statistical hypotheses and the number and nature of the independent and dependent variables (as you will soon learn). At this point, the researcher asks some important questions. First, did the relationships among the variables turn out as expected? And second, are the relationships among the variables due primarily to the effects of the independent variable, or is the obtained relationship due primarily to chance factors? Inferential statistics are used by researchers to help answer these questions.

THE TREATMENT INDEX

To determine if the relationship between the independent and dependent variables was a true effect or more likely due to chance factors, a treatment index can be calculated. The treatment index indicates whether the researcher should reject the null hypothesis. Table 11.3 lists four treatment indices, χ^2, R^2, t, and F.

Understanding the nature, purpose, and rationale behind statistical testing will facilitate your better understanding of the Results section of a quantitative research

TABLE 11.3 **Hypothesis Test Treatment Indices**

Treatment index	Description	Expected value when null is true	Expected value when null is false	Primarily used with these statistical tests
χ^2	Test of association	Depends on sample size	Large relative to that when the null is false	1 Chi square 2 LISREL
R^2 or r^2	Variance accounted for	0.00	Absolute value significantly different from 0.00	1 Correlation 2 Multiple regression 3 Path analysis 4 LISREL
t	Test for differences	0.00	Absolute value of t calculated is typically greater than 1.96	1 t-test 2 Multiple regression 3 Logistic regression 4 LISREL
F	Test for differences	1.00	Value of F calculated is significantly greater than 1.0	1 Multiple regression 2 ANOVA 3 ANCOVA 4 MANOVA 5 MANCOVA 6 Discriminant analysis 7 Canonical correlation 8 Logistic regression

report. A variety of statistical distributions are used to test statistical hypotheses. Those most commonly used are the Z, χ^2, t, and F distributions. There are important differences in each of these distributions but the understanding of a general concept will make you a more informed user of the research report. Granted our overview is simplified, but the concepts are the same, regardless of the statistical procedure used. Look at the normal distribution (this is actually the Z distribution) presented in Figure 11.2. Some possible values for VO_2 $(ml \cdot kg^{-1} \cdot min^{-1})$ have been provided for you. Additionally, the approximate percentage (probability) in specific areas has been illustrated. The mean is 50 and the standard deviation is 5 $ml \cdot kg^{-1} \cdot min^{-1}$. Note that in this distribution it is quite unlikely that a subject would have a VO_2 greater than 60 $ml \cdot kg^{-1} \cdot min^{-1}$. Notice that 50% of the distribution is above 50 $ml \cdot kg^{-1} \cdot min^{-1}$. 34% of the distribution is between 45 and 50 and another 34% between 50 and 55. Let's use the distribution presented in Figure 11.2 to provide a simplified introduction to hypothesis testing. Assume that the VO_2 values presented in Figure 11.2 are accurate for some given population. Additionally, let's assume that you have a method of training that you believe will significantly affect one's VO_2. As indicated above, you must generate a research hypothesis, statistical null, and alternative hypotheses. For this example, these hypotheses are:

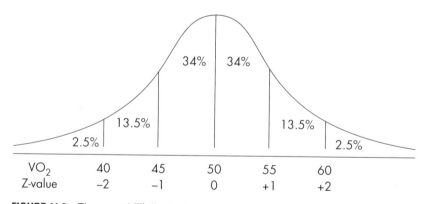

FIGURE 11.2   The normal (Z) distribution.

Research Hypothesis

My method of training will significantly change one's VO_2.

Note that you have purposely not said whether one's VO_2 will become higher or lower.

Null Hypothesis

Your null hypothesis will be that there is no difference in VO_2 as a result of the training program.

Note that this is the same as saying there is no relationship between training method and VO_2. This is the important part! Figure 11.3 illustrates the expected value of the difference between the groups *if there is no training effect.* That is, if your training method does not work and you repeatedly (actually an infinite number of times) conducted your experiment you might obtain the distribution illustrated in Figure 11.3. It is also important to realize that you conduct the experiment only once! Notice that the chances of identifying a mean difference of greater than $+10$ ml $\cdot$ kg^{-1} $\cdot$ min^{-1} or less than -10 ml $\cdot$ kg^{-1} $\cdot$ min^{-1} is very small. Approximately 5% of the time would you expect to obtain a mean difference larger than 10 ml $\cdot$ kg^{-1} if the null is true. Notice also that you are much more likely to obtain a value closer to 0.0 (a null) difference, if the null is actually true.

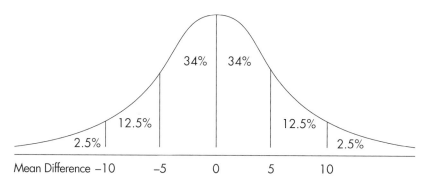

FIGURE 11.3 Illustration of the expected value of the difference between the groups; the expected distribution of the null hypothesis is true.

ALTERNATIVE HYPOTHESIS

The alternative hypothesis states that the two means are not equal (there is a significant difference in VO$_2$ max as a result of training). Thus if a researcher found a large difference between the groups (or $> \pm$ 10 ml $\cdot$ kg^{-1}), it is unlikely that this would occur by chance if the mean difference truly was zero (null). That is, the probability of this outcome is quite small, say less than 5 chances in 100 (or 5/100 or .05). Therefore the researcher rejects the null hypothesis in favor of the alternative hypothesis. Realize, of course, that the researcher could be wrong.

All inferential statistical tests follow the same reasoning. The major difference is that different types of distributions are used to test the probability (likelihood) of the null hypothesis being true. The Z test uses the commonly known normal distribution, the χ^2 distribution looks a bit like the normal distribution but is more positively skewed. The t distribution looks a great deal like the Z distribution (especially when the sample size is large), and the F distribution also approaches the Z distribution when sample size is large. Effectively, the researcher sets up a "falsifiable" hypothesis (the null) and then collects data and makes a decision about the truth of the null (or its alternative) based on the sample data.

Regardless of the distribution used (Z, χ^2, t, or F) and given that the null is assumed to be true, if the researcher finds an extremely rare occurrence, the null hypothesis is rejected in favor of the alternative hypothesis. This is illustrated in Figure 11.4 where in Graph A the means do not differ much, but in Graph B they differ significantly. The researcher who obtains a value that differs little from the null distribution would decide that the null hypothesis is the true state of circumstances and would determine that there is no relationship between the independent and dependent variables under investigation. The researcher who finds a large difference between the means assumed under the null hypothesis and that obtained from the sample data would decide that the null does not actually reflect the true state of circumstances. This researcher (B in Figure 11.4) would reject the null and report that there is a significant relationship between the independent and dependent

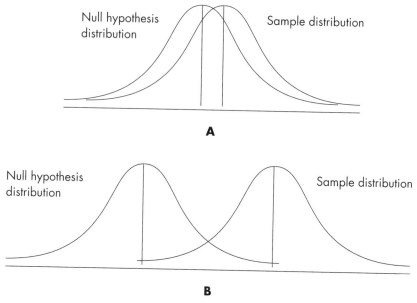

FIGURE 11.4 The null and alternative hypotheses.

variables. This paragraph is important to understanding hypothesis testing and much of the scientific literature. It provides the key and logic to all inferential statistical testing and many very advanced statistical interpretations that research consumers encounter on a daily basis. You are encouraged to reread this paragraph until you understand it fully.

DETERMINING WHICH STATISTICAL PROCEDURE TO USE

Knowing which statistical test to employ for testing the null hypothesis is a function of the number and nature of independent and dependent variables. Nature refers to the level of the measurement scale that the variables reflect (such as nominal, ordinal, interval, or ratio). These scales of measurement were introduced in Chapter 10.

Recall that regardless of the particular inferential statistical test used, the researcher is interested in ascertaining if there is a relationship between independent and dependent

TABLE 11.4 Types of Statistical Analysis

Number of dependent variables	Number of independent variables	Statistical analysis
1 nominal	1 nominal	Chi square
1 interval or ratio	1 nominal	t-test
1 interval or ratio	1 interval or ratio	Pearson Product Moment
1 interval or ratio	2 or more interval or ratio	Multiple regression
1 interval or ratio	1 nominal with 3 or more levels	One-way ANOVA
1 interval or ratio	2 or more nominal	N-way ANOVA
1 interval or ratio	1 or more nominal and 1 or more interval or ratio	ANCOVA
2 or more interval or ratio	1 or more nominal	MANOVA
2 or more interval or ratio	1 or more nominal and 1 or more interval or ratio	MANCOVA
1 or more nominal	2 or more interval or ratio	Discriminant analysis
2 or more interval or ratio	2 or more interval or ratio	Canonical correlation
1 nominal	2 or more interval or ratio	Logistic regression
	Many interval or ratio	Factor analysis

variable(s). While not exhaustive, the statistical tests presented in Table 11.4 are used in a wide spectrum of exercise and sport science research literature. We will present an illustration of each of the statistical analyses and include representative results from the literature.

CHI SQUARE

1 Nominal Dependent Variable

1 Nominal Independent Variable

If the researcher wishes to see if there is a significant association (relationship) between one nominally scaled independent variable and one nominally scaled dependent variable, the appropriate statistical test is a Chi square. Taking the example presented in the box on pp. 302-303, assume that a researcher believes there is a relationship between instructor gender in a conditioning class and the gender of the student enrolled in the class. Essentially, the researcher thinks that women are more likely to enroll in a class if a woman is teaching it and men are more likely to enroll if a man is teaching it. This relationship would be tested with a Chi square test. It is actually a test of whether the proportions of males in each class are equivalent to the proportion of females. The null hypothesis is that there is no difference in the proportions of males and females in the respective classes (that is, there is no relationship between gender of instructor and gender of student). Once the Chi square test is conducted, a probability is presented that indicates whether the proportions differ significantly beyond that which would be expected by chance if the null hypothesis is true. See the abstract box on p. 318 where Kelley and Kelley (1994) investigated the relationship between gender and physical activity. Note that they tested whether the proportion of active males and females was equal.

T-TEST

1 Interval or Ratio
  Dependent Variable

1 Nominal Independent
  Variable

The t-test is used to test if there is a significant relationship between a nominally scaled independent variable with two levels and a dependent variable that is interval or ratio in scale. It is actually a test of whether the means from each of the groups are significantly different or if the difference is small enough to be attributed to chance alone. Another way to express the null hypothesis is to say that the expected mean difference between the two groups is zero when the null hypothesis is true. Again, this is illustrated in the box on pp. 302-303.

There are actually two different types of t-tests (independent and dependent). The difference in the t-test depends on the nature of the experimental design. If the two levels of the independent variable have two different groups of people, the t-test is said to be independent. A study where different subjects are randomly assigned to an experimental group and

Chi Square Use in Exercise Science

Physical Activity Habits of African-American College Students

George A. Kelley and Dristi Sharpe Kelley

The purpose of this study was to examine the physical activity habits of African-American college students enrolled at a historically African-American institution. A total of 253 freshmen (90 males, 163 females) completed self-report measures of physical activity levels and were also assessed on height and weight. Chi-square analyses demonstrated that males (65%) were more active than females (42%). No significant differences existed between the prevalence of overfatness or obesity and activity levels for either males or females. Descriptive statistics showed a trend for groups categorized as more active to participate more frequently in selected physical activities. The authors concluded that freshmen African-American college students, especially females, display low levels of physical activity.

Results

Physical activity levels

Classification of participants' physical activity levels using the LRCPAQ is found in the table below. Overall, males were found to be more active than females, χ^2 (3, $N = 253$) = 14.02, $p < .05$. Post-hoc analysis (very low + low versus moderate + high) demonstrated that more females versus males were very low or low active, χ^2 (1, $N = 253$) = 11.62, $p < .05$. Approximately 42% of males and 65% of females were classified as low or very low active. Analysis of variance tests revealed no statistically significant differences in age, height, weight, or BMI between the LRCPAQ physical activity groups.

Physical Activity Classification of Subjects

Activity level	Males		Females	
	n	%	*n*	%
Very low active	7	8	34	21
Low active	31	34	71	44
Moderately active	34	38	36	22
High active	18	20	22	13

From Kelley GA and Sharpe Kelley D: Research Quarterly for Exercise and Sport 65(3):207-212, 1994.

T-Test Use in Exercise Science

The Physical Activity of Singapore Primary School Children as Estimated by Heart Rate Monitoring

Helen Gilbey and Malcolm Gilbey

Physical activity patterns of Singapore school children aged 9-10 years were assessed by continuous heart rate monitoring. Fifty boys and 64 girls were monitored for three 14-hour periods during normal school days. In addition, 43 boys and 53 girls were monitored for 14 hours on a Saturday. Only 13 children (11.4%) experienced a daily 10-min period of continuous activity at a heart rate ≥140 bpm. Twenty percent of the boys and more than 50% of the girls never achieved a single 10-minute period ≥140 bpm. Boys achieved more periods of moderately intense activity ($p < .01$) than girls on weekdays. Lean girls were more active ($p < .05$) than the obese girls during weekdays. No differences were detected between activity levels on weekdays or on Saturday. The results indicate that Singapore school children in general rarely experience the quantity or quality of physical activity needed for maintenance and development of cardiovascular health and cardiopulmonary fitness.

From Gilbey H and Gilbey M: Pediatric Exercise Science 7(1):26, 1995.

others to a control group is an example of an independent t-test. If the people from group one can be "matched" in some way with people in the second group, the t-test is said to be dependent (or correlated or paired). Test-retest designs (where the same set of subjects make up both groups) are "dependent" in nature. Twin studies, where one twin is in one group and the matching twin is in another group would also be dependent in nature.

The interpretation of the results is exactly the same for each type of t-test. The researcher rejects the null hypothesis if the difference between the means is so large, it is unlikely the null hypothesis is true. The results of an independent t-test are presented in the box above for differences between groups of children.

CONFIDENCE INTERVALS

You may encounter the term "confidence interval" when reading the Results Section. Development of a confidence interval goes "hand-in-glove" with hypothesis testing. While most researchers simply report the statistical significance of the inferential statistics some also include (or report results only with) confidence intervals. The 95% confidence interval is used with the .05 level of significance and the 99% confidence interval is used with the .01 level of significance. Essentially, if the results of the inferential statistics are significant (for example, $p < .05$), the 95% confidence interval does not capture the mean of the theoretical null hypothesis (usually the value of zero). Reporting confidence intervals and significance levels results in exactly the same statistical decision regarding the null hypothesis. Some researchers like to report confidence intervals so that the reader can see whether the null hypothesis was "just" rejected or was "greatly" rejected. Consider the following 95% confidence intervals developed on a t-test where two groups are contrasted and the null hypothesis is that the means do not differ (H_o = zero). The first author reports $p < .05$ and a 95% confidence interval of 0.4 to 10.4. The second author reports $p < .05$ and the 95% confidence interval of 9.4 to 10.4. Note that both researchers reject the null hypothesis at alpha = .05 because the value of zero is not captured in the 95% confidence interval. Note however that the first researcher's 95% confidence interval almost captures 0.00 and the second researcher's 95% confidence interval does not come close to capturing 0.00. Note that both still report statistical significance at $p < .05$.

PEARSON PRODUCT MOMENT

1 Interval or Ratio
  Dependent Variable

1 Interval or Ratio
  Independent Variable

We presented the Pearson Product Moment in Chapter 10 as a descriptive statistic. However, the Pearson Product Moment Correlation can be inferential in nature. That is, a researcher may hypothesize that there is a significant relationship between one interval or ratio scaled independent variable and one interval or ratio scaled dependent variable. This is illustrated in the box on pp. 302-303. The rationale is exactly the same as with other inferential tests. If there is no relationship between the two variables (the null) a researcher would expect to obtain a correlation of r = 0.00 between the two variables. Thus the null hypothesis is centered around a correlation of ρ = 0.00. The researcher gathers data on the two variables from a sample, calculates the correlation, and then decides how likely it would be to find the calculated correlation coefficient if the null hypothesis is true. If this is an unlikely occurrence (given that the null is hypothesized to be true), the null is rejected and the alternative hypothesis is entertained. The alternative hypothesis is that ρ ≠ 0.00. The box below illustrates the results of research using the Pearson Product Moment Correlation. Engelman and Morrow (1991) studied the relationship between two measures of pull-up performance and skinfold measures in elementary children. Notice that the correlations were significantly ($p < .01$) different from zero. The $p < .01$ literally means that if the null

---

Use of Pearson Product Moment in Exercise Science

Reliability and Skinfold Correlates for Traditional and Modified Pull-Ups in Children Grades 3-5

Mary E. Engelman and James R. Morrow, Jr.

Correlations between Pull-Ups and Sum of Skinfolds

Grade		Boys TPU[a]	Boys MPU[b]	Girls TPU	Girls MPU
3	MPU	.60*		.49	
	SKF[c]	-.37	-.36	-.26	-.35
4	MPU	.64		.65	
	SKF	-.40	-.48	-.35	-.46
5	MPU	.63		.71	
	SKF	-.33	-.48	-.41	-.40
3, 4, and 5	MPU	.63		.60	
	SKF	-.36	-.45	-.35	-.43

[a]Traditional pull-up.
[b]Modified pull-up.
[c]Sum of triceps and calf skinfolds.
*All correlations are significantly different from zero ($p < .01$).

From Engelman ME and Morrow JR: Research Quarterly for Exercise and Sport 62(1):88-91, 1991.

hypothesis is true, the probability that correlations of this magnitude would be obtained is less than 1 out of 100 cases.

MULTIPLE REGRESSION

1 Interval or Ratio
  Dependent Variable

2 or More Interval or
  Ratio Independent Variables

The next logical step from the Pearson Product Moment Correlation Coefficient is multiple regression. As evident in Table 11.4, multiple regression is used when two or more interval or ratio scaled independent variables are used to predict (or relate) to a single interval or ratio scaled dependent variable. The researcher's purpose often is to identify the most parsimonious model for accounting for variance in the dependent variable. To do this, the researcher typically hypothesizes that a number of variables are related to the dependent variable but that the independent variables are unrelated to each other. Statistical procedures are then used to develop a regression equation that is used to predict one's score on the dependent variable from the independent variables. Figure 11.5 illustrates different regression models. Each box (A through D) represents the variance of the dependent variable. The various shaded portions indicate the shared variation between the dependent and independent variable(s). Box A is simple regression (Pearson Product Moment Correlation) because there is only one independent variable. Boxes B, C, and D are multiple regression equations with 2, 3, and 4 independent variables, respectively. The area not shaded represents error. The researcher who uses multiple regression desires to reduce the amount of

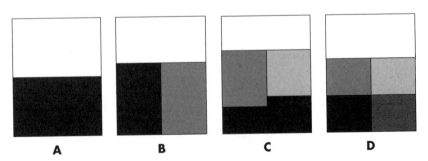

A **B** **C** **D**

FIGURE 11.5 Examples of multiple regression models.

error variance remaining after accounting for variance with the independent variables. The null hypothesis is that there is no relationship ($\rho = 0.00$) between the independent variables and the dependent variable. The alternative hypothesis is that there is a relationship between the independent variables and the dependent variable.

A statistic commonly reported with a multiple regression analysis is the standard error of estimate (SEE) also called the standard error of prediction (SEP), or simply, the standard error (SE). The SEE reflects the amount of error present in predicting the value of the dependent variable from the independent variable(s). Multiple regression and the use of the SEE are best provided by example. Jackson, Pollock, and Ward (1980) developed regression equations for estimating percent fat in women from three skinfold sites and age. The sites are triceps, suprailliac, and thigh. The three skinfolds are summed and used in the multiple regression equation presented in the box below. The regression equations and associated standard errors of estimate were developed for estimating percent fat.

Multiple Regression Use in Development of Skinfold Equations

Generalized Equations for Predicting Body Density of Women

Andrew S. Jackson, Michael L. Pollock, and Ann Ward

Abstract

Previous research with women has shown that body composition regression equations derived from anthropometric variables were population specific. This study sought to derive generalized equations from women differing in age and body composition. The hydrostatic method was used to determine body density (BD) and percent fat (%F) on 249 women 18 to 55 years (X = 31.4 ± 10.8 yrs) and 4 to 44 %F (X = 24.1 ± 7.2 %F). Skinfold fat (S), gluteal circumference (C) and age were independent variables. The quadratic form of the sum of three, four and seven S in combination with age and gluteal C produced multiple correlations that ranged from 0.842 to 0.867 with standard errors of 3.6 to 3.8 %F. The equations were cross-validated on a different sample of 82 women with similar age and %F characteristics. The correlations between predicted and hydrostatically

Continued.

From Jackson AS, Pollock ML, and Ward A: Medicine and Science in Sports and Exercise 12(3):175-182, 1980.

Multiple Regression Use in Development of Skinfold Equations—cont'd

determined %F ranged from 0.815 to 0.820 with standard errors of 3.7 to 4.0 %F. This study showed that valid generalized body composition equations could be derived for women varying in age and body composition, but care need to be exercised with women over an age of forty.

Generalized Regression Equations for Predicting Body Density of Adult Women

Variables	Regression equation	R	Standard error BD	%F
S,S², Age	*Sum of seven skinfolds* BD(1) = 1.0970 - 0.00046971 (X_1) + 0.00000056 (X_1)² - 0.00012828 (X_4)	0.852	0.0083	3.8
S,S², Age	*Sum of four skinfolds* BD(7) = 1.0960950 - 0.0006952)X_2) + 0.0000011 (X_2)² - 0.0000714 (X_4)	0.849	0.0084	3.8
S,S², Age	*Sum of three skinfolds* BD(13) = 1.0994921 - 0.0009929 (X_3) + 0.0000023 (X_3)² - 0.0001392 (X_4)	0.842	0.0086	3.9

Note that the correlation between hydrostatically determined percent fat and the combination of skinfold and age is approximately .85 (actually, .852, .849, and .842). The SEE is approximately 4.0%. This suggests that if by using the multiple regression equation a person's percent fat is estimated to be 20%, the researcher can be 68% confident that the person's actual percent fat is between 24.0% and 16.0% (20% ± 4.0%). Likewise, the researcher can be 95% confident that the subject's percent fat is between 28.0% and 12.0% (20% ± 2 × [4.0%]).

Additionally, researchers using multiple regression often conduct a test of the increase or change in variance accounted for with the inclusion of each subsequent independent variable. This is referred to as a test of R^2 change. Figure 11.6 illustrates

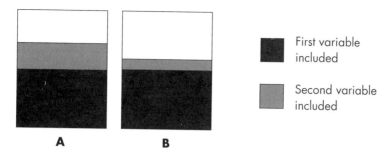

FIGURE 11.6 Example of change in R^2 with multiple regression.

this procedure. Note that both boxes A and B have identical amounts of variance accounted for by the first variable (about 60% for the dark-gray areas). However, the addition of the second variable (the light-gray areas) adds a great deal to the variance accounted for in box A but very little in box B. The researcher would conclude, based on the statistical analysis, that the addition of the second variable to box B does not add significantly to the variance accounted for in the dependent variable. Note again, the null hypothesis for the test of the change in R^2 is the same as for all other statistical tests (for example, that the increase in R^2 is zero). Once evidence is obtained to conclude otherwise (as is indicated here in box A), the researcher will reject the null hypothesis in favor of the alternative hypothesis. As with other inferential tests, the significance level α is reported.

ANALYSIS OF VARIANCE

1 Interval or Ratio
   Dependent Variable

1 Nominal Independent
   Variable with 3 or More
   Levels

One-Way ANOVA

The one-way analysis of variance (**ANOVA**) is a logical extension of the t-test. The t-test is used with two groups. ANOVA is used with an independent variable with three or more groups. A one-way ANOVA is used to analyze data when the researcher has one independent variable (nominal in scale) with three or more levels and one interval or ratio scaled

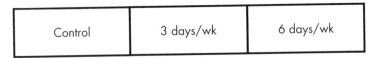

| Control | 3 days/wk | 6 days/wk |

FIGURE 11.7   One-way analysis of variance.

dependent variable. This is illustrated in Figure 11.7 where there are three treatment conditions. This could represent a researcher's interest in whether training 3 days per week differs from those training 6 days per week and those training no days per week. This is also illustrated in the box on pp. 302-303.

A one-way ANOVA results in a test of whether the means of respective levels of the independent variable differ significantly. Once again, the null hypothesis is that the means are equivalent and the alternative hypothesis is that the means are not randomly equivalent. The test statistic for the ANOVA is based on the F distribution. The researcher interprets the probability associated with the test based upon the number of levels of the independent variable and the number of subjects. If the probability of finding mean differences as large as those observed when the null is actually true is very low, the researcher rejects the null hypothesis in favor of the alternative hypothesis.

ANOVA is one of the most commonly used inferential statistics in sport and exercise research. It is essential that you have a basic understanding of ANOVA to help you interpret much of the statistical information found in many research reports. The analysis of variance is used often because it is actually a family of methods that can be used with a wide range of experimental designs. Whether the design has one independent variable, or more than one independent variable, and whether the design is independent groups or repeated measures, there is an analysis of variance that can be used.

Because ANOVA is so widely utilized, we will provide more detail about its use and interpretation than the other statistical procedures presented in this chapter. We are not going to present all of the intricacies of how an ANOVA is calculated from data. There are many statistics books available on the topic if you would like more detail. Rather, we will discuss the result of an analysis of variance, the ANOVA source table, what it represents, and how to interpret the values.

Between Groups Variability

Suppose we conduct an experiment on the effects of aerobic exercise on resting heart rate. The independent variable has three levels: a control group that does not exercise, and two different treatment groups that participate in an aerobic exercise. Subjects are randomly assigned to one of the three groups. Subjects in one group exercise 1 hour a session 3 days each week. The second group exercises 1 hour a session 6 days each week. At the end of 6 weeks of exercise, any differences in resting heart rate that we observe among the three groups can be attributed to two sources:

1 the effect of the independent variable (called the treatment effect)
2 any chance error

We'll call the sum of these two factors **between groups variability:**

Between Groups Variability = Treatment Effect + Error

If aerobic exercise does affect resting heart rate, then we would expect to observe significantly different mean resting heart rates between the three groups of subjects. The difference in heart rate is expressed in the between groups variability value. All other sources of variability are expressed in the chance error value. Chance error includes contributors such as individual differences among subjects, differences in testing conditions like the time of testing, or measurement error attributable to the equipment or the researchers.

Another way to think about the analysis is to consider what would happen if no treatment was administered. In our example, if none of the groups exercised, at the end of the six weeks we would expect the mean resting heart rate for all groups to be approximately the same. We would attribute any measured differences simply to individual differences in the sample (chance error.) Even when the independent variable has no effect, we expect to see slight differences between the groups simply due to chance factors alone. This is the question the researcher has to answer: Is the between groups variability caused by chance error alone, or is the between groups variability a result of the treatment?

Within Group Variability

In addition to between groups variability, we would also expect to observe differences among the subjects within the groups. This variation among subjects who are treated the same is termed **within group variability**. The actual term used for this factor may differ from one source to another (terms such as *residual, error,* and *within* group refer to the same thing). We will use the term *error* in the following examples.

One reason why random selection and assignment procedures are so important is the effect that random procedures have on the within groups variability term. By randomly selecting and assigning subjects to groups, any possible systematic differences that may exist between individuals are expected to average out. We know that separate groups of subjects are bound to be different on the variable that we are measuring, randomization assures that those differences will be randomly distributed among the groups and will be reflected in the within groups term.

When Treatment Effects Are Absent

If aerobic exercise has no effect on resting heart rate, then the differences that we observe between the control group and the treatment groups will be a result of chance error. In other words, if the independent variable has no effect, the treatment index would consist of one estimate of chance error (between group variability) divided by another estimate of chance error (within group variability). Developing a ratio of the Treatment Effect Variability and the Within Variability results in the following:

$$\frac{\text{Treatment Effect Variability} + \text{Within Group Variability}}{\text{Within Group Variability}}$$

Because the independent variable has no systematic effect, the treatment index ratio would be approximately equal to 1.0 when the null hypothesis is true. Note that this is the time when the Treatment Effect Variability is zero. Thus:

$$\frac{\text{A Small or Zero Treatment Effect} + \text{Within Group Variability}}{\text{Within Group Variability}} = \text{A Number Close to 1.0}$$

When Treatment Effects Are Present

Now let's assume that aerobic exercise produces a systematic and true effect on resting heart rate. In this case, we would observe a difference between the mean resting heart rates for the subjects in the exercise groups and the subjects in the control group. When calculating the treatment effect index, the value of the numerator (representing the differences between groups) would contain a value representing the treatment effect plus chance error, divided by the chance error within the groups. That is:

$$\frac{\text{A Large Treatment Effect} + \text{Within Group Variability}}{\text{Within Group Variability}} = \text{A Number Larger than 1.0}$$

In ANOVA, if the null hypothesis is true, the treatment index will be approximately equal to 1.0. If the alternate hypothesis is true, the treatment index will be greater than 1.0 because the treatment effect is expressed in the between groups variability term. In general, the greater the magnitude of the treatment effect, the larger the treatment index will be. The exact value of the index depends on the magnitude of the treatment effect and the amount of within group error. In general, the stronger the treatment effect and the lower the error, the greater the value of the index. If you think of this in terms of a normal distribution, larger treatment indices are near the extreme tails of the distribution and therefore are very unlikely if the null hypothesis is true. If they are unlikely, the researcher rejects the null hypothesis.

Researchers are usually most interested in finding support for the alternate hypothesis. Hypothesis testing, however, actually tests the status of the null hypothesis. To show evidence supporting the alternate hypothesis, we generally hope to be able to reject the null hypothesis. Recall that the null hypothesis predicts an absence of a treatment effect (in other words, no relationship between the independent and dependent variables).

ANOVA SOURCE TABLES
ANOVA Source Table for One-Way ANOVA

Computers are normally used by researchers to compute an analysis of variance. Calculating an ANOVA by hand, in theory,

Source of variation	Degrees of freedom	Sums of squares	Mean square	F-ratio	p-value
Factor A (between groups)	2	206.47	103.24	42.66	.02
Error (within groups)	27	65.40	2.42		
Total	29	271.87			

TABLE 11.5   One-Way Analysis of Variance Source Table

is not difficult. In practice however, hand calculations, particularly with a large data set, can be very time consuming and prone to errors. Whether the ANOVA is calculated by hand or by computer, the result of calculations is an analysis of variance source table. The ANOVA source table contains various information used to obtain the treatment index (the F-ratio) and the associated probability. It is the F-ratio that eventually allows the researcher to evaluate the null hypothesis.

A typical ANOVA source table for a one-way analysis of variance is presented in Table 11.5. The one-way ANOVA is used for experiments with one independent variable and one dependent variable. The source of variation column identifies the sources of variability; between groups variability, within groups variability, and total variability. We have termed the between groups variability as Factor A, it represents the variability primarily due to the effect of the independent variable. The source of variation termed error represents the within groups variability. The degrees of freedom (df) column, is used to determine the minimum F-ratio needed to reject the null hypothesis. The sums of squares column represents the calculated variability for each source of variation. The mean square column represents a value found by dividing the sum of squares term by its degrees of freedom. The F-ratio is the treatment index and is the end product of the analysis. The p-value represents the probability of making a Type I error if the null hypothesis is rejected.

Let's examine a hypothetical numerical example based on our resting heart rate experiment. The independent vari-

TABLE 11.6 Descriptive Statistics for One-Way ANOVA			
Independent variable	n	Mean	Standard deviation
Control group	10	74.9	1.2
3 times per week	10	70.1	1.3
6 times per week	10	68.8	1.4

able is aerobic exercise and has three levels—a control group and two exercise groups. The dependent variable is resting heart rate. We randomly assign 10 subjects to each of the three groups, conduct the exercise program, and measure resting heart rate at the end of the 6-week training period. Means and standard deviations are given in Table 11.6.

Recall that the null hypothesis states the population mean resting heart rates for the three groups will be equal. Our sample means are 74.9 beats per min^{-1} for the control group and 70.1 and 68.8 beats per min^{-1} for the two exercise groups, respectively. The researcher wants to answer the following question: Do the mean scores for the control group and the two exercise groups (which do differ) represent nothing more than samples randomly drawn from the same population, or is the difference between the three means too large to be explained by chance and therefore represents samples drawn from different populations? That is, are the means significantly different (or is there a significant relationship between the exercise and resting heart rate)? The analysis of variance provides the researcher with objective information to make this decision. The ANOVA source table presented in Table 11.5 includes the results of our hypothetical resting heart rate experiment. The two most important values in the ANOVA source table are the F-ratio and the p-value. Either the F-ratio (along with the degrees of freedom) or the p-value (along with the significance level) can be used to make a decision about the status of the null hypothesis.

The f-ratio and the p-value are inversely related. That is, as the F-ratio increases in value (from 1.0 to 10.0) the p-value decreases in value (from 0.5 to 0.05). These values are only for demonstration purposes, but the relationship is real.

The simplest way to make a decision regarding the null hypothesis is to compare the p-value with the significance level set at the beginning of the study. The decision rule is if the p-value is equal to or less than the significance level, reject the null hypothesis. If the p-value is larger than the significance level, fail to reject the null hypothesis. If we set the significance at 0.05, and our obtained p-value is 0.02, we reject the null hypothesis (0.02 < 0.05).

In our example, the calculated F-ratio is 42.62, which is very large. Since the probability is small of obtaining a treatment index this large when the null is true, we reject the null hypothesis at the .05 significance level. Based on this evidence, we can support the alternate hypothesis that persons participating in at least one of our groups do not have resting heart rates that are similar. In other words, aerobic exercise appears to significantly affect resting heart rate.

Indicating Statistical Significance in Tables and Figures

In addition to the written descriptions in the text of the article, researchers commonly use a combination of Tables and Figures to describe the results of the statistical analysis. When a graph is used to illustrate statistically significant results, the Type I error probability (or p-value) is usually also included. Figure 11.8 represents a graph that you may find in a research report. The graph provides the reader with essentially the same information as the written results for the main effect of the exercise group. Notice that the graph combines both descriptive statistics and inferential statistics. The descriptive statistics are indicated by the bars in the graph. The p-value is indicated by the $p < .05$ notation in the graph. When illustrating a result with a graph, the p-value is the only element of the inferential statistic indicated in the graph. The F-ratio and degrees of freedom are only given in the text of the Results section.

Tables are also frequently used in journal articles to summarize statistical information. Similar to Figure 11.8, when statistically significant results are presented in a Table, some form of notation is used to indicate these results. For example, Table 11.7 illustrates the same findings as in the previous graph with additional information about the subjects.

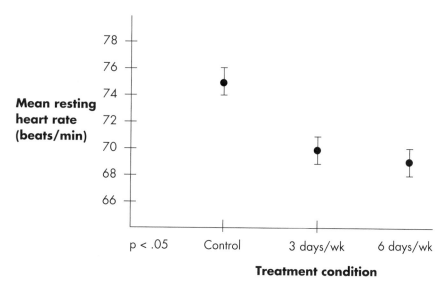

FIGURE 11.8 Graphical representation of ANOVA results.

TABLE 11.7 Tabular Results of Descriptive Statistics					
Means and standard deviations for the subjects in the three groups					
Treatment group	**Number of subjects**	**Age (yrs)**	**Height (cm)**	**Weight (kg)**	**Resting heart rate (beats · min⁻¹)**
Control group	10	21.3 ± 1.3	169 ± 10.5	58.2 ± 8.5	74.9 ± 1.9*
3 days per wk	10	20.9 ± 1.5	162 ± 11.8	57.5 ± 9.4	70.1 ± 1.3
6 days per wk	10	20.5 ± 1.6	165 ± 9.8	59.3 ± 8.4	68.8 ± 1.4

*p<.05

Table 11.7 shows the descriptive statistics for the subjects in the three groups. The asterisk following the resting heart rate alerts the reader to the fact that there was a statistically significant difference for heart rate among the groups. The $p < .05$ notation at the bottom of Table 11.7 indicates the

Type I error probability (p-value) for that difference. Notice, there is no asterisk present for the age, height, and weight. There was no statistically significant difference between the groups for these attributes. For example, if we reject the null hypothesis for age, there would greater than a 5% chance of a Type I inference error. Since we are only willing to accept a 5% or less chance of committing a Type I error if we reject the null hypothesis, we must decide to retain the null hypothesis for age (and height and weight). The actual notation used to indicate statistical significance varies from report to report. When reading a research report, examine the Tables and Figures closely and try to identify how the researchers indicated statistical significance.

MULTIPLE COMPARISON (POST HOC) TESTS

The ANOVA test is often referred to as an "omnibus" test because it is an all encompassing test to determine if the means are different. When the researcher rejects the null hypothesis and thus assumes there is a significant difference among the means, further decisions must be made. The omnibus ANOVA result only tells us that there is a difference among the means, but it does not tell us where the difference lies. In our three-group example, it might be between the exercise group meeting 3 days per week and the control group, and between the exercise group meeting 6 days per week and the control group, but not between the two exercise groups. Multiple comparison procedures (sometimes referred to as post hoc procedures) are used to identify which means are actually different if one rejects the null hypothesis with the omnibus test.

Let's continue with our resting heart rate example. The significant F-ratio tells us we have some significant difference among the three means but the analysis does not tell us specifically where the difference lies. From an examination of Table 11.6, it appears that the resting heart rates for the 3-days-per-week group and the 6-days-per-week group are similar, but these appear to be different from the control group.

Because we need to objectively determine where the statistical difference lies, the next step in the data analysis is the application of a **multiple comparison test.** Multiple comparison techniques are used to make specific comparisons following a significant finding from the omnibus ANOVA. Note that multiple comparison procedures are only necessary when there are more than two levels of an independent variable involved and when the omnibus null hypothesis has been rejected. When examining research in sport and exercise science studies, you will come across several types of multiple comparisons. Some of the more commonly used tests include the Duncan, Dunn, Dunnett, Newman-Keuls, Scheffè, and Tukey. Although these tests vary somewhat in their calculation or criteria, the basic logical underlying theme is the same.

Once again, the key thing to remember is that the null hypothesis for any multiple comparison test is that there is no (null) difference between the means being compared. A particular mean contrast is developed and then the probability of the means being as different as obtained in the sample, when the null is true, is determined. If this probability is small, the null is rejected and the alternative hypothesis is entertained. That is, the researcher concludes that the contrasted means are significantly different.

Multiple comparison procedures can be grouped in three ways. They are either simple (paired) or complex. They are either contrast-based or family-based error rate tests. They are either planned or unplanned. Each of these distinctions needs an explanation.

Simple versus Complex Multiple Comparison Techniques

Simple contrasts involve only two means (a paired comparison). In our resting heart rate example there are three possible pairwise comparisons (3-days-per-week group vs. control group; 6 days per week vs. control group; and 3 days vs. 6 days). A complex comparison involves more than two means in the contrast. From our example, a contrast that compares the average of the two experimental groups to the mean of the control group would be a complex comparison. Multiple comparison procedures used with complex contrasts can also be used to develop simple (pairwise) contrasts. For example, while the Scheffè procedure is a complex multiple comparison procedure, it can also be used to develop contrasts between two means only. However, simple multiple comparisons procedures cannot be used to develop complex contrasts.

Contrast-Based or Family-Based Error Rate

Each multiple comparison procedure has a significance (or alpha) level associated with it (that is, the probability of making a Type I error). However, the probability of making a Type I error can be thought of in two ways. Assume that the researcher is using an alpha level of .05. Some multiple comparison procedures are developed such that *each contrast* has an alpha of .05. Others are developed so that the entire "family" of contrasts has an alpha of .05. As you recall, the alpha level is chosen by the researcher prior to conducting any tests. But, as you might imagine, if a *contrast-based* error rate is chosen and one conducts a large number of contrast tests, the actual alpha level across all of the contrasts will actually exceed the alpha for any one of the contrasts. Regardless of the number of contrasts conducted with a family-based error rate, the alpha level for all of the tests conducted in total is equal to the alpha level chosen. For the family-based error rate, the actual alpha level for any given contrast will be much smaller than the alpha level for the entire family of contrasts. For these reasons, contrast-based error rate multiple comparison techniques are termed more liberal (in alpha) and the family-based error rate multiple comparison techniques are termed conservative (with regard to alpha).

Planned and Unplanned Contrasts

The last distinction we will make about multiple comparison procedures is between planned and unplanned contrasts. Planned contrasts are literally planned before any of the analyses are conducted. The researcher reasons that there are specific hypotheses that are desirable to test and the researcher is not interested in examining other contrasts. Another researcher might be more interested in "data snooping" following a significant omnibus test and thus will conduct several (or many) unplanned tests following a significant omnibus in an attempt to understand the results. As you might expect, the unplanned comparison method must protect against an inflated Type I error rate because of the "data snooping" used by the researcher. Thus a more conservative alpha level is generally associated with unplanned tests to protect the researcher against making a Type I error.

Table 11.8 summarizes some the commonly utilized multiple comparisons procedures.

We will illustrate the results of one of these tests, the Scheffè test, with our resting heart rate example. Recall that we obtained a significant F-ratio with the ANOVA from our hypothetical study with three levels. Because the ANOVA only informs us that there is a significant difference, we need to determine more specifically how groups differ from one another. Table 11.9 presents the results of a Scheffè multiple comparison test based on the means presented in Table 11.7.

TABLE 11.8   Commonly Used Multiple Comparison Tests

Name of test	(S)imple or (C)omplex	(C)ontrast or (F)amily	(P)lanned or (U)nplanned
Duncan	C	F	U
Dunn	S[a]	F	P
Dunnett	S[b]	F	P
Newman-Keuls	S	C	U
Scheffè	C	F	U
Tukey	S	F	U

[a] Dunn is used when the number of contrasts is "small" (for example, $<J(J-1)/4$ where J is the number of levels of the independent variable). See Glass and Hopkins (1984, p. 393).
[b] Dunnett is used when each simple contrast involves a treatment mean and the control group mean.

TABLE 11.9   Results of Scheffè Post Hoc Tests for Resting Heart Rate Experiment

Contrast	Mean difference	Scheffè F-test	p-value
Control vs. 3x	4.8	23.8	$<.05$
Control vs. 6x	6.1	38.4	$<.05$
3x vs. 6x	1.3	1.7	$>.05$

Table 11.9 presents each possible pairwise comparison. Associated with each of the multiple comparison contrasts is a probability similar to that obtained with the omnibus test. The interpretation of the multiple comparison test and probability is exactly like that of the omnibus test. If the contrasted means differ significantly, the null hypothesis for that comparison or contrast is rejected at the specified significance level. In our example, the Scheffè multiple comparison test indicates that the resting heart rate for the two exercise groups do not differ significantly from each other. Furthermore, the control group mean is significantly different from each of those of the exercise groups. Therefore we can conclude that aerobic exercise does affect resting heart rate.

Three other terms may be encountered following a significant omnibus test with ANOVA. The term *orthogonal* refers to contrasts that are independent of one another. Some multiple comparison procedures result in contrasts that are unrelated to one another, and other procedures develop contrasts that are non-orthogonal (related). A *trend analysis* is sometimes conducted in conjunction with an ANOVA. The purpose of a trend analysis is to determine if the changes across levels of an independent variable (typically time or number of trials) can be best described with a linear relationship or some nonlinear description (for example, quadratic, cubic, etc.). The term *Bonferroni* procedure refers to an adjustment made in the alpha (Type I error rate) because of the relatively large number of comparisons or contrasts conducted. The Bonferroni approach is also used when the author wishes to adjust the alpha level because of the number of dependent variables analyzed. For example, researchers may want to use the .05 significance level but because five tests are being conducted, they may choose to adjust the alpha level by dividing the alpha level by the number of tests being conducted. For example, .05/5 = .01. would result in the alpha level for each test being .01 rather than .05.

ONE-WAY ANOVA WITH REPEATED MEASURES (WITHIN SUBJECTS DESIGN)

The repeated measures ANOVA is a logical extension of the dependent (paired) t-test. The dependent t-test has two levels of the independent variable. There can be unlimited levels with a repeated measures ANOVA. Researchers often use a repeated measures or within subjects design. You were introduced to this design in Chapter 6. The researcher tests a single group of subjects on several occasions. Beyond this, the analysis is much like that typically conducted with a one-way ANOVA. One issue that is often presented, however, in the Results section with a repeated measures ANOVA is the test of *sphericity*. The repeated measures ANOVA carries with it specific statistical assumptions. One of these, the sphericity assumption, relates to the underlying structure of the correlations across the various occasions. Suffice it to say that if the sphericity assumption is not met, the researcher is more likely to make a Type I error. However, there are two commonly used ways to adjust the repeated measures ANOVA tests for violation of the sphericity assumption and thus increase the validity of statistical test of the null hypothesis. Should you encounter the names Geisser-Greenhouse or Huynh-Feldt, you can be certain that the researcher was concerned about the sphericity assumption and the possibility of the need to adjust the obtained alpha level to protect against inflating the probability of making a Type I error. The Geisser-Greenhouse and Huynh-Feldt procedures are used to adjust the degrees of freedom and/or the probability so that the possibility of making a Type I error is not inflated.

TWO-WAY ANOVA

Dependent Variable =
   1 Interval or Ratio

2 or More Nominal
Independent Variable

     The two-way ANOVA is a logical extension of the one-way ANOVA. The researcher is now interested in testing the effects of two nominally scaled independent variables. The independent variables can have any number of levels. Consider the example presented in Figure 11.9.

     Note that this is similar to the one-way ANOVA except that we have included a second independent variable (gender). The researcher can now determine if there is an exercise effect, a gender effect, and whether or not the exercise effect is constant across the genders (the interaction). Thus the researcher actually tests three null hypothesis: one for each *main* effect (exercise and gender) and one for the

IV$_1$: Exercise schedule

	Control	3 days/wk	6 days/wk
Male	Control/ male	3 days/ male	6 days/ male
Female	Control/ female	3 days/ female	6 days/ female

IV$_2$: Gender

FIGURE 11.9   Two independent variable experimental design.

interaction (exercise *by* gender). Once again, the ANOVA results are "omnibus" in nature and it may be necessary to follow the ANOVA with a post hoc procedure. This will be the case for any main effect that is significant if there are more than two levels of the independent variable. This is also true if there is a significant interaction. Researchers who obtain a significant interaction typically follow the interaction with a graph that illustrates the nature of the interaction or conduct simple main effects tests which permit the researcher to test for cell differences at various levels of the independent variables.

Figure 11.10 illustrates no interaction in Graph A and an interaction in Graph B. Notice that heart rate differences for men and women are constant at each level of exercise in A but those differences are not equivalent in B.

Let's conduct a two-way analysis of variance by adding a second independent variable, gender, to our resting heart rate example. The 10 subjects in the control group and 10 subjects in each exercise group could be divided by gender so that there are five males and five females in each of the three groups. Now we have a 3 × 2 independent groups design (recall that 3 × 2 means two independent variables, the first, exercise, having three levels and the second, gender, having two levels). Three hypotheses will be tested with this design:

1   Ho$_1$: there is no treatment (exercise) difference in resting heart rate.

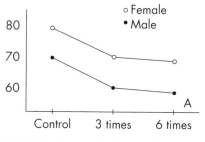
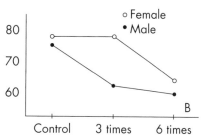

FIGURE 11.10 Graph of interaction.

TABLE 11.10 Two-Way Analysis of Variance Source Table					
Two-way analysis of variance source table					
Source of variation	Degrees of freedom	Sums of squares	Mean square	F-ratio	p-value
Treatment (A)	2	206.47	103.23	40.48	<.0001
Gender (B)	1	3.33	3.33	1.31	0.26
A × B	2	0.87	0.43	0.17	0.84
Error	24	61.20	2.55		
Total	29	271.87			

2 Ho_2: there is no gender difference in resting heart rate.
3 Ho_3: there is no group by gender interaction (the effect of the treatment is constant across the genders).

When this is the case, the ANOVA source table is modified by adding terms to describe each independent variable and interaction among the variables. Notice that the two-way (two independent variables) ANOVA source table presented in Table 11.10 is very similar to the one-way table presented in Table 11.5.

The additions to the table are the two new F-ratios; for the main effect of the second independent variable (factor B), and A × B for the interaction between the first independent variable and the second independent variable. All the other sources of variation remain the same and the methods

TABLE 11.11	Cell Sample Sizes and Means for 3 × 2 ANOVA		
	Males	**Females**	**Total**
Control	5	5	10
	74.4	75.4	74.9
3 days per wk	5	5	10
	70.0	70.2	70.1
6 days per wk	5	5	10
	68.4	69.2	68.8
Total	15	15	30
	70.93	71.6	71.27

for calculating the values are the same as in the one-way ANOVA.

Notice that each of these hypotheses can be thought of as a relationship. Hypothesis 1 investigates the relationship between exercise and resting heart rate. Hypothesis 2 investigates the relationship between gender and resting heart rate. Hypothesis 3 investigates the relationship between gender and exercise and resting heart rate. Hypothesis 3 actually investigates whether the treatment effect (exercise) is constant for both men and women. Table 11.11 presents the means and standard deviations for the six (that is, 3 × 2 = 6) cells in the design.

As was the case with the one-way analysis, next we need to determine if each of the calculated F-ratios for the three tests are large enough for us to reject the three null hypotheses at the .05 significance level. Once again, the most important piece of information in the ANOVA source table is the p-value associated with each null hypothesis.

First we examine the gender by group interaction p-value. The obtained F-ratio is 0.17. Since the probability of such an event is greater than .05 we retain the null hypothesis; there is no evidence of a treatment group by gender interaction. Since there is no significant interaction, we next examine the tests for the main effect of gender and the main effect of exercise.

We retain the null hypothesis for the gender effect because the probability is greater than .05 (actually .26). Based on this, we conclude that there is no evidence showing a difference in resting heart rate between males and females.

The result of the third test, the treatment effect, is nearly identical to the result we obtained with the one-way ANOVA (which we would expect with the same data). Because the p-value is less than .05, we can reject the null hypothesis for treatment. This was the same conclusion we came to with the one-way analysis. Once again, the researcher would have to conduct multiple comparison tests for the treatment effect because there are more than two levels of treatment and the null hypothesis was rejected.

N-WAY ANOVA

1 Interval or Ratio   2 or More Nominal
  Dependent Variable   Independent Variables

We have presented one-way and two-way ANOVA examples. However, the number of factors is theoretically unlimited. The generic term used to describe these factorial designs is "n-way" ANOVA. For example, a four-way ANOVA could be presented as a $2 \times 4 \times 2 \times 3$ ANOVA. This means there are two levels of the first independent variable (gender), four levels of the second independent variables (weeks), two levels of the third independent variable (intensity) and three levels of the last independent variable (frequency). While the design and ANOVA source table is a bit more cumbersome, the interpretation of the statistical tests is nearly identical to that which we have presented with the simpler ANOVAs. Interpretation of the probability statements is identical to that which we have presented for the simpler designs.

ANOVA IN A RESEARCH REPORT

The method of presenting results of an ANOVA varies from report to report and is usually dictated by the requirements of the particular editorial style utilized. At one end of the spectrum complete analysis of variance source tables are printed; at the other end of the spectrum only the Type I error probabilities

Sample Analysis of Variance Write-up

There was no significant gender by group interaction, F(2,24) = .17, p = .84, nor was there a significant main effect for gender, F(1,24) = 1.31, p = .26. There was a signficant difference for treatment group, F(2,24) = 40.48, p< .0001. The means and standard deviations were 74.9 ± 5.1 (control), 70.1 ± 5.4 (3 day week), and 68.8 ± 5.6 (6 day week).

are reported for significant differences. You will usually read this information in parts of the Results section, in the text, and in Tables or Figures. The box above illustrates one style for reporting the results of our two-way analysis of variance in the Results section. This example is representative of the style used by many of the journals in sport and exercise sciences.

Let's examine the ANOVA statistics in the above mentioned box in more detail. The first statistic in the paragraph reads: F(2,24) = .17, p = .84. The symbol, F, indicates that this result is from an ANOVA. The values in the parenthesis, (2,24), are the degrees of freedom. The degrees of freedom and the significance level can be used to determine if the relationship is significant. The calculated F-ratio is .17. Finally, the p = .84 symbol and value indicate the probability of a Type I inference error if the null hypothesis is rejected.

The second statistic in the paragraph reads: F(1,24) = 1.31, p = .26. Again the symbol, F, indicates an ANOVA. The degrees of freedom are, (1,24). The calculated F-ratio equals 1.31. The Type I error probability if the null hypothesis is rejected is .26. Therefore we fail to reject the null hypothesis.

The third statistic in the paragraph reads, F(2,24) = 40.48, p < .0001. The F(2,16) indicates analysis of variance and the degrees of freedom. The calculated F-ratio equals 40.48, and the Type I error probability is < .0001. In this case, the null hypothesis is rejected at the .05 significance level.

The last statistics are the mean and standard deviation for the control and exercise groups. These descriptive statistics are usually written: mean ± standard deviation. The plus and minus symbol, ±, indicates that the next value is the standard deviation.

ANALYSIS OF COVARIANCE (ANCOVA)

1 Interval or Ratio Dependent Variable	1 or More Interval or Ratio and 1 or More Nominal Independent Variables

Analysis of Covariance **(ANCOVA)** is a logical extension of an ANOVA and a multiple regression analysis. Actually, ANCOVA can be viewed as a marriage between an ANOVA and a multiple regression. Note in Table 11.4 that there is a single dependent variable (interval or ratio scaled) but there are now two different types of independent variables. There is at least one independent variable that is nominal in scale and at least one that is interval or ratio in scale. ANCOVA is used to test for mean differences in the levels of the nominal scaled independent variable *after adjustment has been made as a result of perceived differences in the independent variable that is interval or ratio in scale.* Once again, the basic concept is that the researcher is determining if there is a significant relationship between the independent and dependent variables. Research consumers will often encounter words such as, "after adjustment for [the particular interval or ratio scale variable], it was found that the levels of the [nominal scaled independent variable] were significantly different." Additionally, researchers often suggest that a pretest variable is "adjusted for" or "controlled for" to determine if there are differences in the dependent variable at the posttest measurement. ANCOVA is often used when the researcher believes that a particular variable is possibly related to the dependent variable. In fact, the researcher typically believes that the groups to be compared actually differ on the "covariate" (the independent variable that is interval or ratio in scale) and that it is necessary to adjust for any potential influence these initial differences might have on conclusions about the effect of the nominal scaled independent variable on the dependent variable. The use of intact groups (such as classroom research where the students are ability grouped or grouped in some manner) often results in the use of ANCOVA. Researchers often adjust for SES (socioeconomic status) when multiple school sites are used in the research and the schools differ in SES. Once again the null hypothesis, the actual statistical test, and the interpretation of the results

ANCOVA Use in Exercise Science

The Effects of Assigned and Self-Set Goals on Task Performance

B. Ann Boyce and Valerie K. Wayda

This study investigated the effect of three goal-setting conditions (self-set, assigned, and control) and two levels of self-motivation (medium and high) on the performance of females participating in 12 university weight training classes ($N = 252$). The subjects' levels of self-motivation were assessed via Dishman, Ickes, and Morgan's (1980) Self-Motivation Inventory (SMI). The baseline and performance trials were analyzed in a $3 \times 2 \times 10$ (Goal Condition $\times$ Motivation Level $\times$ Trial) ANCOVA design, with repeated measures on the last factor and baseline as the covariate. A significant interaction of goal-setting groups and trials was found. Planned comparisons indicated that the assigned goal group was statistically superior to the control and to the self-set groups from Trial 3 through retention. In addition, the two goal-setting groups were statistically superior to the control group at the seventh through retention trials. The subjects' SMI levels were not found to moderate the effect of goal setting on performance.

From Boyce BA and Wayda VK: Journal of Sport and Exercise Psychology 16(3):258, 1994.

are like all other hypothesis testing situations. The researcher is interested in testing whether the differences (once adjusted for the covariate[s]) differ beyond that which would be expected as a result of chance. Researchers using ANCOVA often report "adjusted means" with their analyses. These means are adjusted for differences in the covariate variable. If the null hypothesis is rejected and there are more than two levels of the significant independent variable, multiple comparison tests are used to identify which levels of the nominal scaled variable differ significantly. The box above illustrates Boyce and Wayda's (1994) use of ANCOVA using the pretest as a covariate.

MULTIVARIATE ANALYSIS OF VARIANCE (MANOVA)

2 or More Interval or Ratio
  Dependent Variables

1 or More Nominal
  Independent Variables

The next logical step in our analysis development is that of Multivariate Analysis of Variance **(MANOVA)**. An important point illustrated in Table 11.4 (on p. 316) is that all the statistical procedures used to this point in our presentation have included only one dependent variable. MANOVA is analogous to ANOVA except that there are *multiple dependent variables.* While the reasoning is relatively simple and the interpretation the same as with other inferential tests, the mathematical sophistication becomes much more involved. A key difference with MANOVA is that there are two or more dependent variables. Note that there may be any number of nominal scaled independent variables. Once again, the researcher is interested in determining if there is a relationship between the independent and dependent variables. Essentially, the researcher is interested in ascertaining if there are differences in a "group" (more than one) of dependent variables as a function of the independent variable(s). The null hypothesis remains the same except the hypothesis mentions the fact there are multiple dependent variables. The alternative hypothesis is that there is a difference somewhere among the multiple dependent variables. Should the null hypothesis be rejected with a MANOVA and the alternative hypothesis entertained, it suggests that there is a difference somewhere in the dependent variables across one or more of the independent variables and/or interactions. The researcher must then conduct some type of post hoc procedure to determine where the difference lies. Some common post hoc multivariate procedures include: (1) post hoc univariate ANOVA tests; (2) discriminant analysis; and (3) contrasts on the dependent variables. See Morrow and Frankiewicz (1979) for a review of this topic in sport and exercise science.

When reading the results of a MANOVA, you may encounter the Greek letter λ (lambda). Lambda is one of the statistics used to test the significance of the null hypothesis. However, the reader will also encounter an F-ratio which is interpreted in exactly the same way as has been described throughout this chapter. The box on pp. 348-349 presents an example of the use of MANOVA. Note that Van Raalte, et al. (1994) utilized three dependent variables (positive, negative, and instructional self-talk and gestures) when comparing two groups (match winners and match losers).

Use of MANOVA in Exercise Science

The Relationship between Observable Self-Talk and Competitive Junior Tennis Players' Match Performances

Judy L. Van Raalte, Britton W. Brewer, Patricia M. Rivera, and Albert J. Petitpas

In sport psychology, there is broad interest in cognitive factors that affect sport performance. The purpose of this research was to examine one such factor, self-talk, in competitive sport performance. Twenty-four junior tennis players were observed during tournament matches. Their observable self-talk, gestures, and match scores were recorded. Players also described their positive, negative, and other thoughts on a postmatch questionnaire. A descriptive analysis of the self-talk and gestures that occurred during competition was generated. It was found that negative self-talk was associated with losing and that players who reported believing in the utility of self-talk won more points than players who did not. These results suggest that self-talk influences competitive sport outcomes. The importance of "believing" in self-talk and the potential motivational and detrimental effects of negative self-talk on performance are discussed.

Self-talk, gestures, and tennis performance

A MANOVA was conducted to compare match winners and losers in terms of positive, negative, and instructional self-talk and gestures. A significant multivariate effect was found, Wilks's lambda = .66, $F(3,20) = 3.42$, $p < .05$, and univariate effects subsequently were examined. Results indicated that winners used significantly fewer negative self-talk and gestures ($M = 23.08$, $SD = 12.63$), than did losers ($M = 40.67$, $SD = 17.49$), $F(1,22) = 7.97$, $p < .02$ ($ES = 1.15$). Winners and losers did not differ in terms of the positive or instructional self-talk and gestures used.

It is possible that match winners used less negative self-talk than did match losers because the winners lost fewer points and therefore had fewer reasons to express negative sentiments. Therefore, analyses of covariance (ANCOVAs) were conducted to compare winners and losers in terms of self-talk used and in terms of the effects of their self-talk and gestures on subsequent points played with total lost points or total won points serving as the covariate.

A MANCOVA comparing match winners and match losers in terms of positive, negative, and instructional self-talk while controlling for total lost points indicated that match losers did not significantly differ from winners in terms of self-talk. Wilks's lambda = .79, $F(3,19) = 1.68$, $p > .05$. This suggests that the

From Van Raalte JL, et al.: Journal of Sport and Exercise Psychology 16(4):400, 407, 1994.

Use of MANOVA in Exercise Science—cont'd

differences between match losers and match winners may not be based on differences in the way that they *generate* negative self-talk.

An ANCOVA comparing match winners and match losers on points lost following negative self-talk while controlling for total lost points indicated that match losers were significantly more likely to lose a point following negative self-talk than were match winners, $F(1,19) = 4.57$, $p < .05$. This suggests that match losers and match winners may differ in the way that they *respond to* negative self-talk. There were no significant differences between winners and losers in their point outcomes following positive self-talk while controlling for total won points.

MULTIVARIATE ANALYSIS OF COVARIANCE (MANCOVA)

2 or More Interval or Ratio Dependent Variables	1 or More Interval or Ratio and 1 or More Nominal Independent Variables

If you have been paying particular attention to the presentation and looking closely at Table 11.4, you should be able to reason through the next topic to be presented. The ANCOVA followed the ANOVA presentation. We then increased the number of dependent variables and presented MANOVA. Thus, the next logical extension should be to include at least one "covariate" independent variable with a MANOVA and this becomes a Multivariate Analysis of Covariance **(MANCOVA).** The rationale here is a marriage between multiple regression and MANOVA. There are multiple dependent variables and the researcher desires to "adjust" for differences that might exist in one or more independent variable that is interval or ratio in scale. Since there are multiple dependent variables, the correct procedure is MANCOVA. Once again, the researcher might present adjusted means. Just like with MANOVA, if the null hypothesis is rejected, post hoc procedures are used to identify the exact nature of the differences that are reflected in the omnibus test. The box on p. 350 presents an example of the use of MANCOVA where Williams, et al. (1994) controlled for choice reaction time

MANCOVA Use in Exercise Science

Visual Search Strategies in Experienced and Inexperienced Soccer Players

A. Mark Williams, Keith Davids, Les Burwitz, and John G. Williams

This study investigated skill-based differences in anticipation and visual search strategy within open-play situations in soccer. Experienced (n = 15) and inexperienced (n = 15) subjects were required to anticipate pass destination from filmed soccer sequences viewed on a large 3-m × 3-m video projection screen. MANCOVA showed that experienced soccer players demonstrated superior anticipatory performance. Univariate analyses revealed between-group differences in speed of response but not in response accuracy. Also, inexperienced players fixated more frequently on the ball and the player passing the ball, whereas experienced players fixated on peripheral aspects of the display, such as the positions and movements of other players. The experienced group fixated on significantly more locations than their inexperienced counterparts. Further differences were noted in search rate, with experienced players exhibiting more fixation of shorter duration. The experienced group's higher search rate contradicted previous research. However, this resulted from using 11 on 11 film sequences, which were never previously used in visual search research. The increased frequency of eye fixations was regarded as being more advantageous for anticipating pass destination during open play in soccer. Finally, a number of practical implications were highlighted.

Because of between-group differences in choice reaction time (see Note 1) and because of the relationship between speed (reaction time) and accuracy (verbal response, computer response) measures (see Note 2), a one-way MANCOVA was used in analyzing group performance scores. In this test, experience (experienced/inexperienced) was the between-subjects variable, choice reaction time the covariate, and response time, verbal response error, and computer response error the three dependent variables.

Notes

1. The results of an independent samples *t*-test revealed statistically significant differences in choice reaction time between the experienced (*M* = 494.64 ms, *SD* = 134.07 ms) and inexperienced (*M* = 405.05 ms, *SD* = 85.51 ms) groups, $t(18) = 2.18$, $p < .05$.

From Williams AM, et al.: Research Quarterly for Exercise and Sport 65(2):127-135, 1994.

when comparing three dependent variables in experienced and inexperienced soccer players.

DISCRIMINANT ANALYSIS (DA)

1 or More Nominal
   Dependent Variable

2 or More Interval or Ratio
   Independent Variables

Notice that the characteristics presented for a discriminant analysis in Table 11.4 are just the reverse of those presented for the MANOVA. Discriminant analysis is essentially a regression equation where the dependent variable is a nominal variable (such as group membership). With a discriminant analysis, the research hypothesis is that the two or more interval or ratio scaled independent variables will significantly discriminate between the levels of the nominal scaled dependent variable. Logical thinking about the MANOVA illustrates that if a researcher identifies a significant MANOVA, one would also identify a significant discriminant analysis, and indeed this is the case. As always, the researcher is interested in knowing if there is a relationship between the independent and dependent variables. The null hypothesis is that the variables do not significantly predict group membership. The alternative hypothesis is that the variables can be used to significantly predict group membership. Researchers who report a significant discriminant analysis then report (1) a regression equation for predicting group membership, and (2) standardized discriminant function coefficients which help to identify which of the independent variables contribute most to group membership within the dependent variable. The box on pp. 352-353 presents the results of a discriminant analysis conducted by Corbin, Feyrer-Melk, Phelps, and Lewis (1994). Note how discriminant analysis was used to develop profiles of anabolic steroid use.

CANONICAL CORRELATION

2 or More Interval or Ratio
   Dependent Variables

2 or More Interval or Ratio
   Independent Variables

The canonical correlation technique is used when a combination of two or more predictor variables are used to

Use of Discriminant Analysis in Exercise Science

Anabolic Steroids: A Study of High School Athletes

Charles B. Corbin, Steven A. Feyrer-Melk, Craig Phelps, and Lisa Lewis

A group of 1,680 high school athletes were studied to determine factors associated with anabolic steroid use. A questionnaire assessed personal factors and steroid use, behavior of others and steroid use, and availability of anabolic steroids. Use rates were 1.1% for females and 2.4% for males. Steroids were more readily available to males, who also reported knowing more steroid users than did females. Older athletes were more likely to consider steroid use, but differences in use rate were not significant from Grade 8 to 12. Using discriminant analysis, significant differences ($p < .001$) were found for profiles of steroid users and nonusers for both males and females. For both males and females, personal factors such as having considered steroid use, a willingness to use them if they were legal, and a willingness to use them if they could insure success in sports were the most useful in classifying athletes as steroid users versus nonusers.

Discriminant function analysis

For males, a profile of independent variables charactrized primarily by personal behavior and availability scores emerged. Scores on the Behavior of Others scale was less important to the profile, as indicated by the standardized functions in the table on p. 353. The difference in the group functions (high positive for users and negative for nonusers) indicates that the profile fits the users and not the nonusers. Thus, male steroid users in this sample can by charactrized by a profile of steroid availability and personal behaviors associated with steroids, including having considered using them, especially if steroids were legal and would guarantee high-level performance.

For females, a profile of independent variables that differentiated anabolic steroid users from nonusers also emerged. Personal Behavior was the principal contributor, as evidenced by the high (.829) standardized function loading (see table on p. 353). Availability and Behavior of Others were significant contributors to the profile, but to a lesser extent. The difference in the group functions (high positive for users and almost zero for nonusers) indicates that the profile fits the users and not the nonusers. Female steroid users in this sample can be characterized by a profile of personal behaviors (having considered using steroids if they were legal and if performance were enhanced) and, to a lesser extent, steroid availability and the behavior of others.

Results of the discriminant analysis can also be used to classify subjects into user groups based on multivariate profiles. Use of this procedure with this sample indicated 89.8% successful classification for males and 93.1% successful

From Corbin CB, et al.: Pediatric Exercise Science 6(2):149, 154-155, 1994.

Use of Discriminant Analysis in Exercise Science—cont'd

classification for females. These classification results must be viewed with caution because the formulas for making the classifications were derived from the same sample that was used in making classifications. Before making generalizations about predicting steroid use with these formulas can be made, the formulas would need to be cross-validated on another sample of teenage athletes.

Discriminant Function Summary

Dependent variable	Males	Females
Standardized function		
Personal behavior	.638*	.829*
Availability	.637*	.296*
Behavior of others	-.123*	.200*
Function centroids		
Users	2.440	3.300
Nonusers	-0.061	-0.038

*Significant contribution to the profile.

predict a combination (two or more) of criterion variables. In other words, this process is used to measure the strength of association between two sets of variables. Canonical correlation is an extension of multiple regression. The difference is that there is now more than one dependent variable. The null hypothesis is that there is no relationship between the set of independent variables and the set of dependent variables. The alternative hypothesis is that the two sets of variables are related. An example of the use of canonical correlation might be to correlate a set of measurements of health-related fitness test items (for example, body composition, endurance run times, muscular strength, etc.) with another set of variables measuring cardiovascular health (such as blood pressure, cholesterol, VO_{2max}, etc.). The box on pp. 354-355 presents Ebbeck and Becker's (1994) research, which related perceived social, contextual, and personal factors to goal orientations in youth sport participants.

FACTOR ANALYSIS

Factor analysis is a multivariate technique having data reduction as its major function. Factor analysis is a method of determining the number of underlying "factors" that are measured by certain variables. Factor analysis is a procedure for reducing many "observed variables" into a few "unobservable but theoretically existent" factors (dimensions). The dimensions consist of variables that are correlated with one another. The researcher can choose to determine derived factors that are orthogonal (unrelated) or oblique (related) depending upon the nature of the questions and the theoretical relationships between and among the

Use of Canonical Correlation in Exercise Science

Psychosocial Predictors of Goal Orientations in Youth Soccer

Vicki Ebbeck and Susan L. Becker

Little is known about the nature of task and ego orientations that are key motivation constructs. The purpose of this study, therefore, was to examine the extent to which perceived social, contextual, and personal factors predicted the goal orientations of youth sport participants. The sample consisted of 166 male and female adolescent soccer players, who completed self-report measures at the end of a 7-week competitive season. A canonical correlation analysis revealed that the set of predictor variables accounted for 24% of the variance in player goal orientations. Higher scores on perceived soccer competence, perceived parent task orientation, and particularly perceived parent ego orientation were primarily associated with higher scores on player ego orientation. In addition, higher scores on perceived soccer competence, perceived parent task orientation, and perceived mastery climate, as well as lower scores on perceived performance climate, were associated with a higher level of player task orientation. These findings are interpreted and discussed in terms of future research directions.

Of primary interest in the present investigation was whether perceptions of social, contextual, and personal factors would predict player goal orientations. A canonical correlation analysis was conducted with self-esteem, perceived soccer competence, perceived mastery climate, perceived performance climate, perceived parent task orientation, and perceived parent ego orientation

From Ebbeck V and Becker SL: Research Quarterly for Exercise and Sport 65(4):355-362, 1994.

Use of Canonical Correlation in Exercise Science—cont'd

comprising the set of predictor variables, and player task and ego orientations comprising the set of criterion variables. This multivariate analysis was deemed most appropriate to determine if the set of predictor variables was related to the set of criterion variables, as well as the amount of variance explained in the criterion variables by the predictor variables. Furthermore, this statistical technique permitted an examination of the expected associations among the different predictor and criterion variables.

Canonical Loadings for the Predictor and Criterion Variables

Variable	Function 1	Function 2
Predictor variables		
Self-esteem	.28	.27
Perceived soccer competence	.36	.32
Perceived mastery climate	.07	.71
Perceived performance climate	.24	-.50
Perceived parent task orientation	.46	.78
Perceived parent ego orientation	.95	-.26
Criterion variables		
Player task orientation	.32	.95
Player ego orientation	.97	-.25

variables being studied. A classic example of the use of factor analysis is presented by Fleishman (1964), in which he reduced dozens of physical fitness measures to nine factors, two involving flexibility, four strength, and one each for coordination, balance, and cardiovascular endurance. Over time, Fleishman's results have been modified by other researchers but his use of this statistical technique still remains a classic example of its applicability. See the box on p. 356 for an example of a factor analysis conducted on body composition and structure measures. This work by Jackson and Pollock (1976) laid the groundwork for much of the skinfold measurements taken in body composition assessment.

Factor Analysis in Exercise Science

Factor Analysis and Multivariate Scaling of Anthropometric Variables for the Assessment of Body Composition

Andrew S. Jackson and Michael L. Pollock

Abstract

This study was designed to identify the body composition factors measured by skinfold fat (S), girth (G), and diameter (D) variables and to provide multivariate scaling models that measure fat (F) and lean body weight (LBW) factors. A total of 7 S, 11 G, and 7D measurements were determined on 83 young women (YW) and 95 young men (YM). Body density (BD) was determined by the hydrostatic technique. All variables were factor analyzed, and F and LBW were used to validate isolated factors. The YM data showed one F factor and two LBW factors. LBW factor I measured muscle mass and bone structure; LBW factor II, bone D. The YW data isolated four factors; the same three of YM plus a second F factor specific to the pelvic girdle. Factor score models were used to develop scaling strategies to measure F and LBW factors. Full models of all 27 variables and restricted models of 14 S, G, and D variables were developed; the correlations between factor scores scaled from the full and restricted models ranged from 0.84 to 0.98. The multiple correlation between factor scores calculated from the restricted models and laboratory-determined F and LBW ranged from 0.90 to 0.94 for YM and from 0.88 to 0.89 for YW. The multivariate scaling models provide a valid field method of measuring body composition.

From Jackson AS and Pollock ML: Medicine and Science in Sports 8(3):196-203, 1976.

EPIDEMIOLOGICAL RESEARCH

Epidemiological research is having a major impact on the quality of life of individuals. Epidemiology is the study of disease and/or disease risk factors and their relationships to morbidity and mortality. There are a number of disease risk factors that are important to those interested in sport and exercise science (for example, physical activity level, fitness level, blood pressure, diet, etc.). Physical activity as a risk factor for cardiovascular disease and a number of other debilitating conditions (such as obesity or diabetes mellitus) has been validated by epidemiologic research. Essentially, epidemiology researchers are interested in differentiating two groups (those with and those without a particular disease). Better yet, epidemiologists are interested in those who die from a given cause and those who do not die from that cause. Epidemiologists want to know if there is increased risk of a particular disease if the potential risk factor under study is present in one group but not in the other (see the box below). The development of odds ratios and relative risk ratios are used to demonstrate the increase or decrease in the prevalence of the disease depending upon whether or not

Epidemiological Statistics in Exercise Science

Physical Fitness and All-Cause Mortality: A Prospective Study of Healthy Men and Women

Steven N. Blair, Harold W. Kohl III, Ralph S. Paffenbarger, Jr., Debra G. Clark, Kenneth H. Cooper, and Larry W. Gibbons

Age-Adjusted All-Cause Death Rates per 10,000 Person-Years of Follow-Up (1970 to 1985) by Physical Fitness Groups in Men and Women in the Aerobics Center Longitudinal Study

Fitness group	Person-years of follow-up	No. of deaths	Age-adjusted rates per 10,000 person-years	Relative risk	95% confidence limits
Men					
1 (low)	14515	75	64.0	3.44*	2.05, 5.77
2	16898	40	25.5	1.37	0.76, 2.50
3	17287	47	27.1	1.46	0.81, 2.63
4	18792	43	21.7	1.17	0.63, 2.17
5 (high)	17557	35	18.6	1.00	. . .
Women					
1 (low)	4916	18	39.5	4.65[†]	2.22, 9.75
2	5329	11	20.5	2.42	1.09, 5.37
3	5053	6	12.2	1.43	0.60, 3.44
4	5522	4	6.5	0.76	0.27, 2.11
5 (high)	4613	4	8.5	1.00	. . .

[*] Test for linear trend, slope = −4.5; 95% confidence limits, −7.1, −1.9.
[†] Test for linear trend, slope = −5.5; 95% confidence limits, −9.2, −1.9.

From Blair SN, et al.: JAMA 262:2395-2401, 1989.

the risk factor is present. The null hypothesis is that there is no relationship between the presence of the risk and the disease development. That is, there is no increase in disease if the potential risk is present. The alternative hypothesis is that the likelihood of developing the disease goes up significantly if the risk factor is present. As stated in the work of Blair, et al. (1989), they indicated that all-cause mortality is related to physical fitness level. Note that the risk of disease is significantly increased when the risk factor (in this case lack of physical fitness) is present.

ADDITIONAL CORRELATIONAL STATISTICS
Path Analysis

Path analysis is used to test hypothesized correlations between variables. Usually the researcher starts with a theory about how a set of variables might be linked to one another. Next, measures of these variables are located or developed. Finally, the path analysis statistics are calculated to determine the strength of the correlations between each of the pairs of variables believed to be causally linked and then these statistics are interpreted as supportive of the hypothesis or not. The null hypothesis is that the variables are uncorrelated and that the paths between variables do not support the theory. The alternative hypotheses consist of statements indicating that the relationships between various variables are significant and meaningful. The box on pp. 359-360 presents Brustad's (1993) path analysis of a theoretical model which examined the role of parental socialization and children's psychological characteristics on children's attraction to physical activity.

LISREL

Linear Structural Relations (LISREL), or structural equation modeling, or confirmatory factor analysis has begun to appear more recently in the sport and exercise science literature. LISREL is, in a sense, a marriage between and among path analysis, correlational analysis, and factor analysis. The researcher presupposes a particular relationship between and among variables. Data are then collected and the researcher attempts to fit the data to the proposed theoretical model. The

---

Path Analysis Example in Exercise Science

Who Will Go Out and Play? Parental and Psychological Influences on Children's Attraction to Physical Activity

Robert J. Brustad

Identifying social and psychological influences affecting children's attitudes about physical activity is an important step in understanding individual differences in children's activity involvement. This study examined the influence of parental socialization and children's psychological characteristics upon attraction to physical activity. Fourth-grade children ($N = 81$) completed questionnaires assessing perceived physical competence and attraction to physical activity. Parents also completed questionnaires assessing their physical activity orientations and level of encouragement of their child's physical activity. A proposed model linking four sets of social and psychological variables was tested through path analysis. The results generally supported the hypothesized model and suggested that parental physical activity orientations, parental encouragement levels, children's gender, and children's perceived physical competence are important influences upon children's attraction to physical activity.

The purpose of this study was to test a conceptual model that links parental physical activity orientations (for example, enjoyment, fitness, importance), parental socialization practices (such as encouragement), and children's self-perceptions with children's attraction to physical activity. The proposed model is presented in the figure on p. 360 and corresponds with the expectancy-socialization research of Eccles and colleagues (8, 9). It is anticipated that parents with favorable orientations toward physical activity will provide their child with more encouragement to engage in it. Higher levels of encouragement will then translate into greater perceived competence. Higher levels of perceived competence will in turn be linked to greater attraction to physical activity. In line with gender related socialization research (8, 9, 14), it is also hypothesized that young males will receive greater encouragement in physical activity than young females and will demonstrate higher perceived competence, thereby indirectly affecting boys' and girls' attraction to physical activity.

Continued.

From Brustad RJ: Pediatric Exercise Science 5(3):210, 212-213, 1993.

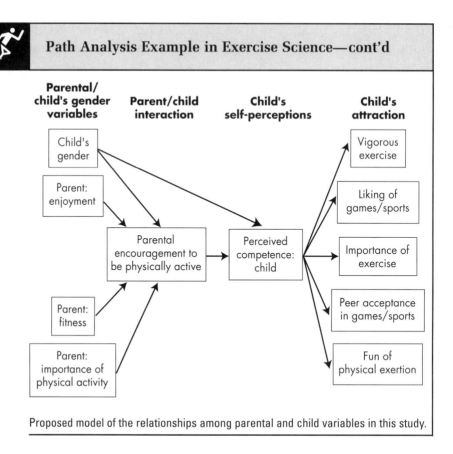

Path Analysis Example in Exercise Science—cont'd

Proposed model of the relationships among parental and child variables in this study.

null hypothesis is that the data do not fit the theoretical model and the alternative hypothesis is that the data fit the model significantly. Attempts are made to redefine the model and refit the data based on preliminary data analysis. Greenockle, Lee, and Lomax (1990) used LISREL to show that prediction of exercise behavior by attitude and subjective norm was significantly mediated by the subject's intention. A summary of the Greenockle, Lee, and Lomax work is presented in the box on p. 361.

OTHER BIVARIATE CORRELATIONS

Researchers occasionally use other correlational statistics. You should be aware that if inference is made and hypothesis testing is the basis for the work and interpretation, the general

Use of LISREL in Exercise Science

The Relationship between Selected Student Characteristics and Activity Patterns in a Required High School Physical Education Class

Karen M. Greenockle, Amelia A. Lee, and Richard Lomax

This study described the activity patterns of students in a high school fitness class and explored the structural relationships between particular student characteristics and their systematically coded exercise behavior. Although percent of time spent jogging was low (18%), with no gains made in cardio-vascular fitness, the amount of time spent jogging, the distance covered, and fitness level were all significantly correlated. A LISREL VI computer program was used to test a structural equation model representing the Fishbein Behavioral-Intention Model. In support of the model, results showed the prediction of exercise behavior by attitude and subjective norm was significantly mediated by intention. Although not significant, it is worth noting that subjective norm was found to be the stronger predictor of intention over attitude. Background variables were found to indirectly influence intention through their signficant influence on attitude and subjective norm. For this sample of 9th and 10th graders, significant others, particularly their peers and teachers, had a stronger impact on behavior than personal attitudes about activity.

From Greenockle KM, Lee AA, and Lomax R: Research and Exercise Quarterly 61(1):59-69, 1990.

procedures and reasoning that we have presented in this chapter will be common to all of these tests. A few uncommonly reported statistics are presented below.

- *Phi Coefficient*—The phi coefficient is used to determine the correlation between two variables that are dichotomies (nominal with two levels of each). Examples might include gender (male or female) and letter winner (yes or no) or two questions on an examination, each scored as correct or incorrect.
- *Rank Biserial Correlation*—This coefficient is used to determine the correlation between a dichotomous variable and an ordinal variable. It would be used, for example, to determine the correlation between gender (male or female) and the rankings resulting from a round robin tennis tournament.

- *Point Biserial Correlation*—This correlational method is appropriate when you wish to determine the correlation between a true dichotomy and a continuous (interval or ratio) variable. It is commonly used to correlate gender (male or female) with any number of continuous variables. Another very common use is in the analysis of written tests where a single item scored dichotomously as correct or incorrect is correlated with the total examination score.
- *Tetrachoric Correlation*—This correlational method is used when the variables involved are assumed to be continuous (interval or ratio) but for some reason the researcher decides to treat them as dichotomous. The artificial dichotomy is typically constructed by selecting a point on the score scale and assigning everyone on one side of the point as "passing" and on the other side as "failing." Passing and failing might be replaced with concepts such as "master" and "nonmaster" or "having the characteristic" and "not having the characteristic." The construction of artificial dichotomies is common in research involving criterion-referenced measurement. For example, establishing the criterion of knocking over seven or more bowling pins on the first ball as a "master" (and, of course, six or less as a "nonmaster") would be an illustration of creating a dichotomy from a continuous variable. Another current example is establishing the point on a health-related fitness test item (the one-mile walk/run) above which an individual needs to score to be considered "healthy." The tetrachoric coefficient might be used to express the correlation between two such health-related fitness test items.
- *Biserial Correlation*—The biserial correlation coefficient is calculated when one variable is an artificial dichotomy and the other is continuous (interval or ratio). This would be used, for example, if you wanted to assess the association between passing or failing a course (this is the artificial dichotomy) and scores on the final examination.
- *Spearman rho Correlation*—Sometimes called the rank-difference correlation coefficient, this procedure is applicable when one or both of the variables are measured at the ordinal level. If one variable is ordinal and one is

continuous, it would be possible to convert the continuous variable to the ordinal level and use the Spearman rho or to treat the ordinal variable as if it were continuous and use the Pearson Product Moment Correlation Coefficient. Judges' rankings, rank in class, ranks resulting from tournaments, and rankings of perceived exertion are all examples of possible variables for which this technique is appropriate.

META-ANALYSIS

Meta-analyses are increasingly being found in the scientific literature. Meta-analytic procedures are used to summarize a large number of quantitative studies and draw conclusions about a particular research hypothesis based on multiple studies. Prior to the use of meta-analysis, researchers would simply read all the studies related to a particular research hypothesis and then draw conclusions based on this qualitative review of the literature. Meta-analytic procedures employ methods where the researcher quantifies the results from the many reviewed studies and then draws conclusions about the research hypothesis based on this quantitative review. The primary dependent variable in a meta-analysis is the "effect size," which represents the effect of the treatment in terms of the number of standard deviation units of difference represented by contrasted groups. Thomas and French (1986) present an excellent review and tutorial on the use of meta-analysis in sport and exercise science. Often, many statistical procedures presented in this chapter are used in conjunction with a meta-analysis (such as t-tests, correlations, ANOVA, and graphical presentations). The results of a meta-analysis on functional capacity in the elderly are presented in the box on p. 364.

MULTIDIMENSIONAL SCALING

Researchers in many fields of inquiry are often faced with the problem of measuring and understanding the relationships between objects when the underlying dimensions are not known. A technique known as multidimensional scaling (MDS) "can help systematize data in areas where organizing

Meta-Analysis in Exercise Science

The Effects of Endurance Training on Functional Capacity in the Elderly: A Meta-Analysis

Abstract

John S. Green and Stephen F. Crouse

In this investigation, meta-analysis was used to delineate exercise induced changes in the VO_{2max} of older individuals and test a null hypothesis of no significant training effects. Parameters included in the analysis were age of the subjects, length of the training regimen, frequency and duration of exercise bouts, pretraining VO_{2max}, posttraining VO_{2max}, and the difference between pretraining and posttraining VO_{2max} (ΔVO_{2max}). Effect size for training-induced improvements in VO_{2max} was calculated, corrected for bias, weighted, and analyzed according to contemporary meta-analysis procedures. The mean effect size was found to be 0.65 standard deviation units, representing an improvement in oxygen consumption of 22.8%. The mean effect size was also significantly different from 0 ($P < 0.0001$), and the null hypothesis was rejected. Stepwise regression analysis indicated that length of training, pretraining VO_{2max}, and duration of training bouts accounted for 59% of the total variation in ΔVO_{2max}. In addition, age was found to be inversely correlated with pretraining VO_{2max} ($r = -0.56$, $P = 0.002$), and ΔVO_{2max} ($r = -0.56$, $P = 0.003$). It was concluded that endurance training significantly increases functional capacity in the elderly, and that the increase is related to subject age, duration of exercise bouts, length of the training regimen, and pretraining VO_{2max}.

From Green JS and Crouse SF: Medicine and Science in Sports and Exercise 27(6): 920-926, 1995.

concepts and underlying dimensions are not well-developed" (Schiffman, Reynolds, and Young, 1981, p. 3). In essence, MDS is a mathematical tool which is used to represent the similarity of objects spatially. These "cognitive maps" can be generated by computer. All that is needed is a set of numbers that expresses most, if not all, combinations of pairs of similarities for a given group of objects. Each object is represented as a point on a spatial map. Objects judged as similar to each other appear close to one another on these maps. Objects judged as dissimilar are represented by points distant from one another.

After a spatial representation is generated, the resulting dimensions can be labeled through visual examination and various property fitting techniques. For example, subjects might be asked to rate the similarity of several pairs of physical activities. MDS analysis of these similarity values would reveal a spatial representation of these activities. Those of high physical intensity might group together at one end of a spatial representation, while those activities of low physical activity might appear toward the other end of the spatial representation. This map would indicate that intensity is an attribute that this subject(s) attends to when perceiving physical activities. Similarly, MDS might yield a spatial representation in which competitive activities group together, away from noncompetitive activities.

One way to label the dimensions is for experts in the area to simply observe and determine what label appears appropriate. As in the example above, it may be obvious that the dimension is determined by the competitive nature of the physical activities. In other cases, the label for a dimension may not be as apparent. In these cases, *property fitting* procedures may be of use. Property fitting is done by having subjects rate each stimulus on certain attributes (such as physical intensity, competitiveness, etc.) which the investigator believes to be salient for the perceiver. These ratings may then be correlated with the dimensional solution. Attributes that correlate strongest with a particular dimension may help to give an indication of characteristics that subjects are perceiving.

ADVANCED TOPICS

You should realize that there are other significance tests available. We have presented those most widely seen in the sport and exercise science literature. However, if you should encounter a particular statistical test (they are often identified by an individual's name), do not be concerned. The rationale and interpretation are likely identical to that we have presented. Research, null, and alternative hypotheses are the basis for each of the statistical tests. The key things are determination of the independent and dependent variables and the probability (p-value) associated with the particular test.

Examples of more advanced analysis include the DM MANOVA and logistic regression analysis. A DM MANOVA is a marriage between a repeated measures (within-subjects) design and MANOVA. In this case, the subjects are measured on more than one occasion and there are multiple dependent measures obtained at each occasion. While very mathematically sophisticated, the purpose and general concept of hypothesis testing with the DM MANOVA is exactly the same as presented throughout this chapter. Schutz and Gessaroli (1987) present an excellent tutorial on the use and interpretation of the DM MANOVA analysis. Logistic regression is related to multiple regression and discriminant analysis. The purpose is to determine variables that predict group membership. The end results are statements of the probability of being in a particular group (for example, diseased, not diseased) based on a profile of predictor variables. Again, there is a research hypothesis and null and alternative statistical hypotheses. The statistical hypotheses have probabilities associated with them just as all the procedures we have presented in this chapter.

SUMMARY

We have presented many different statistical procedures in this chapter. We realize this has been a quick overview. We do not expect that the reader could conduct these statistical tests at this time. However, you should have a reasonable grasp of the concept of hypothesis testing and the interpretation thereof. Nearly all of the procedures mentioned in this chapter find true meaningfulness as a result of hypothesis testing. If you conduct even a cursory review of research in sport and exercise science you will encounter many of these concepts, statistical tests, and procedures. Most researchers utilize more than one of these tests in each of their research reports. Your ability to identify the independent and dependent variables, the purpose of the work, and the null hypothesis will greatly facilitate your reading of the scientific literature. Once again, the key concept is to understand the relationships between the research and statistical (null and alternative) hypotheses and the process of hypothesis testing. If you understand this concept, you will be able to read intelligently much of the scientific literature.

EXERCISES

1 State the null and alternate hypotheses for each of the following experiments:

a A study on the frequency of exercise induced asthma in males and females.

b A study on the pain reduction and flexibility in mild, moderate and severe osteoarthritis patients following hydro-exercise.

c A study on the amount of delta-wave sleep in low, moderate, and high fitness level subjects who exercise at moderate levels for 15 minutes, 45 minutes or 75 minutes a day.

d A study on strength gains in adolescent (13-16 years), young adult (23-26 years), and middle-age adult (33-36) subjects who train setting either their own goals or train following the goals set by a strength and conditioning coach.

2 Try to list some of the variables that might predict college graduation rates. Of these variables, which do you think would be the most important predictors and which would only be relatively minor predictors?

3 A study was done to test whether diet affected strength gains for individuals in a strength training program. One groups of subjects had a diet with 10% protein, a second group had a diet with 15% protein, and a third group had a diet with 25% protein. The dependent variable was strength gain. A .05 significance level was used to evaluate the results.

a Is the dependent variable measured on the nominal, ordinal, interval, or ratio scale?

b Which descriptive statistic would you use in this study?

c Which inferential statistic would you use to test the differences among the groups?

d What are the null and alternate hypotheses?

e What is the probability of a Type I inference error if the null hypothesis is rejected?

f What would have to occur for the researchers to make a Type II inference error?

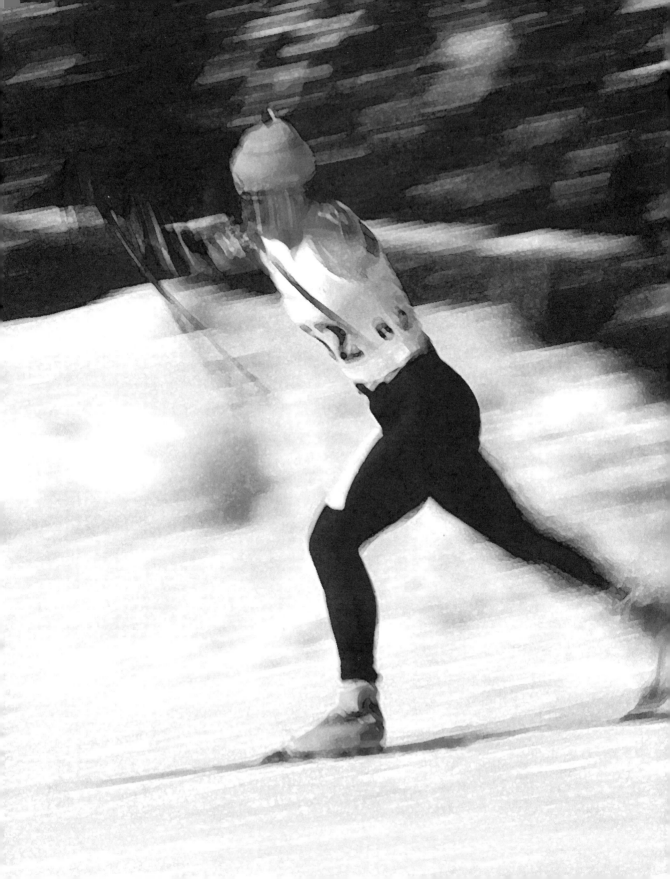

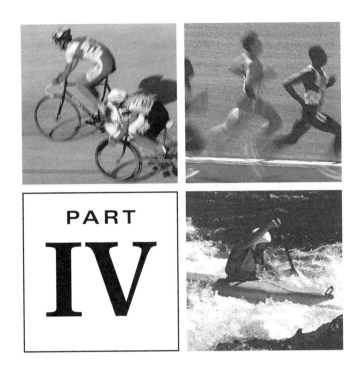

Discussion

12   Conducting Research

Conducting Research

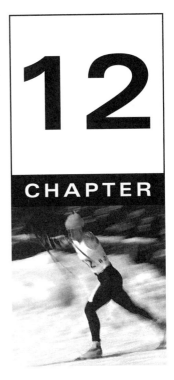

12

CHAPTER

LEARNING GOALS

After reading this chapter you will be able to:

1 Describe the purpose of the Discussion section of a research report.

2 Explain why writing creatively is important to an effective Discussion section.

3 Describe the general goals of a research proposal and how a well-designed proposal makes conducting research more efficient and effective.

4 Define the term *objectivity*.

5 List the main sections of a research proposal.

6 Explain how pilot studies assist the research process.

7 Explain why it is important for researchers to control both subject and experimentalist expectations.

8 Explain the difference between single-blind and double-blind methods.

9 Discuss why replication is important and explain the difference between exact and conceptual replication.

10 Explain the difference between *limitation* and *delimitation*.

11 Explain the purpose of informed consent in research.

12 Outline the steps in the peer review process.

TERMS

Research proposal
Pilot study
Single-blind
Double-blind
Delimitation
Limitation
Informed consent
Peer review

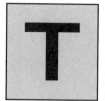he key to an effective research Discussion section is to tie the purpose, methods, and results together to convey to the reader the importance of what the researcher has learned. The Discussion section answers the question, "So what?" regarding the research question(s). This is true regardless of the nature of the research report. That is, the Discussion section serves the same purpose whether the work is quantitative or qualitative in nature. Essentially, the Discussion section is the culmination of the author to creatively transmit the results and findings in a way that convinces the reader that important new understanding has emerged as a result of the current research process. Creativity and insight are the researcher's most valuable assets when completing the Discussion section. The box on pp. 373-375 contains an excellent example of the important role that the Discussion section plays in a research report.

While the editorial in the box speaks specifically to the written research report, similar comments can be made about the oral or poster presentation that a researcher might develop. In a brief (typically 12-15 minutes) oral report the researcher must succinctly summarize the purpose and methods, and then focus on the results and a good discussion of what the research means to the audience. Likewise, the poster presenter must be able to "discuss" the implications of the research to interested parties who provide lively interaction with the author. While the audiences in both oral and poster settings are interested in the purpose and methods, their interest is often focused on the results and discussion. Thus the discussion is of vital importance to the researcher.

Since this text is not actually a research study, we will use this Discussion chapter to present issues that researchers and authors must consider as they conduct the research process. As much as possible, we have presented these issues in a chronological order, similar to that which the researcher will encounter during the research process. Additionally, there are topics presented in this chapter that simply do not fit nicely in the general research report format that has been used in this text. Collectively, these topics are important to the research process and communication to the scientific community.

Editor's Viewpoint: Do You Know the Way to San José?

Maureen R. Weiss

Okay, I own up to it. As many of my friends will attest, I have a terrible sense of direction. Even as a native Californian, I can relate quite well to Dionne Warwick's words, "Do you know the way to San José? I've been away so long, I've lost the way." The fact is that I think my bad sense of direction is mostly due to a lack of attention and especially a failure to take the time to consult a road map. It has occurred to me after nearly two years as Editor that there is a strong relationship between a good road map and writing the Results and Discussion sections of an article.

In my editorial viewpoint, "Who's on first, What's on second?" (June 1994), I indicated that the data analysis section of the Method serves as a "road map" for how the data will be analyzed in accordance with the research questions or hypotheses. Continuing with this analogy, it is critical that the Results systematically lead the reader to the desired answers (such as location) posed by the research questions and allow for the most direct, unambiguous route in determining "what did the authors find?" in relation to the study's rationale. Leading the reader through a meandering set of side streets and alleys will only delay the estimated time of arrival, if one arrives at all! Similarly, the Discussion must help the reader arrive at the desired address by providing a step-by-step account of "what do these statistical results mean?" in terms of theoretical and practical significance, as well as future research directions (such as the next address to be visited). Finally, it is important to understand that the Results and Discussion sections are reached using the same highway and not two completely unrelated circuitous routes.

The first quality of the Results road map should be its readability. We have all experienced the struggle of trying to learn the "take-home message" by trying to filter through lots of numbers. We have also been left hanging on this message when there is not a sentence or two translating what these numbers mean. For instance, I have seen some Results in which a higher order interaction is reported in statistical terms[1] (for example, F value, degrees of freedom, p level), but the authors failed to then systematically interpret which levels of which independent variables differed and in what direction. Along these same lines, authors are encouraged to enhance the readability of their findings by visually displaying the results of an interaction—a principle that Cohen (1990) labeled "simple is better" (p. 1305). Most of us would view this recommendation simply as "a picture is worth a thousand words."

A second quality of the Results, one that also enhances readability, is the ample use of subheadings when there are multiple analyses—these in themselves provide a form of road map. For example, the first crossroads in many studies should be documenting the reliability of instrumentation, measures, or coders used with the study sample. Despite this important aspect, it is often a source of inaccuracy or confusion (Morrow and Jackson, 1993). According to Morrow and Jackson, it is the authors' responsibility to select the appropriate reliability estimate, report on how the estimate was calculated, and translate the obtained estimate in terms of the measure's acceptability. Another component of many Results sections is a subheading of descriptive statistics such as

---

[1]Feingold (1989) warns that a statistical interaction should not be mistaken with a social interaction. The former often makes life unpleasant while the latter usually makes life very pleasant.

Continued.

From Weiss MR: Research Quarterly for Exercise and Sport 66(1): iii-v, 1995.

measures of central tendency and variability for the entire sample, as well as correlations among variables to determine whether multicollinearity exists.[2] In the event of very high correlations among selected variables, the authors should clearly spell out how this problem was handled (for example, which variables were removed or combined). The notion of subheadings continues with the main analyses and their follow-up procedures.

A third quality of the Results is that it answers the question, "What are the appropriate statistics to answer my research questions?" Although there is no black-and-white answer to this question, generally a "group difference" research hypothesis is tested using some type of ANOVA procedure (for example, ANOVA, MANOVA, repeated measures analysis), whereas a question of "relationships among variables" is tested with some form of regression procedure (such as multiple regression, path analysis, structural equation modeling). Although this may appear rather straightforward, I have seen authors unnecessarily incorporate several different types of analyses (for example, both ANOVA and regression procedures) without a clear sense of why these multiple analyses were conducted in relation to the research questions posed. I call this practice "statistical overkill" as it focuses more on the number and types of statistical methods used than directly and unambiguously selecting the most appropriate procedure for testing the original hypotheses.

Related to the issue of appropriate statistics is whether all relevant information associated with a particular procedure has been reported. Along with the required statistics denoting the test of significance (such as F value, degrees of freedom, p level), it is also crucial to follow up this standard reporting with things like: (a) which groups differed (main effect), or which groups differed at which trial

blocks (interaction)? (b) in what direction are these differences? (c) what are the group means and standard deviations (refer to a table or figure)? and (d) what is the strength of the statistical significance (such as effect size)? In two excellent papers (Cohen, 1990; Thomas, Salazar, and Landers, 1991), the authors cogently demonstrate the misleading conclusions one can draw based on $p<.05$ alone, rather than going beyond statistical significance to interpret the finding as weak, moderate, or strong in terms of meaningfulness. Reporting an effect size (of which there are several types) is perhaps the most frequent request given to authors who are invited to revise and resubmit. The most current APA manual (1994) encourages the reporting of effect size information.

Finally, given that all relevant information is reported for a statistical procedure (such as factor analysis, canonical correlation), are the results interpreted accurately? For example, is an interaction given priority in interpretation over main effects? What do these findings mean in nonstatistical terms? Does the visual of the interaction depict the associated verbal description? Are the correct variables reported as "significant" using univariate Fs and/or discriminant coefficients following a MANOVA? Are the statistically significant findings ($p<.05$) complemented by noting the effect size (for example, η^2, R^2, redundancy index)? The preceding paragraphs outline several of the concerns that are commonly encountered by reviewers and editors, and authors can be proactive in their preparation of manuscripts by attending to these issues.

Now that we've reached the midpoint of our destination, I conclude with the critical remainder of the journey—the Discussion. Readers must be provided with the necessary information to ensure that the bottom-line conclusion is driven home. As Editor, I sometimes have seen authors deliver a strong Introduction, Method, and Results but then "run out of gas" when it comes to the Discussion. Although the rationale of the study, methodology, and key results have already been communicated, the

---

[2]Feingold (1989) cautions that multicollinearity is only a life-threatening condition in the case when a graduate student's thesis employs many redundant measures.

interpretation of the results must be linked back to the original study rationale and significance. That is, one should be able to trace the path of their journey from start to finish. Essential elements of the Discussion for reaching the final destination of the article include: (a) a brief reiteration of the purpose of the study, (b) a summary of the results in relation to research hypotheses, (c) discussion of the obtained findings relative to pertinent studies mentioned in the Introduction, (d) theoretical implications of the study findings, (e) practical implications (if appropriate), (f) future directions along this line of research, and (g) a concluding paragraph to bring closure to the trip by ensuring that the readers have learned the take-home message.

The Results and Discussion sections, like their predecessor sections, are crucial for clearly and systematically communicating "What did we find?" and "What does this mean?" The road map for the Results should be as readable as possible, employ the use of subheadings, use the most appropriate statistics to address study hypotheses, report all relevant information to determine significance and meaningfulness of the findings, and interpret the statistical findings accurately. The Discussion road map serves to highlight the statistical information in verbal form and attempts to bring closure to the article by spelling out how the results support or do not support study hypotheses, providing theoretical and practical implications, suggesting future research directions, and concluding on a spirited and strong note.

By following the trip ticket I have provided here, I can ensure that reviewers and readers will respond most favorably to your article. Of course, laying out the road map like this will most likely help you plan subsequent trips to similar or different vacation spots. Now that I've figured out these particular maps—the Results and Discussion—how *do* I get to San José? Help!

Conducting research can be a complex and time consuming process. Similar to other complicated projects, careful advance planning greatly increases the likelihood that the outcome will be satisfactory. Researchers plan and prepare studies using two important methods: written research proposals and pilot studies.

RESEARCH PROPOSALS

Once the research report is finalized, it is relatively easy for the researcher to write a proposal "post hoc" (after the fact). However, the **research proposal** is actually written before any of the work is conducted. Thus the researcher must have a thorough understanding of the previous work conducted, the methods that will be used, and an expectation for what the ultimate results will be. This is often difficult to do, particularly for the novice researcher.

Written research proposals are prepared for a variety of purposes. Researchers pursuing funds for a study are required to submit a written proposal to the granting agency. Graduate students are required to submit a proposal to a faculty committee for advice and official approval of the project. Undergraduates may submit a proposal to an instructor for a project associated with a course. Research projects involving human subjects are reviewed to assure safe and ethical treatment of the participants. In all cases, the research proposal serves as a blueprint or road map to help the researcher communicate, organize, and conduct a study. A well-developed proposal serves the researcher well. If the proposal is well-developed, the researcher needs only to follow the blueprint. (With a full understanding, of course, that detours and changes to the blueprint must often be made.)

No matter what the purpose, research proposals all tend to be similar in content even though the appearance of the proposal and the amount of detail will vary depending on the intended reviewers. For example, proposals written for U.S. Government agencies such as the National Institutes of Health are very structured and detailed whereas proposals for a human subjects review board are less detailed and focus on the treatment of the subjects. Proposals typically include the following sections: the research question, hypotheses, variables, subjects, experimental design, statistical analysis, and budget, equipment, and materials. Each of these sections is briefly described below.

The Research Question

The starting point for any proposal is a description of the question under investigation. For students, developing the question is often the most difficult step. Sources for ideas are class lectures, textbooks, group discussions, research articles, professional presentations, or perhaps from suggestions made by a professor. For experienced researchers, the question usually stems logically from previous work or knowledge in the field. Asking the research question is usually not difficult for experienced researchers. For them, finding the means to perform the research is sometimes the most difficult step.

Describing the research question also provides the investigator with the opportunity to provide background information on the current state of knowledge in the area and a justification for why the question deserves attention. In addition, any theoretical concepts associated with the question may be described and developed.

Hypotheses

When stating the null and research hypotheses, the researcher defines the conditions under which decisions will be made based on the evidence gathered. The null and research hypotheses are usually explicitly stated in proposals written by students. Student proposals are intended, in part, to demonstrate to the supervising committee that the student clearly understands the hypothesis testing process. More experienced researchers may only describe the research hypothesis because an understanding of the hypothesis testing process by the reader is assumed.

Variables

Research proposals contain a section where the independent, dependent, and control variables are defined and described. Operational definitions for the independent variables are given including the number of levels of each independent variable for both manipulated and subject independent variables. Each dependent variable is also defined and measurement methods to be used are described. The control variables are also identified and explanations for why it is important to control these factors are given.

Subjects

When human or animal subjects are studied, the proposal contains detailed information about the subjects. This information includes the number of subjects, their relevant characteristics, and how they will be selected and assigned to groups. This section may also include the results of statistical calculations used to estimate the number of subjects that will be necessary for the intended research (a "power" analysis).

Experimental Design

In the experimental design section the experimental methodology that will be used in the study is identified. For example, the researcher will describe if an independent groups or a repeated measures design will be used and why.

Statistical Analysis

This section of the proposal identifies the descriptive and inferential statistical methods that will be used to analyze the data. The choice of inferential statistical methods, particularly for students but also for many experienced researchers, can be difficult. Many researchers employ or consult with professional statisticians to help select the most appropriate analytical methods.

Budget, Equipment, and Materials

The budget section is a crucial element of many research proposals. For large research projects, the budget can be quite complex. Equipment, salaries, benefits, indirect costs, payments to subjects, and other items are included in budgets. Budgets for projects conducted by students are normally not nearly as complex, but are still important.

PILOT STUDIES

A **pilot study** is a small scale trial run of a study conducted to test and refine the procedures that the researcher intends to use in the larger scale study. A pilot study can provide valuable information allowing the researcher to make modifications prior to initiating the full study. For example, a pilot study can reveal if the subjects understand and follow the instructions properly, if equipment and procedures are working properly, or if the independent variables are effective. Data gathered in the pilot study can be used to estimate whether or not the results of the full study will meet the research hypotheses and expectations. Students are particularly encouraged to conduct pilot work. This provides an opportunity to test and refine procedures and see what "goes wrong." As Murphy has stated, "If two things can go wrong, they both will and the worst will go wrong first." Thus much can be learned from pilot studies. All novice researchers are particularly encouraged to conduct pilot studies.

CONTROLLING EXPECTATIONS

The researcher is concerned about threats to the internal validity of the study. Two particular threats are subject and researcher expectations, which may cause bias on the part of study participants and invalidate the results. Researchers must address issues that could effectively cause the research to be faulty or open to criticism.

Subject Expectations

When working with human subjects, researchers are careful to avoid biasing the subjects' responses by inadvertently giving the subject too much information about the nature of the study. The goal of most studies is to observe behavior as it naturally occurs under certain conditions. In some experiments, if the subjects have too much information, they may not behave naturally. They may intentionally alter their behavior either because they think the researchers want them to behave in a certain way, or they may intentionally misbehave for mischievous reasons. In any case, since the behavior is unnatural, the results will be less meaningful. Researchers have an ethical obligation to provide subjects with enough information so that any prospective subject can make an informed choice concerning study participation. At the same time, the researcher has to balance this with the need to avoid biasing the subjects by providing too much information. As a result, certain tradeoffs are sometimes made between completely informing subjects and protecting the nature of the study. Subjects should always be completely informed about experimental procedures and any associated risks to their physical or psychological well being. Information concerning the differences between the treatment groups, or the hypotheses under investigation is usually not initially disclosed to subjects, but may be disclosed once their participation is completed.

Recall from the Methods section the three basic types of experimental design: independent groups, repeated measures, and mixed group. One potential disadvantage of repeated measures and mixed group designs is that because the subjects receive multiple treatments and measurements, they can eventually ascertain important information which might unnaturally influence their behavior. One of the advantages of the independent groups design is that the subjects only experience one treatment condition, and therefore are less likely to gain unintended information as a result of their participation.

Although independent groups designs may be used to help control subject expectations, repeated measures or mixed model designs are more appropriate in some studies for other overriding reasons. For example, in many motor behavior studies, factors that affect learning motor skills are the focus of the research. When learning is investigated, repeated measures or mixed model designs are often the most appropriate design choice. As a group of subjects practice a movement task, the rate of learning is measured over successive practice sessions. In this way the researcher can examine any changes in the subjects' performance with increasing numbers of practice trials.

A second way to control subject expectations is to use placebo groups. A placebo is a "fake" treatment that is administered to some of the subjects so that the psychological effects of the treatment can be assessed. Placebos are commonly used in medical and drug research when one group of subjects is administered a pill containing the ingredients under investigation and a second group is administered a pill with no active ingredients. Comparisons can then be made between the subjects in each group to assess the psychological and physiological effects of the agent under investigation.

Suppose a researcher wanted to conduct an experiment of the effects of caffeine on endurance exercise capacity. The experimental design could have four groups of subjects: Group 1 expects to receive a caffeine tablet and does receive a caffeine tablet; Group 2 expects to receive a caffeine tablet and receives a placebo; Group 3 expects to receive a placebo and receives a placebo; and Group 4 expects to receive a placebo tablet and receives a caffeine tablet. With this design, the researcher could examine the belief (psychological effect) that caffeine enhances exercise capacity versus the fact (physiological effect) that caffeine enhances exercise capacity.

Researcher Expectations

Since researchers are naturally well aware of the purpose of a study, they readily develop expectations concerning how the subject should behave under certain conditions. Recall our discussion on the basic assumptions of the scientific method in the Introduction section. The need for objectivity on the part of the researcher was one of the important assumptions we described.

Researchers, however, can have all of the same human strengths and weaknesses that everyone else has, and are susceptible to opinions, beliefs, and biases even though they are aware that they should maintain an objective point of view.

A commonly cited example of the effects of researcher expectations is the study by Rosenthal (1966). Rosenthal instructed groups of students to train rats to run a maze. He led the students to believe that some of the rats were very good at learning maze tasks—the "bright-maze rats"—and that other rats were poor maze learners—the "dull-maze rats." There was, in fact, no known systematic difference in the actual learning capacity of the two groups of rats. Nevertheless, the student researchers concluded that the bright-maze rats out performed the dull-maze rats in learning the maze task. Rosenthal maintained that the causal factor was how the students interacted with each group of rats depended on their expectations for each group. The differences were subtle and unintentional, but still affected how they trained the rats and judged their performance. Table 12.1 illustrates the results of this study.

Another famous case illustrating the powerful effects of expectancies is described by Gould (1981). During much of the 1800s in both Europe and the United States, there was a strong belief that intelligence was a strictly inherited attribute and that there was a strong positive association between brain size and intelligence. That is, the larger the brain, the greater the intelligence. Gould describes the case of Samuel George Morton who was a well-known scientist and physician living

TABLE 12.1 **Researcher Expectations**						
	Days					
Experimenter sample	**1**	**2**	**3**	**4**	**5**	**Mean**
Research assistant	1.20	3.00	3.80	3.40	3.60	3.00
"Maze-Bright"	1.33	1.60	2.60	2.83	3.26	2.32
"Maze-Dull"	0.73	1.10	2.23	1.83	1.83	1.54
"Bright" > "Dull"	+0.60	+0.50	+0.37	+1.00	+1.43	+0.78
t	2.54	1.02	0.29	2.28	2.37	4.01
p (one-tail)	.03	.18	.39	.04	.03	.01

From Rosenthal K: Experimentor effects in behavioral research, New York, 1966, Meredith Publishing Company.

in Philadelphia during that time. Morton was very interested in this issue and had collected and studied a large number of human skulls worldwide. Morton measured the internal capacity of the skulls to show that different ethnic groups (at that time people actually regarded the ethnic groups as separate races) were more or less intelligent than another group by virtue of cranial capacity. His bias was that Caucasian males (the group to which he was a member) had the greatest cranial capacity, and therefore were innately the most intelligent. Gould describes how Morton's methods, calculations, and interpretations of his measurements seemed to confirm this hypothesis. Gould argues in Morton's defense, that there is no evidence of fraud or the deliberate misrepresentations on Morton's part. Rather, Gould concluded that, "All I can discern is an a priori conviction about racial ranking so powerful that it directed his tabulations along preestablished lines. Yet, Morton was widely hailed as the objectivist of his age . . ." (Gould, 1981, p. 69). These two examples illustrate that sometimes it is very difficult to reject our long-held beliefs and opinions. Yet the scientific method requires us to do so.

Several methods are commonly used to help control researcher expectations. One of the most important methods of doing so is treating all subjects in the same way (such as how subjects are instructed, how measurements are made, and how events are interpreted).

Single-blind methods shield the subjects from group assignment information. That is, the subjects do not know if they are in a control (or placebo group), or if they are in one of the treatment groups. **Double-blind** methods shield both the subjects and the researchers who interact with the subjects from group assignment information. Researchers are less likely to view a subject's behavior from a biased perspective if they have no knowledge concerning which group a particular subject is assigned.

GENERALIZING FINDINGS

As you read research reports in sport and exercise sciences, you may notice that the subjects in many studies are college students. In fact, it has been shown college undergraduates were used as the subjects in about 70% of the research published during 1980 to 1985 in social psychology (Sears, 1986). Sears found that most subjects were college freshmen and sophomores enrolled in introduction to psychology courses. A concern is how well this narrowly defined group of people represents the general population. For example, college students in general are young, intelligent, willing to participate, and able to follow instructions well. Conversely, many college students are not yet physiologically or psychologically fully mature and are still in the process of defining a required self-identity.

Although many sport and exercise investigations are conducted with "normal" subjects (no special characteristics required), many other investigations have focused on groups of people with particular attributes. For example, athletes such as weight lifters, endurance athletes, or sports team members, children at varying stages of development, the elderly, and the disabled or injured have all been the population of interest in sport and exercise research.

Generalizability of results is important to both the researcher and the research reader. The researcher has a particular population in mind to which generalization is desired. The reader also has a particular population in mind. It is best if these two populations are identical (or nearly so). It is central to valid reading of research results for the reader not to infer beyond the limits of logical generalization.

Research by Neufer, et al. (1987) provides an example illustrating this point. An abstract of this work is presented in the box on p. 384. The researchers examined the effect of two reduced training schedules for college-level competitive swimmers during the off-season. All subjects were highly conditioned collegiate swimmers. They were divided into three groups: one group did not train during the 4-week testing period, the second group trained once a week, and the third group trained 3 times a week. The researchers measured physiological responses such as lactic acid production and oxygen uptake capacity at the beginning of the study and at 1 week, 2 weeks, and 4 weeks. At the same time, they also measured performance variables such as stroke rate, stroke distance, and swimming power. They found that training 3 times a week effectively helped the swimmers maintain fitness levels comparable to levels achieved during the swimming season. Our question here is, to whom can these results

Effect of Reduced Training on Muscular Strength and Endurance in Competitive Swimmers

P. Darrell Neufer, David L. Costill, Roger A. Fielding, Michael G. Flynn, and John P. Kirwan

Abstract

Following 5 months of competitive training (~9,000 yards $\cdot$ d^{-1}, 6 d $\cdot$ wk^{-1}), three groups of eight male swimmers performed 4 wk of either reduced training (3,000 yard $\cdot$ session^{-1}) or inactivity. Two groups reduced their training to either 3 sessions $\cdot$ wk^{-1} (RT3) or 1 session $\cdot$ wk^{-1} (RT1), whereas the third group (IA) did no training. Measurement of muscular strength (biokinetics swim bench) showed no decrement in any group over the 4 wk. In contrast, swim power (tethered swim) was significantly decreased ($P<0.05$) in all groups, reaching a mean change of −13.6% by week 4. Blood lactate measured after a standard 200-yard (183 m) front crawl swim increased by 1.8, 3.5, and 5.5 mM over the 4 wk in groups RT3, RT1 and IA, respectively. In group RT1, stroke rate measured during the 200-yard swim significantly increased ($P < 0.05$) from 0.54 ± 0.03 to 0.59 ± 0.03 strokes $^{-1}$ while stroke distance significantly decreased ($P < 0.05$) from 2.50 ± 0.08 to 2.29 ± 0.13 m $\cdot$ stroke^{-1} during the 4-wk period. Both stroke rate and stroke distance were maintained in group RT3 over the 4 wk of reduced training. Group IA was not tested for stroke mechanics. Whereas maximal oxygen uptake decreased significantly ($P<0.05$) over the 4 wk in group RT1 (4.75 to 4.62 1 $\cdot$ min^{-1}), no change in maximal oxygen uptake was observed in group RT3. These results suggest that aerobic capacity is maintained over 4 wk of moderately reduced training (3 sessions $\cdot$ wk^{-1}) in well-trained swimmers. Muscular strength was not diminished over 4 wk of reduced training or inactivity, but the ability to generate power during swimming was significantly reduced in all groups.

From Neufer PD, et al.: Medicine and Science in Sports and Exercise 19(5):486, 1987.

legitimately be generalized? In the author's words, "In summary, this study has demonstrated that a reduction in training to an energy requirement equal to approximately 30% of prior training results in little or no decrement in VO$_2$max in well-trained male collegiate swimmers (p. 490)." The operative phrase here is well-trained male collegiate swimmers. They did not study female swimmers, bicyclists, or runners, for example, so they directed their conclusions to the population studied. Of course we can theorize that similar conclusions could be drawn with other populations, but without actually conducting an investigation, we must confine our conclusions to the population studied.

When reading a research article, it is very important to identify who the subjects are because that may limit how legitimately the findings can be generalized to other groups. All findings are limited to a certain extent by the characteristics of those individuals who served as the subjects. In general, as the definition of the population under investigation is increasingly delimited, the more confined the findings will be to like populations. However, we should be careful to not needlessly confine findings based solely on the characteristics of the subjects. For example, the conclusions drawn with college students should not necessarily be limited only to other college students if there is no compelling reason for doing so.

REPLICATION

Recall from the Introduction section that one of the tenants of the scientific method is replication. If the results of a study can be convincingly replicated, the credibility of those results is strengthened. Results from studies that cannot be reliably replicated must be viewed with caution. Replications that support original findings also strengthen the external validity of research. As you know, the Methods section of the research report is written for the purpose of providing all necessary information so that a study can be reasonably replicated. Replications of previous research may be conducted generally in two ways: exact replications and conceptual replications.

Exact Replication

If a researcher is interested in conducting an exact replication of a previous study, the researcher strives to reproduce all possible relevant aspects of the study to determine if the same findings can be obtained. Of course, most research cannot be exactly replicated. It would be unlikely, for example, that a researcher could gain access to the same subjects who served in a given study. Even if the same subjects could be recruited, their original behavior could not be replicated exactly. And, of course, they would be "contaminated" by having been in the first study. Rather, the researcher reproduces the same procedures, utilizes similar equipment, gathers the data under similar conditions, and recruits subjects with the same relevant characteristics.

Exact replications are comparatively rare. Unless the findings of a study are so surprising or unexpected that obvious doubts may arise, it is uncommon for someone else to invest the time and efforts to exactly reproduce a previous study. In general, exact replications do not advance the body of knowledge.

Conceptual Replication

Perhaps the best way to demonstrate how well the results of a study can be generalized is by conducting conceptual replications of previous research. Conceptual replications are studies that are modeled on previous research, but with certain aspects of the original study modified such as the experimental design or the population investigated, by adding or changing variables, or by modifying some combination of these. For example, recall the Quadagno (1991) study described in the Methods section where women weight lifters and swimmers were studied. To enhance the external validity of the original findings, a similar study could be conducted with different athletes. Rather than college athletes, perhaps high school athletes in the same sports, or college athletes in different sports could serve as subjects. If similar results are obtained, the original findings are strengthened and broadened to a wider range of individuals or environments.

An example of a conceptual replication in sport and exercise research can be found in the study by Goode and Magill (1986) who conceptually replicated an earlier study conducted by Shea and Morgan (1979) on motor skills learning. Shea and Morgan conducted a study in a research laboratory investigating the effects of unpredictable practice sequences on motor skills learning utilizing a special device termed a knock-down barrier. They found that when practicing motor skills following an unpredictable practice sequence, learning increased as compared to practicing following a predictable practice sequence. A few years later, Goode and Magill (1986) conducted a very similar experiment. Rather than conducting a laboratory experiment, they conducted a field experiment using students in badminton classes. In their study, the effect of practicing three badminton serves following either a predictable practice sequence or an unpredictable practice sequence was investigated. Both the Shea and Morgan study and the Goode and Magill study investigated the effects of unpredictable practice sequences on motor skills learning. In effect, Goode and Magill conducted a conceptual replication of the earlier research.

Shea and Morgan and Goode and Magill both found that unpredictable practice sequences benefited learning when compared to predictable practice sequences. Goode and Magill could have exactly replicated Shea and Morgan's original study, but advances in our understanding of practice and skills acquisition would not have been as enriched. It was beneficial to our understanding to build on the previous research rather than to duplicate it.

LIMITATIONS AND DELIMITATIONS

Researchers must consider **delimitations** and **limitations** to their work. Delimitations are constraints that the researcher places upon the work. For example, a researcher might delimit the work to children between the ages of 6 and 10 or delimit the work to female, freshman college students. Limitations are "shortcomings" that are encountered when the work is conducted. Limitations are typically placed on the researcher because of the nature of the data collection procedures. For example, if an experiment on physiological adaptations to exercise is conducted at high altitude, the researcher is limited to the extent that the adaptations might to some extent depend on altitude. To draw conclusions, the researcher must accept that the environment might affect the findings. The research might be limited by the quality of the equipment used or by the representativeness of survey respondents.

INFORMED CONSENT

The principle of **informed consent** specifies that prospective subjects should receive an accurate appraisal of the demands, the risks, and the benefits they may experience as a participant in a study. The informed consent principle was developed after World War II when, at the Nuremberg Trials, the extent of the human experimentation conducted by the Nazis on people against their will was made public (Robinson and Neutens, 1987). The following informed consent policy statement is quoted from the APA guideline for "Research with Human Participants," (1990, p. 394):

> Except in minimal-risk research, the investigator establishes a clear and fair agreement with research participants, prior to their participation, that clarifies the obligations and responsibilities of each. The investigator has the obligation to honor all promises and commitments included in the agreement. The investigator informs the participants of all aspects of the research that might reasonably be expected to influence willingness to participate and explains all other aspects of the research about which the participants inquire. Failure to make full disclosure prior to obtaining informed consent requires additional safeguards to protect the welfare and dignity of the research participants. Research with children or with participants who have impairments that would limit understanding and or communication requires special safeguarding procedures.

Currently, the U.S. government requires local review of all research projects that involve human subjects at any institution receiving federal funds. The researcher submits to an Institutional Review Board (IRB) a summary of the proposed project detailing the reasons for using human subjects and an assessment of potential risks and benefits. The board is responsible for reviewing proposals and issuing approval decisions. Several informed consent issues are presented below.

Informed consent issues are important to both the researcher and the study participants. Each researcher's home institution has developed procedures that must be followed to protect the rights of individuals. The box on p. 389 provides examples of the types of questions that must be addressed before actually conducting the study. A key factor throughout the informed consent approval process is that researchers *cannot* grant themselves approval to conduct a study. The authority to conduct a study rests ultimately with each IRB. Researchers typically make early contact with the IRB so that study approval is not delayed.

DECEPTION

Researchers examining human behavior have been presented with a dilemma for many years: some research questions are

> **Typical Information Requested by an Institutional Review Board**
>
> **1** Include copies of all questionnaires, surveys, etc.
> **2** Identify the sources of potential subjects.
> **3** Describe the procedures used in the study.
> **4** Describe the informed consent procedures to be used.
> **5** Include a copy of all informed consent materials.
> **6** Indicate steps taken to insure confidentiality, when appropriate.
> **7** Describe the potential benefits to subjects.
> **8** Describe the physical, psychological, and/or social risks involved.

difficult or impossible to answer if the subjects are aware beforehand exactly what is being investigated. Therefore deception is sometimes used by providing only general information designed not to reveal the exact nature of the investigation. Deception is not to be used if the hidden information presents actual risk to the subject. The following deception policy statement is quoted from the APA guideline for "Research with Human Participants," (p. 394):

> Methodological requirements of a study may make the use of concealment or deception necessary. Before conducting such a study, the investigator has a special responsibility to (i) determine whether the use of such techniques is justified by the study's prospective scientific, educational, or applied value; (ii) determine whether alternative procedures are available that do not use concealment or deception; and (iii) ensure that the participants are provided with sufficient explanation as soon as possible.

The experiments conducted by Milgram (1965) are commonly cited as an example of the use of deception in research. The participants in Milgram's experiments were led to believe that they were serving in learning and memory research. In fact, the researchers were actually investigating the willingness of people to follow the instructions of an authority figure even though the actions may be disturbing. The subjects were told that a second subject (the learner) would be memorizing and then recalling word-pairs. The first subject's task was to administer an electric shock each time the learner failed to correctly recall a word-pair. The subjects were not aware of the fact that the learner was actually a member of the research team, and that no electric shocks were ever delivered. During the experiment, the subject sat at a panel with switches labeled 15-volts, 30-volts, 45-volts, up to 450-volts. Every time the learner made an error, the subject was instructed to administer a shock, beginning with 15-volts, and then increase the voltage for each successive mistake. The learner gave dramatized reactions to the phony shocks ranging from very slight reactions at low voltages, to loud screams and painful looking antics at high voltages. The subjects could withdraw from the experiment at any time, but were encouraged to continue. Surprisingly, over 60% of the subjects delivered fake shocks up to the 450 volt limit demonstrating the strong influence of an authority figure over the behavior of others.

Consider the effects that full disclosure would have had on the subjects in this experiment. If the subjects were aware that the shocks and the responses were not real, the intended psychological stress would have been effectively eliminated and their behavior would have been different. To adequately study this behavior, the researchers felt it was essential to deceive the subjects so that natural responses could be elicited.

DISCLOSURE

Closely linked to informed consent principle is the disclosure principle. Upon completing their participation in a study, the nature of the research should be explained to the participants. This is particularly important if any deception was involved. Many universities consider disclosure an important educational tool. Students who serve as participants can gain an appreciation of research if the study is explained to them. The following disclosure policy statement is quoted from the APA guideline for "Research with Human Participants," (p. 395):

> After the data are collected, the investigator provides the participant with information about the nature of the study and attempts to remove any misconceptions that may have arisen. Where scientific or humane values justify delaying or withholding this information, the investigator incurs a special responsibility to monitor the research and to ensure that there are no damaging consequences for the participant.

CONFIDENTIALITY

Protection of the right to privacy is another aspect of the ethical treatment of participants. Participants are afforded anonymity, particularly if the research is sensitive or potentially embarrassing. In addition, when publishing research, authors normally do not include information that can be used to identify or trace any particular person. The following confidentiality policy statement is quoted from the APA guideline for "Research with Human Participants," (p. 395):

> Information obtained about a research participant during the course of an investigation is confidential unless otherwise agreed upon in advance. When the possibility exists that others may obtain access to such information, the possibility, together with the plans for protecting confidentiality, is explained to the participant as part of the procedure for obtaining informed consent.

VOLUNTARY PARTICIPATION

Students are commonly recruited as study participants and may be given class credits for participating. Introduction to psychology courses in particular have a long history of recruiting subjects this way. Participants, however, should have the freedom to choose to not participate or to withdraw from the study. This is particularly true in exercise research where participants may be asked to exert themselves at strenuous levels. Participants who believe the activities are too strenuous or stressful should not be forced to continue. Losing participants complicates research for the experimentalist, but the welfare of the participants is always the first priority. The following voluntary participation policy statement is quoted from the APA guideline for "Research with Human Participants," (p. 395):

> The investigator respects the individual's freedom to decline to participate in or withdraw from the research at any time. The obligation to protect this freedom requires careful thought and consideration when the investigator is in a position of authority or influence over the participant. Such positions of authority include, but are not limited to, situations in which research participation is required as part of employment or in which the participant is a student, client or employee of the investigator.

ANIMAL RESEARCH

The use of animals in research procedures has recently been criticized. Issues include the use of nonhuman models for conducting research, cruelty to animals, animal care, and alternative data sources. Many researchers in exercise science utilize animal models in their work. The U.S. government has developed specific guidelines for the care and use of laboratory animals. The following box presents a summary of the issue from the perspective of the American College of Sports Medicine.

Policy Statement of the American College of Sports Medicine on Research with Experimental Animals

The ability of science to enhance the well-being of humans and animals depends directly on advancements made possible by research, much of which requires the use and availability of experimental animals. Therefore, all who propose to use animals for research, education, or testing purposes must assume the responsibility for their general welfare. It is essential to recognize and to appreciate that the intent of scientific research is to provide results that will advance knowledge for the general and specific benefits of humans and animals. To accomplish these goals, the American College of Sports Medicine (ACSM) will support research of high scientific merit that includes the use of experimental animals.

Before the college will consider supporting research projects, the College must receive written assurances from the institution that the policies and procedures detailed in the *Guide for the Care and Use of Laboratory Animals* as published by the U.S. Department of Health and Human Services and proclaimed in the Animal Welfare Act (PL89-544, PL91-979, and PL94-279) are policy of the institution. Furthermore, the ACSM endorses the rules, procedures, and recommendations for the care of laboratory animals as advocated by the American Association for Accreditation of Laboratory Animal Care (AAALAC). Support for research and publication of research findings by the ACSM require that the institution where the research was conducted confirm it has filed a National Institutes of Health assurance and/or has AAALAC approved facilities.

From: Medicine and Science in Sports and Exercise 27(7):vii, 1995.

ETHICS

Researchers and scientists want their work to be of the highest ethical standard. One's personal and professional reputation rests in the ethical standards demonstrated in the completion of the scientific process. Thus researchers take special care to assure their readers that the work was conducted with the highest degree of integrity. Unfortunately, there are incidents where researchers and their work are questioned. Safrit's (1993) "Oh what a tangled web we weave" provides an excellent commentary (and many examples) of unethical activities by exercise and sport science researchers.

A recent study from Belgium raises a particularly interesting question in health promotion. Since the early 1980s, the Belgian government has conducted an extensive AIDS education program in that country. In 1988, the government reported that the program was successful—that most gay men understood how HIV was transmitted and consistently practiced safer sex. These findings were based on the results of surveys conducted by government health department officials targeted at the gay population. An American anthropologist living in Belgium at the time was not convinced that the surveys were completely accurate and sought additional evidence by conducting his own research. The researcher met gay men in local bars and bathhouses, had sex with them, and later recorded their tendencies for high-risk or low-risk behaviors. He maintains that he never actually engaged in high-risk behaviors, but he did allow things to progress to the point where those behaviors appeared to be the next step. He concluded that the government's findings were seriously flawed—many gay men were still engaging in high-risk behaviors and they were lying about it to the government officials (Burdick, 1993).

As you might expect, the researcher's ethics and methods have been questioned. For example, is it ethical for a researcher studying sexual behavior to have sex with the subjects when the subjects were not aware of his real motives? The researcher asserted that in this situation, his unorthodox methods were necessary because the men were lying on the surveys rather than admitting to high-risk behaviors. He also argued that controlling AIDS is such a compelling issue that it is more important to understand what is really occurring than worrying about ethical concerns. A second ethical issue was the lack of informed consent. When given informed consent, the subject is fully apprised about the nature of the research and is given the opportunity to decline participation. The researcher, in this case, felt that giving informed consent would have ruined the opportunity to gain valid and truthful information.

Ethical issues aside, if you were criticizing the findings, what concerns might be mentioned that could have biased the results? For one, since he conducted his research in bars and bathhouses, he may have met men who were more promiscuous, and less likely to be safe than other gay men who were either in monogamous relationships, or who didn't use public places to meet people for the purpose of having sex. Secondly, his appearance and behavior may have unintentionally influenced the men that he met to perceive him as a "low-risk" partner, and therefore they may have sensed less need to be cautious. Consequently, he may have unintentionally but systematically excluded those men whose practices were less promiscuous or less risky. He may have met disproportionally more men who generally behaved less safely. Clearly, generating reliable and meaningful information in this area is a difficult problem. His findings suggest that the government is underestimating the rate of dangerous behaviors in the gay population. At the same time, ethical issues aside, one could argue that these results may be overestimating the rate of the same behaviors.

This unusual example illustrates some of the ethical concerns confronting researchers when working with human subjects. Researchers are expected to conform to established ethical principles concerning the treatment of human subjects. The following general ethical treatment of human subjects policy statement is quoted from the APA guideline for "Research with Human Participants," (p. 394):

> In planning a study, the investigator has the responsibility to make a careful evaluation of its ethical acceptability. To the extent that the weighing of scientific and human values suggests a compromise of any principle, the investigator incurs a corresponding serious obligation to seek ethical advice and to observe stringent safeguards to protect the rights of human participants.

RESEARCH DISSEMINATION

Researchers initiate their activities with an altruistic motive. They desire to influence their profession and society, and add to the body of knowledge in their respective fields. The researcher must choose which methods best provide the means to disseminate the work once data are collected, analyzed, and conclusions are drawn. Most researchers want their work published in a form that makes it retrievable worldwide. Additionally, researchers want their work to have the greatest impact possible and to receive the most recognition from scholarly peers. Thus researchers (or the research team) will typically decide to submit their work for peer review and possible publication in the journal which they believe meets these intended goals. Researchers try to decide which prestigious journal publishes work similar in nature to that which was conducted and submit the work here first. Should the manuscript not be accepted for publication, the researchers then decide which journal is the "next best" on the list. The following box summarizes the factors used to decide to which journal the work should be submitted.

The peer review process can generally take up to a year and the lag time from acceptance to publication may take another year. Thus it may be nearly 2 years (or more) before completed research actually appears in the peer reviewed literature. Therefore researchers typically seek additional means through which to disseminate their work before the peer

---

Factors Researchers Consider When Deciding to Which Journal to Submit a Manuscript

1 The nature of the current work
2 The typical kinds of research the journal publishes
3 The reputation of the journal
4 Whether or not the journal is "peer reviewed"
5 Who the editor-in-chief (or section editor) is
6 The time delay typically encountered in the review process
7 The lag time delay from acceptance to actual publication
8 The journal's circulation (how many, who, and where)

review process or while the peer review process is being conducted. This venue is typically through personal presentation at a scholarly meeting. Recall from Chapter 3 that professional organizations generally have regional and national meetings on an annual or biannual basis. "Calls for papers" are distributed to the membership and through other means (such as inserts in professional journals) where researchers are encouraged to submit their work for evaluation and possible presentation at the meeting. The format may be an oral or poster presentation. The oral presentation format typically involves a 12-15 minute presentation where the author provides a brief overview of the importance, purpose, methods, results, and discussion of the work. Approximately 3-5 minutes are then permitted for the audience to interact with the presenter and ask questions about the work. The poster presentation format consists of the researcher creating a series of pages (typically 10-15) that are then posted on a large bulletin board during a specified time during the professional meeting. Poster sessions are generally "thematic" in nature in that several (or many) posters on related topics are presented concurrently. The total amount of time varies from meeting to meeting (2-3 hours). The research is summarized in charts, graphs, and so forth. The author must then be available to interact with those attending the poster session to answer questions. The time that the author is available is typically one half of the time that the poster is available for viewing. Simplicity, brevity, interpretability, and understandability are the key features of a good poster presentation. Figure 12.1 provides an overview of a typical poster presentation. The main sections presented on a poster typically include an abstract, purpose, methods, results, and conclusions. Poster presenters attempt to use figures, graphs, and charts to present an interesting display and summary of the research.

THE PEER REVIEW PROCESS

The **peer review** process is generally the same regardless of the journal to which the researcher submits a manuscript for possible publication. A key element that all researchers should consider are the "guidelines for contributors" that are typically published in selected issues of the journal to which

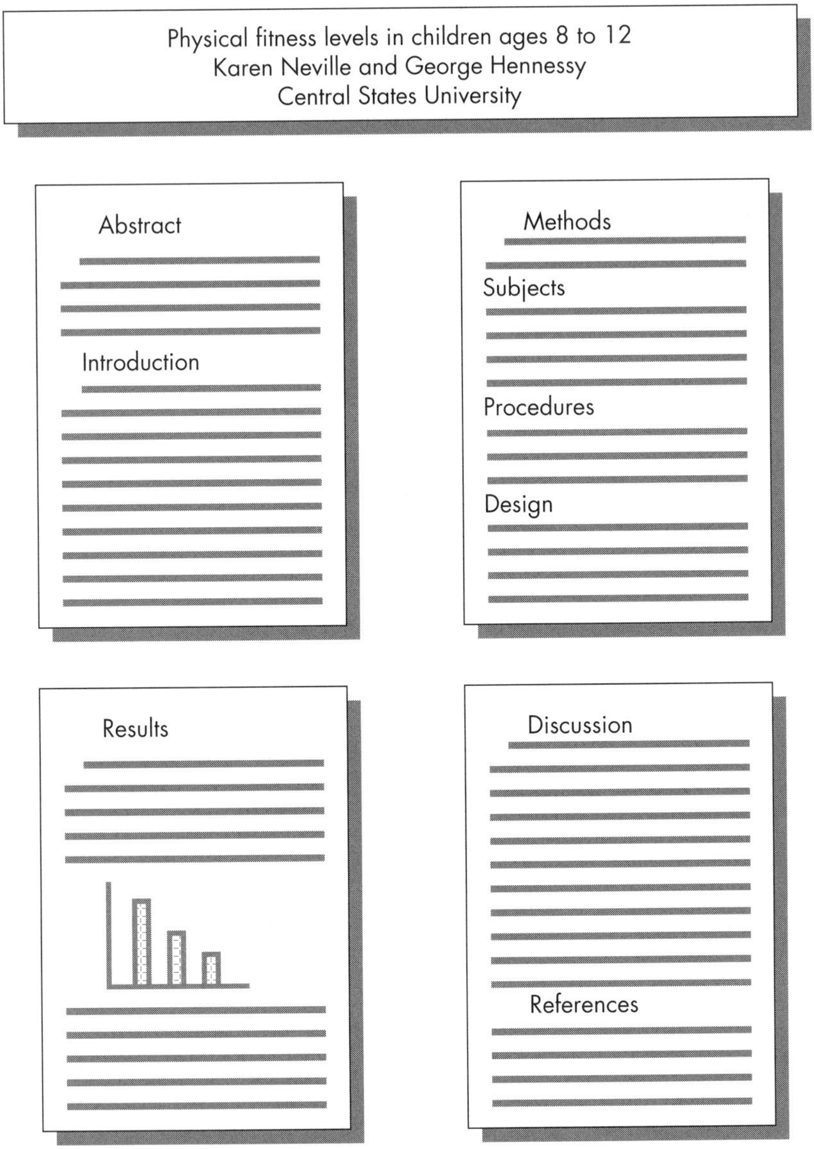

FIGURE 12.1 Sample poster presentation design.

they are planning to submit a manuscript. The guidelines tell the researcher much about what the editor expects to receive from the researcher. The box on p. 398 provides a listing of some of the important considerations typically found in guidelines for contributors.

Common Elements Presented in Guidelines for Contributors

1 The types of manuscripts considered for publication
2 Copyright information
3 Specific elements required by the journal (such as informed consent statements, author signatures, etc.)
4 The editor's address
5 The editorial style used by the journal
6 The number of copies to submit
7 A brief description of the review process
8 The order of presentation for the manuscript (such as title page, content, references, tables, figures, etc.)
9 Specific statements that may be required in the researcher's submission letter (for example, the work is not previously published nor submitted elsewhere, etc.)

The author should follow the guidelines as closely as possible. Editors and reviewers value the scientific quality of the manuscript over the substance of the editorial style that is used by the author. However, reviewers expect a common format when reviewing for a particular journal and major deviations from the required format will lead to difficulty in conducting an objective review or to an outright rejection by the editor.

The editor (or section editor, in some cases) identifies content and/or methodological experts who have conducted similar or related work. The submitted manuscript is then forwarded for review. Sometimes the reviewers and authors are "blinded" to one another in that neither knows the identity of the other. Other journals use a single-blinded review (where the author does not know who the reviewer is but the reviewer knows who the author is), and others use a totally open review process so that both the author and the reviewers can be identified by one another. Once reviewers are identified by the editor, a copy of the manuscript is forwarded to the reviewer who is asked to conduct a "timely evaluation of the scientific quality of the work." Timely typically refers to the fact that the review is to be returned to the editor within approximately 30 days. Once all reviews have been received by the editor, the editor consolidates the reviews and makes a final decision on the appropriateness for publication. The decision can range from "publish it as is" (only rarely is this the first evaluation of a manuscript), to "needs required revisions based on the reviewers' comments" (the more typical response), to outright "rejection."

SUMMARY

This Discussion chapter presented important issues that affect research that may not be obvious to you, such as proposals, pilot studies, the informed consent process, the peer review process, and other factors. These are issues that are not normally discussed at length in a research report, but are very necessary to the research process.

The Discussion is the second to last section of a research report followed by the references. In the Discussion, the author's goal is to convince the audience that the findings that have emerged from the current research are both interesting and important. While the research question and methods are of interest, the results and discussion are usually the most important parts of a report and are therefore particularly vital.

Conducting research can be a complex and time consuming process, but when conducted well, the results can be very rewarding. Research reports, either in the form of a written paper, an oral presentation, or a poster presentation are the primary methods of disseminating new information that emerges from research. In this text we have used the research report as a model for the organization of the information. The purpose of doing so was to reinforce the importance of the report in furthering knowledge.

EXERCISES

1 Prepare a research proposal for one of the following studies:
   a the effects of static and dynamic stretching on delayed on-set muscle soreness;
   b the effects of specific or variable practice on basketball free throw shooting;
   c the effects of rewards on exercise adherence.
   State the research question, and identify the independent, dependent, and control variables. Specify the subject selection process. Choose an experimental design. Determine the appropriate descriptive and inferential statistical methods, and plan a budget.

2 Design a conceptual replication of the Neufer, Costill, Fielding, Flynn, and Kirwan (1987) study discussed in this chapter. Think in terms of subjects, methods, and experimental design.

3 Explain how you would apply each of the APA research guidelines in your proposed replication of the Neufer, et al. study.

4 As a managing editor of a scientific journal, describe how you would decide whether or not to publish a research report.

Sports and Exercise Science Measures

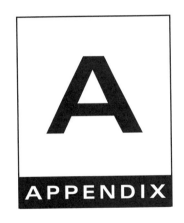

COMMON SPORT AND EXERCISE MEASURES

The areas of investigation within sport and exercise sciences are quite extensive because responses of the human body to physical activity can be examined at many levels (from cellular to whole society). For example, biomechanists measure mechanical forces such as the velocity, rotation, and acceleration of objects. Exercise physiologists measure oxygen consumption rates, metabolic rates, and lactic acid levels in individuals. Motor behaviorists measure performance variables such as response latencies and response errors. Sociologists "measure" social trends, activities, and consequences.

Not only are a wide range of variables measured, measurements can also be taken at different points during a movement. For instance, response latency measurements are made just prior to movement, many biomechanical or physiological measurements are made during movement, and many learning and psychological measurements are made immediately following movement. Fig. A.1 shows the four phases of movement during which many sport and exercise sciences measurements are made.

This section of the textbook presents definitions of commonly measured variables in biomechanics, exercise physiology, and motor learning. As you read research reports and your textbooks in these areas, you will encounter many of these terms.

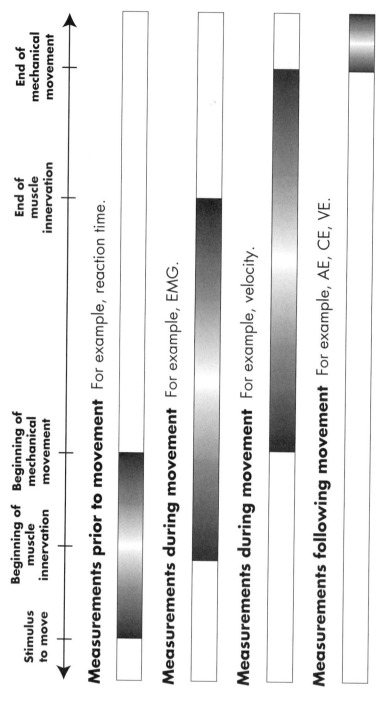

FIGURE A.1 Common sports and exercise science measurement intervals.

COMMON BIOMECHANICS MEASURES

Acceleration: The time rate change in velocity.

Angular momentum: The quantity of angular motion determined by the product of the object's angular velocity and its moment of inertia.

Angular power: The time rate of change of angular work determined by the product of the torque and the angular velocity.

Angular speed: The angular distance traveled divided by the time period over which the angular motion occurred.

Angular velocity: The time rate change of angular displacement.

Angular work: The product of torque applied to an object and the angular distance over which the torque is applied.

Axis of rotation: The point about which a body rotates.

Center of gravity: The point at which all the body's mass seems to be concentrated.

Digitization: The process of applying x-y coordinates to points on a film or video image.

Energy: The capacity to do work.

Equilibrium: A balanced state in which there is no movement or no change in the movement because the sum of the forces and torques acting on the object is zero.

Force: An interaction between two objects in the form of a push or pull that may or may not cause motion.

Impulse: The product of the magnitude of a force and its time of application.

Inertia: The resistance of a body to a change in its state of motion.

Kinematics: The area of study that examines the spatial and temporal components of motion.

Kinetics: The branch of mechanics that deals with the forces that act on a system.

Mass: The amount of matter of which an object is composed.

Moment of inertia: The resistance of a body to angular acceleration.

Motion: The progressive change in position of an object.

Movement: A change in place, position, or posture occurring over time and relative to some point in the environment.

Muscle power: The product of the net muscle movement and the angular velocity of the joint.

Position: The location of an object or a point on the object with respect to a designated reference point in the environment.

Power: The quantity of work done per unit time.

Pressure: Force per unit area.

Projectile angle: The angle at which a projectile is released.

Projectile height: The difference between the height at which a projectile is released and the height at which it lands.

Projectile velocity: The velocity at which a projectile is released.

Radius of rotation: The linear distance from the axis of rotation to a point on the rotating segment.

Shear force: A force that acts in parallel to a surface.

Stability: The resistance to a disturbance on the body's equilibrium.

Strain energy: The capacity to work by virtue of the deformation of an object.

Torque: The product of the magnitude of a force and the perpendicular distance from the line of action of the force to the axis of rotation.

Trajectory: The flight path of a projectile.

Translation: Motion in a straight or curved path where different regions of the object move the same distance in the same time interval.

Vector: A quantity that is defined by both magnitude and direction.

Velocity: The time-rate change in position.

Weight: The force of the earth's gravitational attraction to a body's mass.

Work: The product of the force applied to a body and the distance through which the force is applied.

COMMON EXERCISE PHYSIOLOGY MEASURES

Aerobic metabolism: In the presence of oxygen.

Aerobic power: Synonymous with terms such as cardiovascular endurance capacity or maximal oxygen uptake.

Anaerobic metabolism: In the absence of oxygen.

Anaerobic threshold: That intensity of workload or oxygen consumption in which anaerobic metabolism is accelerated.

Anthropometry: Measurements of the physical body (i.e., height, weight, girth, etc.).

Arteriovenous oxygen difference: The difference in oxygen content of arterial and mixed venous blood.

Atrophy: Loss of body tissue or size.

Basal metabolic rate: The rate at which energy is expended for only the basic metabolic processes of the body; usually expressed in kilocalories per hour.

Blood pressure: The force that drives blood through the circulatory system.

Body density: Body weight divided by body volume.

Body mass index: The ratio of body weight divided by height.

BTPS: Body temperature, pressure, saturated.

Calorie: The amount of heat necessary to raise the temperature of one gram of water 1° Celsius.

Cardiac cycle: Contraction (systole) and relaxation (diastole) of the heart.

Cardiac output: The amount of blood pumped by the heart in one minute; the product of stroke volume and heart rate.

Diastolic volume: The amount of blood that fills the ventricles during diastole.

Dynamometer: A device for measuring muscular strength.

Effective blood volume: The volume of blood available to exercising muscles.

Efficiency: The ratio of work output to work input.

Electrocardiogram (ECG): A recording of the electrical activity of the heart.

Electromyogram (EMG): A recording of the electrical activity of muscles.

Ergometer: A device such as a treadmill used for measuring physiological effects of exercise.

Fatigue: A state of decreased efficiency resulting from physical work.

Flexibility: The range of motion of a joint or combination of joints.

Hyperthermia: Increased body temperature.

Hypertrophy: An increase in the size of a cell or muscle.

Inspiratory capacity (IC): Maximal volume of air inspired from resting expiratory level.

Kilocalorie: The amount of heat necessary to raise the temperature of 1 kilogram of water 1° Celsius.

Lean body mass: Body weight minus the weight of body fat.

Maximum heart rate reserve: The difference between resting heart rate and maximum heart rate.

Maximum oxygen consumption (VO$_2$ max): The greatest rate of oxygen consumption attained during exercise at sea level; usually expressed in liter per minute or milliliters per kilogram body weight per minute; represents the maximal rate of aerobic metabolism.

MET (metabolic equivalent unit): A measurement scale used to estimate the metabolic cost of physical activity relative to resting metabolic rate; 1 MET = 3.5 ml of oxygen consumed per kilogram of body weight per minute.

Minute ventilation: The amount of air inspired or expired in one minute.

Muscular endurance: The ability of a muscle to perform repeated contractions against a light load for an extended period of time.

Net oxygen cost: The amount of oxygen, above resting rates, required to perform a given amount of work.

Oxygen debt: The amount of oxygen consumed during recovery from exercise.

Oxygen deficit: The time period during exercise in which the level of oxygen consumption is below that necessary to supply all the ATP required for the exercise.

Perceived exertion: A subjective measurement scale for rating exercise intensity. Commonly measured on a 1 to 20 point scale where 0-9 indicates very light to light intensity, 10-15 indicates moderate to high intensity, and 16-20 indicates very intense to maximum intensity physical effort.

Percent body fat: Total body fat expressed as a percentage of body weight.

Pulse pressure: The mathematical difference between systolic and diastolic blood pressure.

Relative body fat: The ratio of fat weight to total body weight.

Residual volume: Volume of air remaining in the lungs at the end of maximal expiration.

Respiratory exchange ratio: The ratio of the amount of carbon dioxide produced and the amount of oxygen consumed.

Respiratory quotient: The ratio of carbon dioxide produced in the tissues to the oxygen consumed by the tissues.

STPD: Standard temperature, pressure, dry.

Stroke volume: The amount of blood pumped by the left ventricle of the heart beat.

Tidal volume: Volume of air inspired or expired per breath.

Total lung capacity: The sum of vital capacity and residual lung volume.

Ventilatory efficiency: The amount of ventilation required per liter of oxygen consumption.

Vital capacity: Maximal volume of air forcefully expired after maximal inspiration.

COMMON PERCEPTUAL-MOTOR MEASURES

Response Latency Measures

Motor time: The interval from the first change in EMG to the start of the physical movement.

Movement time: The interval from the start of movement to the completion of the movement.

Premotor time: The interval from the presentation of a stimulus to the first change in EMG.

Reaction time: The time interval from the presentation of a stimulus to the onset of the physical movement. A reaction time is the sum of the premotor time plus the motor time.

Response time: The time interval from the presentation of a stimulus to the termination of the movement. A response time is the sum of reaction time plus movement time.

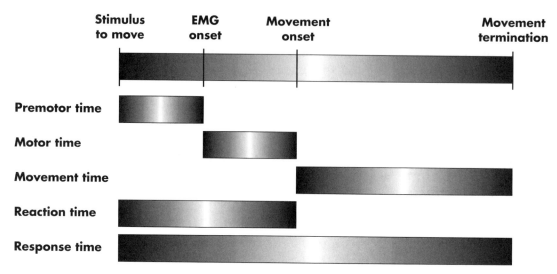

FIGURE A.2 Response time fractions.

RESPONSE ERROR MEASURES

Absolute error (AE): A measure of movement error without regard to the direction of the error. AE is an average.

Constant error (CE): A measure of movement error with regard to the direction of the error. CE is an average.

Variable error (VE): A measure of movement variability. VE is a standard deviation.

Total variability (E): A measure of movement accuracy. E is the square root of the sum of VE² plus CE².

$$AE = \frac{\Sigma |X - C|}{N}$$

$$CE = \frac{\Sigma (X - C)}{N}$$

$$VE = \sqrt{\left[\frac{\Sigma (X - C)^2}{N}\right] - CE^2}$$

$$E = \sqrt{CE^2 + AE^2}$$

where

x = the measured value
c = the criterion (or target)
n = the number of trials

FIGURE A.3 Response error formulas.

Sample Survey
and Cover Letter

Neville Marketing Research
4901 Osage St.
College Park, MD 20740

August 25, 1995

Dear Student:

Neville Marketing Research is conducting a survey on the athletic apparel preferences of college students. The purpose of this letter is to ask you to participate in this survey by completing and returning the enclosed questionnaire. Your participation is important because the results will be used by a local retailer to help develop an athletic apparel and marketing program designed to meet the preferences of college students.

Your participation in this survey is voluntary and all responses will be kept strictly confidential. No attempts will be made to sell you anything should you agree to participate. To encourage your participation, a $25 gift certificate to an athletic apparel store in your area will be mailed to you upon receipt of your completed survey. Simply print your name and address on the enclosed postcard and return it, with the completed questionnaire, in the enclosed envelope.

If you have any questions regarding any aspect of this survey, or if you would like a copy of the findings, please feel free to contact me at the address provided above.

Please mail the completed survey by **September 5, 1995**.

Thank you for your time and assistance; your participation in this survey is truly appreciated.

Sincerely,

Carol Anne Hennessy, Research Assistant

Enclosures

The purpose of this survey is to investigate factors affecting athletic apparel preferences by college students. The first three sections focus on store preferences, sales personnel, and merchandise. The remaining two sections focus on individual shopping preferences and demographics.

Please complete all five sections according to the directions provided.

SECTION I. THE FOLLOWING QUESTIONS PERTAIN TO STORE PREFERENCES.

Please circle the number that best approximates your agreement with the given statements.

strongly disagree	disagree	neutral	agree	strongly agree

1. The number of customer services provided by a store determines where I prefer to shop for athletic apparel.

   1   2   3   4   5

2. I prefer to shop for athletic apparel only at the most conveniently located stores.

   1   2   3   4   5

3. The opinions of others influence my preference for an athletic apparel store.

   1   2   3   4   5

4. The assortment of color and style coordinated athletic apparel are important factors in my store preference.

   1   2   3   4   5

5. The expertise of the sales personnel in athletic apparel is an important factor in my store preference.

   1   2   3   4   5

6. I prefer to shop in stores that carry specific athletic apparel brands (e.g., Adidas, Nike, Wilson, etc.).

   1   2   3   4   5

7. The shopping environment is an important factor in my choice of athletic apparel store.

   1   2   3   4   5

8. I am willing to pay higher prices for athletic apparel in a store that provides good customer service.

   1   2   3   4   5

	strongly disagree	disagree	neutral	agree	strongly agree

9. Price is an important factor in where I decide to shop
    for athletic apparel.

      1   2   3   4   5

10. Shopping enjoyment is a major factor in my store
    preference.

      1   2   3   4   5

11. Merchandise return policy is an important factor in my
    store preference.

      1   2   3   4   5

Please rate the athletic apparel stores listed below concerning
the following attributes:

  Use the scale provided below.

  1 = Poor
  2 = Fair
  3 = Good
  4 = Excellent
  * = Not familiar with this store

Attributes	Foot Locker	Nike World	R.E.I.	E.M.S.	Herman's
Efficiency of salespeople					
Attitude of salespeople toward the customer					
Store atmosphere					
Return policy					
Apparel quality					
Selection					
Prices					
Sales and promotions					

Where do you usually obtain information about sales and promotions for athletic apparel? (Check the *three* most common sources)

____ newspaper ads	____ fliers inserted in newspapers
____ television ads	____ magazines
____ radio ads	____ friends
____ personal mailings	____ at the store
____ resident mailings	____ catalogs
____ other _____	

SECTION II. THE FOLLOWING QUESTIONS ADDRESS YOUR OPINIONS AND ATTITUDES TOWARD SALES PERSONNEL.

Please circle the number that best approximates your agreement with the given statements.

	strongly disagree	**disagree**	**neutral**	**agree**	**strongly agree**

1. I appreciate a sales clerk who gives an honest appraisal of the garments.

        1   2   3   4   5

2. Aggressive sales personnel bother me.

        1   2   3   4   5

3. I prefer to purchase athletic apparel from a sales clerk who is of the same gender as myself.

        1   2   3   4   5

4. I appreciate suggestions from sales clerks.

        1   2   3   4   5

Please rank the following sales personnel characteristics, from 1 to 6, in order of importance to you. Use **1** to indicate the **least important** characteristic, and use **6** to indicate the **most important** characteristic. Use each number only once.

____ Fashion sense

____ Knowledge of the best clothing for different athletic activities

____ Genuine interest in the customer

_____ Apparel knowledge: clothing quality, properties, and care

_____ Good judgment on when to approach and assist customers

_____ Ability to remember customers' sizes, tastes, and needs

SECTION III. THE FOLLOWING QUESTIONS PERTAIN TO ATHLETIC APPAREL.

Please circle the number that best approximates your agreement with the given statements.

strongly disagree	**disagree**	**neutral**	**agree**	**strongly agree**

1. Quality is the most important factor in my decision to purchase an athletic apparel item.

   1   2   3   4   5

2. I prefer athletic apparel made from natural fibers (cotton, wool, etc.).

   1   2   3   4   5

3. I prefer athletic apparel made from man-made fabrics (CoolMax, Supplex, etc.).

   1   2   3   4   5

4. Quality is more important than price in my decision to purchase athletic apparel.

   1   2   3   4   5

5. Fabric and fiber content are important considerations in my athletic apparel purchase decisions.

   1   2   3   4   5

6. Place of manufacture is an important consideration for me in athletic apparel (U.S.A., Mexico, etc.).

   1   2   3   4   5

7. Fit is the most important consideration in athletic apparel.

   1   2   3   4   5

8. Function is the most important consideration in athletic apparel.

   1   2   3   4   5

	strongly disagree	disagree	neutral	agree	strongly agree

9. Brand name is the most important consideration in athletic apparel.

	1	2	3	4	5

10. Style is the most important consideration in athletic apparel.

	1	2	3	4	5

Please rank the following items, from 1 to 6, in order of importance to you. Use **1** to indicate the **least important** characteristic and **6** to indicate the **most important** characteristic. Use each number only once.

____ Fit
____ Function
____ Brand name
____ Style
____ Fabric
____ Price

SECTION IV. THE FOLLOWING QUESTIONS CONCERN INDIVIDUAL SHOPPING BEHAVIORS.

Please write-in or check the most appropriate responses.

1. How many times a month on average do you shop for athletic apparel <u>for yourself</u>?
   ____ zero
   ____ 1-2
   ____ 3-4
   ____ 5-7
   ____ 8 or more

2. How many times a month on average do you shop for athletic apparel <u>for others</u>?
   ____ zero
   ____ 1-2
   ____ 3-4
   ____ 5-7
   ____ 8 or more

3. On average, how much money do you spend on <u>total</u>, clothing purchases each month? $_____

4. Of the money you spend each month for clothing, what percentage is spent on nonathletic apparel?
   _____%
   What percentage is spent on athletic apparel?
   _____%

5. If you spend more money on clothing purchases for another individual than you spend on yourself, what is that individual's relationship to you?
   _____ (i.e., husband, girlfriend, son, etc.)

6. Based on your shopping behavior over the past 2-3 years, at what store would you say:
   you made the majority of your clothing purchases for yourself?_____
   you made the majority of your clothing purchases for other people?_____

7. When do you prefer to shop for athletic apparel? Please rank the following times in order of preference from 1 to 4, with **1** indicating the time **least preferred**, and **4** indicating the time **most preferred**.

   ____ Monday-Friday, during the day
   ____ Monday-Friday, evenings
   ____ Saturday
   ____ Sunday

SECTION V. PLEASE PROVIDE THE FOLLOWING INFORMATION.
Demographics

1. Age _____
2. Gender: _____ male _____ female
3. Race: _____ African-American _____ Asian
   _____ Hispanic _____ Caucasian
   _____ Other
4. Class Standing: ____ Freshman
   ____ Sophomore
   ____ Junior
   ____ Senior

5. Average number of times per week that you exercise:
   a. specifically for fitness _____
   b. for recreation   _____

6. Indicate each <u>fitness</u> activity that you participate in regularly (once a week or more on average depending on the season) with a check (√):
   ____ Jogging
   ____ Weight lifting
   ____ Swimming
   ____ Bicycling
   ____ Rowing
   ____ Aerobics
   ____ Hiking/walking
   ____ Calisthenics
   ____ Others_____

7. Indicate each <u>recreational</u> activity that you participate in regularly (once a week or more on average depending on the season) with a check (√):
   ____ Softball/baseball
   ____ Basketball
   ____ Tennis/racquetball/squash/handball
   ____ Golf
   ____ Alpine skiing
   ____ Cross-country skiing
   ____ Water skiing
   ____ Surfing/windsurfing
   ____ Climbing
   ____ Others_____

ANOVA Tables

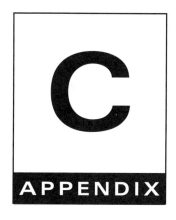

C

APPENDIX

TABLE C.1   One-Way Analysis of Variance Source Table

Source of variation	Degrees of freedom	Sums of squares	Mean square	F-ratio	p-value
Factor A	df_A	SS_A	MS_A	F_A	P_A
Error	df_E	SS_E	MS_E		
Total	$N-1$	SS_T			

TABLE C.2   One-Way Analysis of Variance Source Table

Source of variation	Degrees of freedom	Sums of squares	Mean square	F-ratio	p-value
Factor A	$A-1$	SS_A	$\dfrac{SS_A}{df_A}$	$\dfrac{MS_A}{MS_E}$	P_A
Error	$N-A$	SS_E	$\dfrac{SS_E}{df_E}$		
Total	$N-1 = (A-1) + (N-A)$	$SS_T = (SS_A) + (SS_E)$			

TABLE C.3 Two-Way Analysis of Variance Source Table

Source of variation	Degrees of freedom	Sums of squares	Mean square	F-ratio	p-value
Factor A	df_A	SS_A	MS_A	F_A	P_A
Factor B	df_B	SS_B	MS_B	F_B	P_B
A × B interaction	$df_{A\times B}$	$SS_{A\times B}$	$MS_{A\times B}$	$F_{A\times B}$	$P_{A\times B}$
Error	df_E	SS_E	MS_E		
Total	df_T	SS_T			

TABLE C.4 Two-Way Analysis of Variance Source Table

Source of variation	Degrees of freedom	Sums of squares	Mean square	F-ratio	p-value
Factor A	$A-1$	SS_A	$\dfrac{SS_A}{df_A}$	$\dfrac{MS_A}{MS_E}$	P_A
Factor B	$B-1$	SS_B	$\dfrac{SS_B}{df_B}$	$\dfrac{MS_B}{MS_E}$	P_B
A × B interaction	$(A-1)(B-1)$	$SS_{A\times B}$	$\dfrac{SS_{A\times B}}{df_{A\times B}}$	$\dfrac{MS_{A\times B}}{MS_E}$	$P_{A\times B}$
Error	$(A)(B)(n-1)$	SS_E	$\dfrac{SS_E}{df_E}$		
Total	$N-1^*$	SS_T^{**}			

$N-1^* = (A-1) + (B-1) + (A-1)(B-1) + (A)(B)(n-1)$
$SS_T^{**} = SS_A + SS_B + SS_{A\times B} + SS_E$

Library of Congress Classification System

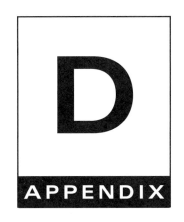

APPENDIX

Most university and college libraries follow the Library of Congress Classification System to organize books, journals, magazines, and other materials. The Library of Congress system separates all knowledge into 21 subjects or classes. Each class is identified by a letter of the alphabet and is further subdivided into subclasses by the addition of a second letter, and specific topics within a class or subclass by a letter/number notation. No two items have exactly the same call number.

     The following is a partial list of the Library of Congress Classification System limited to fields related to sport and exercise science. Your school library should have the complete classification system available in the reference or information area.

  A   **General Works**
       Encyclopedias, reference books, periodicals, etc.
  B   **Philosophy-Religion**
       BF Psychology
  G   **Geography, Anthropology, Folklore, etc.**
       GV Recreation
  H   **Social Sciences**
       HA Statistics
       HM-HX Sociology
  L   **Education**
  Q   **Science**
       QC Physics
       QD Chemistry
       QL Zoology

    QM Human Anatomy
    QP Physiology
R Medicine
    RC Sports Medicine

You will find that most journals and books in sport and exercise studies are classified under the BF, GV, L, QP, and RC headings.

Most Call Numbers have four lines: The first line is made up of a letter or letters, the second line is always a number, the third line is a combination of a letter and a number, and the fourth line is the publication date. The example below, a GV call number, is used to show you what each element of the Call Number indicates.

Book: **Hill, Christopher, R. (1992) Olympic Politics**
Call Number at Kansas State University:

GV
721.5
.H54
1992

GV   (G) First letter is the general subject (Geography, Anthropology, Folklore, etc).
        (V) Second letter is the subclass (Recreation).

721.5   Numbers indicate the specific topic of the subject.

.H54   The letter/number combination identifies this particular book, and is based on the first letter of the author's last name.

1992   The year published.

Abscissa The horizontal or x-axis on a graph.

Alpha error (α) The probability of committing a Type I inference error. This ranges from nearly zero to nearly 100 percent.

Alternative hypothesis The hypothesis predicting a significant difference among groups. The opposite of the null hypothesis.

Analysis of covariance (ANCOVA) A type of analysis of variance used when a statistical control variable is included in the design of the study.

Analysis of variance (ANOVA) An inferential statistical procedure commonly used to test for differences among group means used in designs with one or more independent variables.

Anthropomorphizing Explaining animal behavior using terms associated with human behaviors such as reasoning, envy, or love.

A Posteriori test (post hoc test) Comparisons between treatment conditions that are not planned prior to conducting a study.

Applied research Research designed to solve practical problems or supply answers to immediate questions.

A Priori contrast Comparisons between groups that are planned prior to conducting a study.

Archival research Research based on existing information that does not actively require the generation of new data.

Association The relationships among variables. The association between variables can be strong or weak and negative or positive.

Authority Knowledge based on the acceptance of information provided by authoritative individuals or entities.

Baseline A measurement of behavior during the period just prior to the introduction of the experimental treatment. For example, resting heart rate prior to beginning an aerobic exercise session.

Basic research Research designed to gain knowledge—not necessarily intended to solve practical problems.

Behavioral measures Measurements obtained from observations of behaviors such as reaction time, anxiety, or strength.

Beta error (β) The probability of committing a Type II inference error.

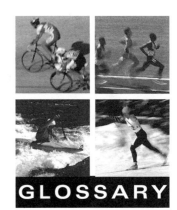

GLOSSARY

Between groups deviation The deviation of a treatment mean from the overall mean in a data set. Used to calculate the between groups sum of squares in analysis of variance.

Between subjects design An experimental design where separate groups of subjects are assigned to each treatment condition. See independent groups design.

Biased sample An unrepresentative sample drawn from a population that may result in incorrect conclusions or inferences about the population.

Bimodal A distribution of scores with two most frequently occurring scores.

Bivariate A measure containing two variables. Height and weight, for example.

Block A series of trials. A block might have five trials, and the design of the study might have 10 blocks. Blocks are usually treated as an independent variable.

Block randomization The subject assignment method whereby subjects are randomly assigned to treatment conditions or blocks.

Carryover effect A potential problem with repeated measures designs where effects of one treatment affect responses to subsequent treatments.

Case study An in-depth description of the behavior of a single subject or small group of subjects. A type of descriptive research.

Categorical data A set of measurements that is classified into categories based on having or not having a particular attribute. When the data are qualitative, categories are often expressed as proportion or percentage. For example, percentage of professional endurance athletes classified as either marathon runners, cyclists, or triathletes.

Ceiling effect The condition that results from a task in which most subjects achieve high scores and some limitations are present to prevent scores from going above a certain point. Ceiling effects can make it difficult to discriminate among levels of performance. See floor effect.

Cell The junction of a row and column in a table. Usually contains a discrete data value or a mean.

Central tendency Measures that indicate the middle point(s) in a distribution of scores. The most common measures of central tendency are the mode, median, and mean.

Closed question A category of survey questions with limited answer options.

Cluster sampling A sampling method in which groups of connected individuals (clusters) are selected for the purpose of serving as subjects in a study.

Coefficient of determination (r^2) The percent of the variation in the dependent variable that is accounted for by the independent variable.

Coercion Inducing subjects to continue participating in an investigation even though they would prefer not to.

Cohort A group of subjects categorized based on some characteristic. Age is a common cohort category.

Concurrent validity The degree to which an instrument correlates with a criterion measure. Test and criterion measurements are made at the same time.

Confidence interval A range of values from a sample that will likely capture the value of a population parameter. 90%, 95%, or 99% confidence intervals are commonly reported in research reports.

Confounding The effect of any uncontrolled variable in an investigation. The presence of a confounding variable may threaten the internal validity of the investigation.

Construct validity Measurement validity associated with tests of psychological constructs such as motivation, anxiety, or creativity.

Content validity The extent to which an instrument adequately samples the subject matter it was designed to measure.

Continuous variables A variable that may take any value within a defined range of values—that is, a variable that is capable of any amount of subdivision.

Control group An untreated group(s) in an investigation. Control groups provide a condition against which the treatment groups(s) can be compared.

Control variable Any variable fixed at constant levels throughout an experiment.

Correlation coefficient (r) A statistical value that describes the relationship between two variables.

Correlation research The study of two or more variables observed under natural conditions.

Counterbalancing A method of controlling for possible order effects in a repeated measures design. Accomplished by systematically or randomly varying the order of the conditions in the investigation.

Criterion variable A variable used to predict the value of a second variable. For example, a submaximal exercise test can be used to estimate maximum work capacity.

Critical value A specific value that must be exceeded to reject the null hypothesis.

Cross-sectional design A research method in which subjects of differing ages are studied at only one point in time. See longitudinal design.

Data Factual information obtained in an investigation. Data may be qualitative (descriptive) or quantitative (numerical) in form.

Datum A single unit of data.

Debriefing The explanation of the investigation given to the subjects following their participation.

Degrees of freedom The number of scores that are free to take any value. In hypothesis testing, degrees of freedom and significance levels are used to determine critical values.

Demand characteristics Clues that may provide subjects with unintended information about the purpose of the investigation.

Dependent variable The variable measured in an investigation.

Descriptive research Investigations designed to describe behavior as it naturally occurs.

Descriptive statistics A branch of statistics that describes the properties of a set of data (for example, the mean and standard deviation).

Dichotomous classification A variable with only two values (for example, yes and no or true and false).

Differential mortality The term used to describe the act of subjects dropping out of a study for some systematic reason. A threat to internal validity.

Discrete variables A characteristic whose value when pictured on a number line consists only of isolated points; for example, the number of students in a class.

Dispersion The extent to which the scores in a distribution deviate from the middle score. Usually expressed by the standard deviation.

Double-blind methods An experimental design in which neither the subjects nor the investigators know which subjects are assigned to which treatment conditions.

Ecological validity The degree to which the conditions of a study simulate real world conditions.

Empirical Information obtained through the direct observation of events.

Error variance Random variability in a data set originating from sources other than the effect of the independent variable.

Experiment A scientific procedure whereby variables are manipulated and then measurements on other variables are taken. Experiments are conducted to investigate cause-and-effect relationships.

Experimental design A specific plan that describes the design of an investigation.

Experimenter bias (expectancy) The intentional or unintentional influence that an experimenter may exert on an investigation.

External validity The degree to which the results from an investigation (particularly laboratory experiments) generalize to other settings (ecological) and people (populations).

Extraneous variables Uncontrolled variable(s) that may generate rival (confounding) explanations of the findings of an investigation.

Factor An alternate term for the term independent variable.

Factor analysis A statistical procedure using correlations to determine whether a set of variables can be reduced to a lesser number of variables to make a prediction.

Factorial design An experimental design with two or more independent variables.

Floor effect A condition resulting from a task on which most subjects find it difficult to achieve a score or some limiting factor prevents scores from going below a given point. See ceiling effect.

Frequency distribution An arrangement of data where the frequency of scores similar in value is tabulated by placing like scores in groups called intervals.

Frequency polygon A type of graph that uses lines to link values.

F-table A table listing critical values of F organized by degrees of freedom and significance levels.

F-test (analysis of variance) An inferential statistic used to test statistical hypotheses.

Gopher A computer program that helps organize information found on the Internet.

Grand mean The mean calculated using all scores in a data set.

Haphazard sampling (accidental sampling) A type of selection procedure based on convenience rather than proper sampling procedures.

Hawthorne effect The term used to describe the effect of being a subject in an investigation that may affect natural behavior.

Histogram A graph with columns placed along the horizontal axis that vary in height to indicate frequency or percentage.

History The effect of extraneous events that may affect the findings from an investigation. A threat to internal validity.

Html Hypertext mark up language.

Http Hypertext transfer protocol.

Hypothesis An assertion about what may be true in a given situation. Implies insufficient of presently attainable evidence and therefore is a tentative explanation.

Independent groups design An experimental design where separate groups of subjects are assigned to each treatment condition. See between subjects designs.

Independent variable The manipulated variable in an experiment.

Individual difference The natural physical and/or behavioral diversity among people, animals, or objects.

Inferential statistics A branch of statistics used to evaluate the accuracy of statements about population characteristics based on information gathered from sample data.

Informed consent The approval given to a researcher by the subject prior to participating in a study. Researchers are required to disclose facts concerning the nature of a study and advise the subject as to any potential risks.

Instructions Information provided to subjects prior to their participation in an experiment. Uniform presentation of instructions helps control for demand characteristics or experimenter bias.

Instrumentation decay Unplanned changes in equipment that go unrecognized by the researcher. A threat to internal validity.

Interaction The combined effect of two or more independent variables on the dependent variable.

Internal validity The degree to which extraneous variables have been controlled in an investigation. The technical quality of an investigation.

Interval measurement scale A measurement scale with order and equal interval widths for which a score of zero is arbitrary.

Interviewer bias The inappropriate influence that an interviewer may have on a respondent.

Intuition Knowledge based on personal beliefs, observations, or hunches.

Invasive methods Measurements that require devices that directly record responses inside the body.

In vitro In the test tube. The study of living tissue outside of the body.

In vivo In the body. The study of living tissue in the body.

Latin square design An arrangement of symbols in the form of a square so that each symbol occurs once in each row and column. Used in counterbalancing repeated measures designs.

Law Implies a statement of order and relation in nature that has been found to be in variable under the same conditions.

Levels of a factor The specific value or characteristic of each level of an independent variable.

Likert-type scale A closed question scale with three or more response alternatives.

Longitudinal design A research method in which the measurement of subjects of the same age are studied over a long period of time. See cross-sectional design.

Main effect The effect of an independent variable on a dependent variable. A term commonly associated with factorial design.

Manipulation check A test to determine if the independent variable has the anticipated effect on the dependent variable.

Matched random design Subjects are matched based on certain characteristics and then each of the matched subjects are randomly assigned to different treatment conditions.

Maturation Naturally occurring but unwanted changes in an individual over time that may affect the results of an investigation. A threat to internal validity.

Mean The arithmetic average of a set of scores.

Mean square A term calculated by dividing the sum of squares by the corresponding degrees of freedom. Used in ANOVA.

Measurement The process of assigning numerical or symbolic values to members of a group for the purpose of distinguishing among the members on the basis of the degree to which they possess the characteristic being assessed.

Measurement error The degree to which a measured score deviates from its true value.

Measurement scales Four levels of measurement: nominal, ordinal, interval, and ratio.

Median The 50th percentile of a distribution of scores.

Mixed design An experimental design combining independent and repeated conditions.

Mode The most frequently occurring value in a distribution of scores.

Multiple regression A statistical technique that employs several independent variables to estimate values of the dependent variable.

Multivariate analysis of variance (MANOVA) A statistical technique used to test for differences between more than one dependent variable.

Naturalistic observation Unobtrusive recording and description of behavior under natural conditions.

Negative relationship An association between variables for which high scores for one variable are paired with low scores for a second variable.

Nominal scale A level of measurement that permits only the making of statements of sameness or difference.

Noninvasive technique Measurement processes that do not require direct measures of internal responses.

Nonparametric statistics A family of statistical tests that is not based on assumptions concerning the distribution of the data set.

Norm Average scores obtained from previous studies against which current information can be compared.

Normal distribution A specific frequency distribution that has known mathematical properties and is used in many statistical procedures.

Null hypothesis The statistical hypothesis that predicts that the variables under investigation are not related to the population. See alternative hypothesis.

Numerical data set A set of measurements that is expressed in numerical form. For example, percent body fat values, or maximum oxygen uptake values.

Occam's razor The principle that states that explanations should be kept as simple as possible and with the fewest assumptions.

One-tailed test An inferential test that places the rejection region at one end of a distribution. See two-tailed test.

Open-ended questions Survey questions that do not place any limitations on the possible range of responses. Normally short-answer questions.

Operational definition A detailed description of the variables used in an investigation. Particularly the independent and dependent variables.

Order effect The possible effect on measurement when treatment conditions always follow the same order. A threat to internal validity in repeated measures designs.

Ordinal scale A level of measurement that permits the ordering of scores in addition to statements of sameness or difference.

Ordinate The vertical (y-axis) of a graph.

Parameter A characteristics of a population (such as μ, σ).

Parametric statistics A family of statistics that involves assumptions about population parameters and the distribution of scores.

Parsimony The principle that the simpler of two otherwise equally acceptable explanations is preferable. See Occam's razor.

Pearson's r The correlation statistic that expresses the direction and strength of the relationship between two variables.

Pilot study A small scale study conducted to test the methods and procedures before embarking on a large-scale study.

Placebo A chemically inert substance.

Point estimate A single value based on sample information that is used to estimate the corresponding population value.

Population All members of a defined group.

Positive correlation When high scores on one variable are paired with high scores on a second variable.

Post hoc test A statistical technique to compare treatment conditions that were not planned prior to conducting a study.

Power The probability of correctly rejecting the null hypothesis when the null hypothesis is false $(1-\beta)$.

Prediction A statement about the likely outcome of an event.

Predictor variable A variable used to predict the value of another variable.

Pretest-posttest design An experimental design in which subjects are tested prior to administration of the treatment condition (pretest) and then again following the treatment (posttest).

Probability The likelihood that a given event will occur.

p-value The smallest significance level at which H_o can be rejected.

Qualitative research A method of collecting subjective data generally involving the investigator as the primary data collecting agent.

Quantitative research A method of collecting data generally involving valid and reliable measuring instruments as the primary data collecting agent.

Quasi-experimental design A type of experimental design used to reduce as many threats to internal validity as possible when it is not possible to conduct a true experiment.

Quota sampling A sampling technique whereby subgroups within a population are first identified and then sampled.

Random assignment Procedures used to assign subjects to conditions in an experiment based on independent and equally likely selection procedures.

Ratio scale A level of measurement that permits the making of statements of equality of ratios, such as one variable is twice another, in addition to statements of sameness or difference, greater or less than, and equality of intervals.

Reactivity The possible unwanted influence of the act of measuring or observing the behavior of subjects.

Regression equation A statistical method used to predict the most likely value of one variable from the known value of a second variable.

Regression to the mean The condition exhibited when extreme scores on the first measurement move in the direction of the mean on the second measurement. A threat to internal validity.

Rejection region The area containing all values for which H_o would be rejected.

Reliability The extent to which a measurement process yields the same result when used repeatedly under similar conditions.

Repeated measures design A design in which the same group of subjects serves in all treatment conditions. See within subjects designs.

Replication The act of repeating a study to determine the degree to which the original findings can be duplicated.

Representative sample A sample that accurately reflects the population from which it is drawn.

Robust The property of a statistical test that results in valid conclusions despite violations of the assumptions underlying the test.

Sample A subset of a population.

Sample size (N) The number of individual data points in a distribution or the number of subjects in a study.

Sampling Procedure for selecting members from a population to serve as subjects in an investigation.

Sampling distribution The frequency distribution of a statistic resulting from calculating the statistics from a vary large number of samples taken in a consistent manner from the population.

Sampling error The difference between the value of a sample statistic and a true population value as a result of chance measurement errors.

Scatter plot A graph used to plot the relationship between two variables.

Science A systematic method of building knowledge founded on principles designed to protect the objectivity and reliability of information.

Self reported measure An assessment of a variable based on responses given by a subject, such answers to survey questions.

Single-blind method An experimental procedure designed to limit bias in subjects' responses by withholding group assignment information from the subjects.

Single subject design An experiment where data are gathered from only one subject.

Standard deviation The average deviation of scores from the mean (square root of the variance).

Standard error of the mean The standard deviation of a sampling distribution of means.

Standard score A general term indicating any of several converted raw scores.

Statistical analysis Mathematical based methods used to organize, describe, and interpret data sets.

Statistical hypotheses Hypotheses stating the possible relationship between population parameters. Normally stated using the null and/or alternative forms.

Statistics A characteristic of a sample.

Stratified random sampling A sampling procedure during which a population is first divided into groups or strata, and then random samples are drawn from each group.

Subject contamination Unintended knowledge about the purpose of an investigation that may alter the behavior of the subjects.

Subjective rating The assignment of a score to a response or situations based on personal opinion.

Sum of squares The sum of squared deviations of scores from their mean.

Survey research Method used for gathering information, opinions, or beliefs from large numbers of people using questionnaires and interviews.

Theory A statement or set of statements designed to explain or integrate a set of related facts or information. Implies the existence of a range of evidence supporting the theory and thus the likelihood of truth.

Treatment effect The influence on behavior that is attributed to the independent variable in an experiment.

Treatments Conditions in an experiment that are under the control of the experimenter.

Trial A single response obtained from a subject in the form of a score or data point.

True score The value of a measured variable with no measurement error or bias present.

Two-tailed test A statistical test that places one-half of the rejection region at each end of the distribution. See one-tailed test.

Type I error A decision to reject the null hypothesis when the null hypothesis is actually true.

Type II error A decision to accept the null hypothesis when the null hypothesis is actually false.

Unbiased statistic A statistic whose expected value is equal to the population parameter it estimates.

Validity The extent to which a measurement tool actually measures the intended trait or attribute.

Variability The amount of dispersion of scores about the midpoint of a distribution.

Variable Any characteristic or condition that can assume different values.

Variance A unit of measure of score variability.

Veronica A computer program that helps search for information on the Internet.

Within subjects design An experiment in which the same subjects serve in all treatment conditions. See repeated measures designs.

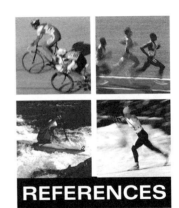

Acevedo, E. O., Rinehardt, K. F., and Kraemer, R. R. (1994). Perceived exertion and affect at varying intensities of running. *Research Quarterly for Exercise and Sport, 65,* 372-376.

American College of Sports Medicine. (1995). Policy statement of the American College of Sports Medicine on research with experimental animals. *Medicine and Science in Sport and Exercise, 27(1),* vi.

American Psychological Association. (1990). Ethical principles of psychologists. *American Psychologist, 45,* 390-395.

————. (1994). *Publication manual of the American Psychological Association* (4th ed.). Washington, DC: APA.

Ansorge, C. J., and Scheer, J. K. (1988). International bias detected in judging gymnastic competition at the 1984 Olympic Games. *Research Quarterly for Exercise and Sport, 59,* 103-107.

Bahl, S. M., Hamilton, S., and Ormesher, P. (1993). A study of the nutrition knowledge of allied health students. *Health Values, 17,* 3-8.

Blair, S. N. (1993). 1993 C. H. McCloy research lecture: Physical activity, physical fitness, and health. *Research Quarterly for Exercise and Sport, 64,* 365-376.

Blair, S. N., et al. (1989). Physical fitness and all-cause mortality: A prospective study of healthy men and women. *JAMA, 262,* 2395-2401.

Bogdan, R., and Biklen, S. K. (1982). *Qualitative research for education: An introduction to theory and methods.* Boston: Allyn and Bacon.

Boyce, B. A., and Wayda, V. K. (1994). The effects of assigned and self-set goals on task performance. *Journal of Sport and Exercise Psychology, 16,* 258-269.

Brustad, R. J. (1993). Who will go out and play? Parental and psychological influences on children's attraction to physical activity. *Pediatric Exercise Science, 5,* 210-223.

Burdick, A. (1993). Going all the way. *The Sciences, 33(2),* 8-9.

Calfas, K. J., et al. (1994). Physical activity and its determinants before and after college graduation. *Journal of Medicine, Exercise, Nutrition, and Health, 3(6),* 323-334.

Campbell, W. G. (1978). *Form and style: Theses, reports, term papers.* Boston: Houghton Miffin.

CBE Style Manual Committee. (1983). *CBE style manual: A guide for authors, editors, and publishers in biological sciences* (5th ed.). Bethesda, MD: CBE.

Corbin, C. B., et al. (1994). Anabolic steroids: A study of high school athletes. *Pediatric Exercise Science, 6,* 149-158.

Cornacchia, H. J., and Barrett, S. (1993). *Consumer health: A guide to intelligent decisions.* St Louis: Mosby-Year Book.

Cotten, D. J. (1990). An analysis of the NCYFS II modified pull-up test. *Research Quarterly for Exercise and Sport, 61(3),* 272-273.

Council of Biology Editors. (1978). *Council of Biology Editors style manual: A guide for authors, editors, and publishers in the biological sciences* (4th ed.). Arlington, VA: CBE.

Curry, T. J. (1991). Fraternal bonding in the locker room: A profeminist analysis of talk about competition and women. *Sport Sociology Journal, 8,* 119-135.

Dawber, T. R., Kannel, W. B., and Lyell, L. P. (1963). An approach to longitudinal studies in a community: The Framingham study. *Annals of New York Academy of Sciences, 107,* 539-556.

REFERENCES

de Vries, H. A. (1966). Quantitative electromyographic investigation of the spasm theory of muscle pain. *American Journal of Physical Medicine, 45,* 119-134.

Eastman, S. T., and Riggs, K. E. (1994). Televised sports and ritual: Fan experiences. *Sociology of Sport Journal, 11,* 249-274.

Ebbeck, V., and Becker, S. L. (1994). Psychosocial predictors of goal orientations in youth soccer. *Research Quarterly for Exercise and Sport, 65,* 355-362.

Engleman, M. E., and Morrow, J. R., Jr. (1991). Reliability and skinfold correlates for traditional and modified pull-ups in children grades 3-5. *Research Quarterly for Exercise and Sport, 62,* 88-91.

Estes, S. (1994). Knowledge and kinesiology. *Quest, 46,* 392-409.

Fehlandt, A., and Micheli, L. (1995). Acute exterional anterior compartment syndrome in an adolescent female. *Medicine and Science in Sport and Exercise, 27(1),* 3-7.

Fleishman, E. A. (1964). *The structure and measurement of physical fitness.* Englewood Cliffs, NJ: Prentice Hall.

Fraser, G. E. (1994). Diet and coronary heart disease: Beyond dietary fats and low-density-lipoprotein cholesterol. *American Journal of Clinical Nutrition, 59 (suppl),* 000S-00S.

Friden, J., Kjorell, U., and Thornell, L. E. (1984). Delayed muscle soreness and cytoskeletal alterations: An immunocytological study in man. *International Journal of Sports Medicine, 5,* 15-18.

Gabbard, C., Kirby, T., and Patterson, P. (1979). Reliability of the straight-arm hang for testing muscular strength among children 2 to 5. *Research Quarterly, 50,* 735-738.

Gallup, G. (1948). *A guide to public opinion polls.* Princeton, NJ: Princeton University Press.

Gantz, W., and Wenner, L. A. (1995). Fanship and the television sports viewing experience. *Sociology of Sports Journal, 12,* 56-74.

Gilbey, H., and Gilbey, M. (1995). The physical activity of Singapore primary school children as estimated by heart rate monitoring. *Pediatric Exercise Science, 7,* 26-35.

Gilster, P. (1993). *The Internet navigator.* New York: John Wiley and Sons, Inc.

Glass, G. V, and Hopkins, K. D. (1984). *Statistical methods in education and psychology* (2nd ed.). Englewood Cliffs, NJ: Prentice Hall.

Glass, G. V, McGraw, B., and Smith, M. L. (1981). *Meta-analysis in social sciences.* Beverly Hills, CA: Sage Publications.

Goode, S. L., and Magill, R. A. (1986). The contextual interference effect in learning three badminton serves. *Research Quarterly for Exercise and Sport, 57,* 308-314.

Goodgame, D. (1994, September 14). Better off dead? *Time Magazine,* 40-42.

Gould, D., Finch, L. M., and Jackson, S. A. (1993). Coping strategies used by national champion figure skaters. *Research Quarterly for Exercise and Sport, 64,* 453-468.

Gould, S. J. (1981). *The mismeasure of man.* New York: W.W. Norton and Co.

Green, J. S., and Crouse, S. F. (1995). The effects of endurance training on functional capacity in the elderly: A meta analysis. *Medicine and Science in Sport and Exercise, 27(6),* 920-926.

Greenockle, K. M., Lee, A. A., and Lomax, R. (1990). The relationship between selected student characteristics and activity patterns in a required high school physical education class. *Research Quarterly for Exercise and Sport, 61,* 59-69.

Guttmann, A. (1978). *From ritual to record.* New York: Columbia University Press.

Hale, B. D. (1982). The effects of internal and external imagery on muscular and ocular concomitants. *Journal of Sport Psychology, 4,* 379-387.

Hartley, A. A., and Hartley, J. T. (1984). Performance changes in champion swimmers aged 30 to 84 years. *Experimental Aging Research, 10(3)*, 141-147.

Heagy, B. S. (1993). Kinsimative analysis of male olympic cross-country skiers using the open field skating technique. Thesis (M.S.). Oregon State University, Corvallis, Oregon.

High, D. M., Howley, E. T., and Franks, B. D. (1989). The effects of static stretching and warm-up on prevention of delayed-onset muscle soreness. *Research Quarterly for Exercise and Sport, 60,* 357-361.

Hird, J. S., et al. (1991). Physical practice is superior to mental practice in enhancing cognitive and motor task performance. *Journal of Sport and Exercise Psychology, 13,* 281-293.

Hooper, S. L., et al. (1994). Markers for monitoring overtraining and recovery. *Medicine and Science in Sports and Exercise, 27,* 106-112.

Howe, C. Z. (1988). Using qualitative structured interviews in leisure research: Illustrations from one case study. *Journal of Leisure Research, 20,* 305-324.

Jackson, A. S., and Pollock, M. L. (1976). Factor analysis and multivariate scaling of anthropometric variables for the assessment of body composition. *Medicine and Science in Sports, 8,* 196-203.

Jackson, A. S., Pollock, M. L., and Ward, A. (1980). Generalized equations for predicting body density of women. *Medicine and Science in Sports and Exercise, 12,* 175-182.

Jackson, A. W., and Solomon, J. (1995). One-mile walk test: Reliability, validity, norms, and criterion-referenced standards for young adults. *Medicine, Exercise, Nutrition, and Health, 3,* 317-322.

Johnson, B. D., and Johnson, N. R. (1995). Stacking and "stoppers": A test of the outcome control hypothesis. *Sociology of Sports Journal, 12,* 105-112.

Kane, M. J., and Disch, L. (1993). Reproduction of male power in the locker room: The "Lisa Olson incident." *Sociology of Sport Journal, 10,* 331-352.

Katz, J. F., et al. (1985). Psychological consequences of an exercise training program for a paraplegic man: A case study. *Rehabilitation Psychology, 30,* 53-58.

Kelley, B. C., and Gill, D. L. (1993). An examination of personal/situational variables, stress appraisal, and burnout in collegiate teacher-coaches. *Research Quarterly for Exercise and Sport, 64,* 94-102.

Kelley, G. A., and Kelley, K. S. (1994). Physical activity habits of African-American college students. *Research Quarterly for Exercise and Sport, 65,* 207-212.

Kelly, K. P., et al. (1995). Cocaine and exercise: Physiological responses of cocaine-conditioned rats. *Medicine and Science in Sports and Exercise, 27(1),* 65-72.

Klein, A. (1986). Pumping iron: Crisis and contradiction in body building. *Sport Sociology Journal, 3,* 112-133.

Klein, R. D. (1983). How to do what we want to do: Thoughts about feminist methodology. In G. Bowles and R. D. Klein (Eds.), *Theories of women's studies* (p. 89). London: Routledge and Kegan Paul.

Knudson, D. (1991). Effect of string type and tension on ball vertical angle of rebound in static tennis impacts. *Journal of Human Movement Studies, 20,* 39-47.

Kollath, J. A., et al. (1991). Measurement errors in modified pull-ups testing. *Research Quarterly for Exercise and Sport, 62,* 432-435.

Komi, P. V., and Buskirk, E. R. (1972). Effect of eccentric and concentric conditioning on tension and electrical activity of human muscle. *Ergonomics, 15,* 417-434.

Lancy, D. F. (1993). *Qualitative research in education: An introduction to the major traditions.* White Plains, NY: Longman Publishers.

Leddy, M. H., Lambert, M. J., and Ogles, B. M. (1994). Psychological consequences of athletic injury among high-level competitors. *Research Quarterly for Exercise and Sport, 65*, 347-354.

Lee, T. D., and Magill, R. A. (1985). Can forgetting facilitate skill acquistion? In D. Goodman, R. B. Wilberg, and Franks, I. M. (Eds.), *Differing perspectives in motor learning, memory and control* (pp. 3-22). Amsterdam: North-Holland.

Locke, L. F. (1989). Qualitative research as a form of scientific inquiry in sport and physical education. *Research Quarterly for Exercise and Sport, 60*, 1-20.

McCracken, H. D., and Stelmach, G. E. (1977). A test of schema theory of discrete motor learning. *Journal of Motor Behavior, 9*, 193-201.

McElroy, M., and Cartwright, K. (1986). Public fencing contests on the Elizabethan stage. *Journal of Sport History, 13*, 193-211.

———. (1982). Sport literature, literary criticism, and historical inquiry. *North American Society for Sport History Proceedings*, 11-13.

Messner, M., and Solomon, W. S. (1993). Outside the frame: Newspaper coverage of the Sugar Ray Leonard wife abuse story. *Sociology of Sport Journal, 10*, 119-134.

Milgram, S. (1965). Some conditions of obedience and disobedience to authority. *Human Relations, 18*, 57-76.

Monroe, D. A. (1995). Fear of personal fitness and discrimination towards obesity. *Research Quarterly for Exercise and Sport, 66(1)*, A-41.

Mood, D. (1971). Test of physical fitness knowledge: Construction, administration and norms. *Research Quarterly, 42*, 423-429.

Moore, D. S. (1991). *Statistics: Concepts and controversies*. New York: W.H. Freeman and Company.

Morrow, J. R., Jr., and Frankiewicz, R. G. (1979). Strategies for the analysis of repeated and multiple measures designs. *Research Quarterly, 50*, 297-304.

Morrow, J. R., Jr., and Jackson, A. W. (1993). How 'significant' is your reliability? *Research Quarterly for Exercise and Sport, 64*, 352-355.

Nelson, J. K., Yoon, S. H., and Nelson, K. R. (1991). A field test for upper body strength and endurance. *Research Quarterly for Exercise and Sport, 62*, 436-441.

Neufer, P. D., et al. (1987). Effect of reduced training on muscular strength and endurance in competitive swimmers. *Medicine and Science in Sports and Exercise, 19(5)*, 486-490.

Newcomb, S. (1903). The outlook for the flying machine. *The Independent, 55*, 2508-2512.

Newell, K. M. (1990a). Physical education in higher education: Chaos out of order. *Quest, 42(3)*, 227-242.

———. (1990b). Kinesiology: The label for the study of physical activity in higher education. *Quest, 42(3)*, 269-278.

Noble, L., and Walker, H. (1994). Baseball bat inertial and vibrational characteristics and discomfort following ball-bat impacts. *Journal of Applied Biomechanics, 10*, 132-144.

Oriard, M. (1983). On the current status of sport fiction. *Arete: The Journal of Sport Literature, 1*, 7-20.

Paffenbarger, R. S., et al. (1986). Chronic disease in former college students: Physical activity, all-cause mortality, and longevity of college alumni. *New England Journal of Medicine, 314*, 605-613.

Palmer, S. L. (1992). A comparison of mental practice techniques as applied to the developing competitive figure skater. *The Sport Psychologist, 6*, 148-155.

Park, R. J. (1991). Physiology and anatomy are destiny: Brains, bodies and exercise in nineteenth century American thought. *Journal of Sport History, 18*, 31-63.

————. (1992). The rise and demise of Harvard's B.S. program in anatomy, physiology, and physical training: A case of conflicts of interest and scarce resources. *Research Quarterly for Exercise and Sport, 63,* 246-260.

Payne, V. G., and Morrow, J. R., Jr. (1993). Exercise and VO$_2$max in children: A meta-analysis. *Research Quarterly for Exercise and Sport, 64,* 305-313.

Polit, A., and Bizzi, E. (1979). Characteristics of motor programs underlying arm movements in monkeys. *Journal of Neurophysiology, 42,* 183-194.

Poppleton, W. L., and Salmoni, A. W. (1991). Talent identification in swimming. *Journal of Human Movement Studies, 20,* 85-100.

Post, W. S., Larson, M. G., and Levy, D. (1994). Impact of left ventricular structure on the incidence of hypertension: The Framingham Heart Study. *Circulation, 91(1),* 179-184.

Quadagno, D., et al. (1991). The menstrual cycle: Does it affect athletic performance? *The Physician and Sportsmedicine, 19(3),* 121-124.

Ragsdale, D., Kotarba, J. A., and Morrow, J. R., Jr. (1992). Quality of life of hospitalized persons with AIDS. *IMAGE: Journal of Nursing Scholarship, 24,* 259-265.

Rich, B. S., et al. (1993). Inguinal mass in a college football player: A case study. *Medicine and Science in Sports and Exercise, 25,* 318-320.

Riess, S. A. (1994). From pitch to putt: Sport and class in Anglo-American sport. *Journal of Sport History, 21(2),* 138-184.

Robinson, L., and Neutens, J. J. (1987). *Research techniques for health sciences.* New York: Macmillian.

Rosenthal, K. (1966). *Experimenter effects in behavioral research.* New York: Appleton-Century-Crofts.

Ryan, E.D., and Simons, J. (1983). What is learned in mental practice of motor skills? A test of the cognitive-motor hypothesis. *Journal of Sport Psychology, 5,* 419-426.

Safrit, M. J. (1993). Oh what a tangled web we weave. *Quest, 45,* 52-61.

Schiffman, S., Reynolds, M., and Young, F. (1981). *Introduction to multidimensional scaling: Theory, methods, and applications.* New York: Academic Press.

Schmidt, R. A. (1975). A schema theory of discrete motor skill learning. *Psychological Review, 82,* 225-260.

Schutz, R. W., and Gessaroli, M. E. (1987). The analysis of repeated measures designs involving multiple dependent variables. *Research Quarterly for Exercise and Sport, 58,* 132-149.

Sears, D. O. (1986). College sophomores in the laboratory: Influences of a narrow data base on social psychology's view of human nature. *Journal of Personality and Social Psychology, 51,* 515-530.

Sekiya, H., et al. (1994). The contextual interference effect for skill variations from the same and different generalized motor program. *Research Quarterly for Exercise and Sport, 65,* 330-338.

Shank, M. D., and Haywood, K. M. (1987). Eye movements while viewing a baseball pitch. *Perceptual Motor Skills, 64,* 1191-1197.

Shea, J. B., and Morgan, R. L. (1979). The contextual interference effects on the acquisition, retention, and transfer of a motor skill. *Journal of Experimental Psychology: Human Learning and Memory, 5,* 179-187.

Slowikowski, S. S., and Newell, K. M. (1990). The philosophy of kinesiology. *Quest, 42(3),* 279-296.

Smart, R. (1966). Subject selection bias in psychological research. *Canadian Psychologist, 7,* 115-121.

Smith, L. T., Jr. (1984). Versions of defeat: Baseball autobiographies. *Arete: The Journal of Sport Literature, 2,* 141-158.

Standards for educational and psychological tests. (1985). Washington, DC: American Psychological Association.

Stull, G. A., Christina, R. W., and Quinn, S. A. (1991). Accuracy of references in Research Quarterly for Exercise and Sport. *Research Quarterly for Exercise and Sport, 62,* 245-248.

Sundgot-Borgen, J. (1993). Prevalence of eating disorders in elite female athletes. *International Journal of Sport Nutrition, 3,* 29-40.

Thomas, J. R., and French, K. E. (1986). The use of meta-analysis in exercise and sport: A tutorial. *Research Quarterly for Exercise and Sport, 57,* 196-204.

Twain, M. (1938). Letters from the earth. B. DeVoto (Ed.), Greenwich, CT: Fawcett Publications.

Van Raalte, J. L., et al. (1994). The relationship between observable self-talk and competitive junior tennis players' match performances. *Journal of Sport and Exercise Psychology, 16,* 400-415.

Weiller, K. H., and Higgs, C. T. (1994). The all American girls professional baseball league, 1943-1954: Gender conflict in sport. *Sociology of Sport Journal, 11,* 289-297.

Weiss, M. R. (1994a). Editor's viewpoint: Who's on first, what's on second? *Research Quarterly for Exercise and Sport, 65(2),* iii-iv.

————. (1994b). Editor's viewpoint: Why ask "Why"? *Research Quarterly for Exercise and Sport, 65(1),* iii-iv.

————. (1995). Editor's viewpoint: Do you know the way to San José? *Research Quarterly for Exercise and Sport, 66(1),* iii-v.

Wessinger, N. P. (1994). "I hit a home run!" The lived meaning of scoring in games in physical education. *Quest, 46,* 425-439.

Whitehurst, M., and Menendez, E. (1991). Endurance training in older women. *Physician and Sportsmedicine, 19(6),* 95-102.

Wiggins, D. K. (1980). The play of slave children in the plantation communities of the old south, 1820-1860. *Journal of Sport History, 7(2),* 21-39.

————. (1991). Prized performers, but frequently overlooked students: The involvement of Black athletes in intercollegiate sports on predominantly White university campuses, 1890-1972. *Research Quarterly for Exercise and Sport, 62,* 164-177.

Williams, A. M., et al. (1994). Visual search strategies in experienced and inexperienced soccer players. *Research Quarterly for Exercise and Sport, 65,* 127-135.

Williamson, K. M. (1993). A qualitative study on the socialization of beginning physical education teacher educators. *Research Quarterly for Exercise and Sport, 64,* 188-201.

Wyshogrod, D. (1985). Current treatment of obesity exemplified in a case study. *Journal of Behavior Therapy and Experimental Psychiatry, 16,* 151-157.

A

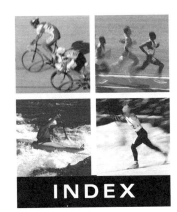

INDEX